Recent Progress in Otolaryngology

Recent Progress in Otolaryngology

Editor: Chad Downs

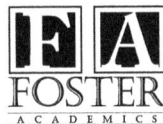

FA FOSTER
ACADEMICS

www.fosteracademics.com

www.fosteracademics.com

FA
FOSTER
ACADEMICS

Cataloging-in-Publication Data

Recent progress in otolaryngology / edited by Chad Downs.
      p. cm.
Includes bibliographical references and index.
ISBN 978-1-63242-566-9
1. Otolaryngology. I. Downs, Chad.
RF46 .R43 2018
617.51--dc23

© Foster Academics, 2018

Foster Academics,
118-35 Queens Blvd., Suite 400,
Forest Hills, NY 11375, USA

ISBN 978-1-63242-566-9 (Hardback)

Contents

Preface

As a sub-type of medical sciences otolaryngology deals with the surgery of nose, ears and throat to cure them of disorders. This area also includes curing diseases in the skull and neck area. This book traces the progress of this field and highlights some of its key concepts. It unravels the recent studies in the field of otolaryngology. The aim of the book is to present researches that have transformed this discipline and aided its advancement. Those in search of information to further their knowledge will be greatly assisted by this text.

This book is a comprehensive compilation of works of different researchers from varied parts of the world. It includes valuable experiences of the researchers with the sole objective of providing the readers (learners) with a proper knowledge of the concerned field. This book will be beneficial in evoking inspiration and enhancing the knowledge of the interested readers.

In the end, I would like to extend my heartiest thanks to the authors who worked with great determination on their chapters. I also appreciate the publisher's support in the course of the book. I would also like to deeply acknowledge my family who stood by me as a source of inspiration during the project.

Editor

Persistent Down-Beating Torsional Positional Nystagmus: Posterior Semicircular Canal Light Cupula?

Akihide Ichimura[1,2] and Koji Otsuka[1]

[1]*Department of Otorhinolaryngology, Tokyo Medical University, 6-7-1 Nishishinjuku, Shinjuku-ku, Tokyo 160-0023, Japan*
[2]*Ichimura ENT Clinic, 2-11-10 Nishiwaseda, Shinjuku-ku, Tokyo 169-0051, Japan*

Correspondence should be addressed to Akihide Ichimura; amt1004@viola.ocn.ne.jp

Academic Editor: Nicolas Perez-Fernandez

A 16-year-old boy with rotatory positional vertigo and nausea, particularly when lying down, visited our clinic. Initially, we observed vertical/torsional (downward/leftward) nystagmus in the supine position, and it did not diminish. In the sitting position, nystagmus was not provoked. Neurological examinations were normal. We speculated that persistent torsional down-beating nystagmus was caused by the light cupula of the posterior semicircular canal. This case provides novel insights into the light cupula pathophysiology.

1. Introduction

In the head-hanging position, positional down-beating nystagmus (p-DBN) generally occurs in patients with a cerebellar nodulus lesion [1]. Several authors have recently reported that nystagmus of benign paroxysmal positional vertigo of the anterior semicircular canal (A-BPPV) is observed as a down-beating component with or without a torsional component in the head-hanging position on Dix-Hallpike test [2–4]. In A-BPPV, nystagmus is typically observed as transient positional nystagmus with latency and habituation [2–4]. We report a case of a patient with persistent torsional DBN in the head-hanging position, without central nervous system findings, on the Dix-Hallpike test. We speculated that persistent torsional DBN was not caused by A-BPPV but by the light cupula of the posterior semicircular canal. The condition of this light cupula, characterized by a lower specific gravity than the endolymph, reportedly explains direction-changing characteristics of the first phase of positional alcohol-induced nystagmus with changes in head positions [5, 6]. Several authors have reported that persistent geotropic direction-changing positional nystagmus with the neutral position when turning the head to either side in the supine position occurred because of the light cupula of the horizontal semicircular canal [7–9]. We found that the condition of the light cupula may occur not only in the horizontal but also in the posterior semicircular canal.

2. Case Report

A 16-year-old boy with rotatory positional vertigo and nausea particularly when lying down and at the time of rising visited our clinic on the next day of onset. He denied any hearing loss, tinnitus, headache, or facial neurological symptoms. Past medical, surgical, and family history and head trauma were unremarkable. There was no dysdiadochokinesis, dysmetria, or tremors. Gait was not ataxic, and there was no spontaneous or gaze-evoked nystagmus. Pure tone audiogram, neurological, and eye movement examinations, including the eye-tracking test, saccades, and drum optokinetic nystagmus test, were normal. Brain magnetic resonance imaging (MRI) and magnetic resonance angiography (MRA) findings were normal. The positional and positioning nystagmus test, including the supine head roll and bilateral Dix-Hallpike tests, was recorded using an infrared charge-coupled device camera. The supine head roll test revealed DBN with the torsional component toward the left without latency in straight and right supine positions (Figure 1). The duration of the positional nystagmus was observed for >90 s. The Dix-Hallpike test of the right head-hanging position provoked

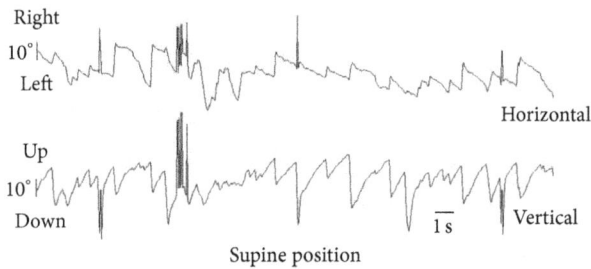

FIGURE 1: Video-oculographic recording of torsional down-beating nystagmus in the supine position in the head roll test. The vertical component is observed to be down-beating (slow phase velocity 16.5°/s, 84 beats/min) on the vertical recording. The torsional component is observed as a horizontal component beating toward the left on the horizontal recording. Video-oculography was performed using the public domain software ImageJ and a Windows computer [10].

DBN with the torsional component toward the left for >30 s. In the supine position with the head turning to the left, both left head-hanging and sitting positions on the Dix-Hallpike test did not provoke nystagmus. After 5 days, nystagmus and vertigo disappeared without medical or physical treatment.

The authors have obtained written informed consent from participant's guardian.

3. Discussion

We speculated that persistent torsional DBN occurred because of the light cupula of the right posterior semicircular canal in the patient.

Persistent geotropic direction-changing positional nystagmus with the neutral position when turning the head to either side in the supine position reportedly occurred because of the light cupula of the horizontal semicircular canal [7–9]. In the neutral position, the deflectable cupula is almost positioned perpendicular to the gravitational direction without any deflection; therefore, nystagmus is not induced in the neutral position [7–9]. The pathophysiology of the light cupula remains unclear, and there are no reports regarding the light cupula of the posterior semicircular canal. However, Ichijo [8] conjectured that the cupula is deflected by the buoyancy of attached light debris, which has lower specific gravity than the endolymph, such as monocytes and lymphocytes. Furthermore, an increase in the specific gravity of the endolymph may lead to the light cupula [7, 9]. This indicates that the light cupula of the posterior semicircular canal is extremely rare because light debris is more difficult to sink into the ampulla of the posterior semicircular canal in the lower position than into the ampulla of other semicircular canals in sitting and supine positions, if the light cupula is due to the buoyancy of attached light debris.

In the light cupula of the posterior semicircular canal, persistent DBN with the torsional component toward the unaffected ear was observed in the affected ear-down position in the supine head roll test, because this position causes ampullopetal deflection of the cupula according to Ewald's third law (Figure 2(a)). Furthermore, nystagmus was not observed in sitting and unaffected ear-down supine positions, because the direction of the deflectable cupula was almost positioned perpendicular to the gravitational direction without any deflection (Figure 2(b)). These positions without nystagmus are regarded as neutral positions in the light cupula of the posterior semicircular canal. Therefore, we speculated that positional nystagmus in our patient was due to the light cupula of the posterior semicircular canal and diagnosed that the right ear was affected.

Several studies have reported that nystagmus of A-BPPV had down-beating component with or without a torsional component in the head-hanging position on the Dix-Hallpike test [2–4]. A-BPPV is generally accompanied by positional nystagmus with typical characteristics of latency, crescendo, and transience [2–4]. Moreover, persistent torsional DBN in the head-hanging position on the Dix-Hallpike test reportedly occurred by the anterior canal cupulolithiasis, a rare variant of A-BPPV [11–13]. However, the pathophysiology of nystagmus also involves the anterior canal cupulolithiasis, which raises several concerns. First, in patients with persistent torsional DBN, reversal of nystagmus was not observed while shifting from the head-hanging to sitting position. Second, nystagmus was not observed as persistent positional nystagmus in the sitting position. In anterior canal cupulolithiasis, the debris should rest on the cupula in the sitting position because the direction of the deflectable cupula is almost positioned to the gravitational direction in the sitting position; this theoretically induces persistent upbeating torsional nystagmus because of ampullopetal deflection of the cupula according to Ewald's third law. There are no reports regarding anterior canal cupulolithiasis with persistent upbeating torsional nystagmus in the sitting position, indicating that cupulolithiasis is not the cause of nystagmus.

Vannucchi et al. reported that torsional DBN in the head-hanging position in the Dix-Hallpike test also occurred because of a rare variant canalolithiasis of the posterior semicircular canal [14]. Their hypothesis involved the debris being in the highest part of the posterior canal in the sitting position and dislodging toward the ampulla in the long arm in the bilateral Dix-Hallpike positions [14]. However, it is difficult in this theory to explain persistent torsional DBN because of canalolithiasis, and nystagmus is not observed while shifting from the head-hanging to the sitting position.

P-DBN in the head-hanging position, with or without slight positional vertigo, is indicative of a cerebellar nodulus lesion and may be caused by multiple sclerosis, ischemia, intoxication, craniocervical malformation, or cerebellar degeneration [1]. However, neurological examination and brain MRI/MRA findings were normal in the patient. The patient was 16 years old and did not experience any gaze-evoked nystagmus. Nystagmus and rotatory vertigo disappeared after 5 days. Thus, we speculated that central nervous system disorders do not cause nystagmus.

In conclusion, we speculated that persistent torsional DBN in our patient was due to the light cupula of the posterior semicircular canal. We determined that the condition of the light cupula probably occurred not only in the horizontal but also in the posterior semicircular canal. These findings prove useful for elucidating the light cupula pathophysiology.

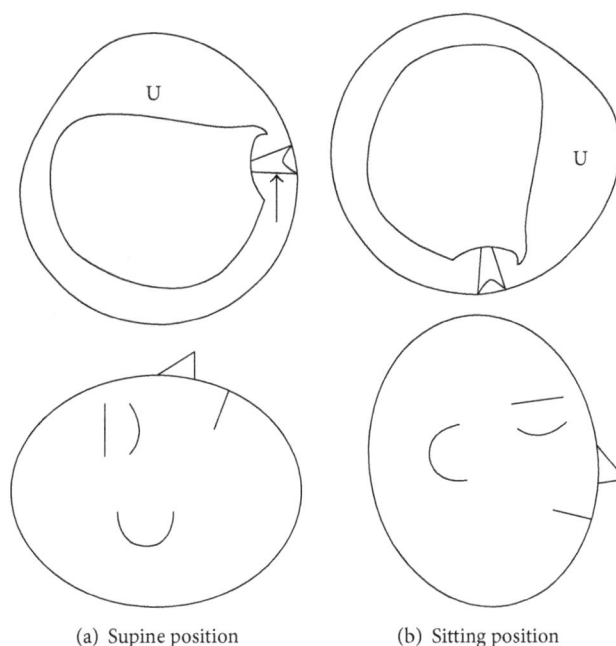

(a) Supine position (b) Sitting position

FIGURE 2: A light cupula of the right posterior semicircular canal. Arrows indicate the deflection of the cupula. U: utricle.

Competing Interests

The authors declare that they have no competing interests.

References

[1] T. Brandt, "Positional and positioning vertigo and nystagmus," *Journal of the Neurological Sciences*, vol. 95, no. 1, pp. 3–28, 1990.

[2] J. A. Lopez-Escamez, M. I. Molina, and M. J. Gamiz, "Anterior semicircular canal benign paroxysmal positional vertigo and positional downbeating nystagmus," *American Journal of Otolaryngology—Head and Neck Medicine and Surgery*, vol. 27, no. 3, pp. 173–178, 2006.

[3] D. A. Yacovino, T. C. Hain, and F. Gualtieri, "New therapeutic maneuver for anterior canal benign paroxysmal positional vertigo," *Journal of Neurology*, vol. 256, no. 11, pp. 1851–1855, 2009.

[4] S. Park, B. G. Kim, S. H. Kim, H. Chu, M. Y. Song, and M. Kim, "Canal conversion between anterior and posterior semicircular canal in benign paroxysmal positional vertigo," *Otology and Neurotology*, vol. 34, no. 9, pp. 1725–1728, 2013.

[5] G. Aschan, M. Bergstedt, L. Goldberg, and L. Laurell, "Positional nystagmus in man during and after alcohol intoxication," *Quarterly Journal of Studies on Alcohol*, vol. 17, no. 3, pp. 381–405, 1956.

[6] K. E. Money, W. H. Johnson, and B. M. Corlett, "Role of semicircular canals in positional alcohol nystagmus," *American Journal of Physiology*, vol. 208, pp. 1065–1070, 1965.

[7] K. Hiruma and T. Numata, "Positional nystagmus showing neutral points," *ORL: Journal for Oto-Rhino-Laryngology and Its Related Specialties*, vol. 66, pp. 46–50, 2004.

[8] H. Ichijo, "Persistent direction-changing geotropic positional nystagmus," *European Archives of Oto-Rhino-Laryngology*, vol. 269, no. 3, pp. 747–751, 2012.

[9] C.-H. Kim, M.-B. Kim, and J. H. Ban, "Persistent geotropic direction-changing positional nystagmus with a null plane: the light cupula," *The Laryngoscope*, vol. 124, no. 1, pp. E15–E19, 2014.

[10] T. Ikeda, M. Hashimoto, and H. Yamashita, "Analysis and display of nystagmus using ImageJ. Based on the material for the standard examination of equilibrium," *Equilibrium Research*, vol. 68, no. 2, pp. 92–96, 2009.

[11] L. E. Jackson, B. Morgan, J. C. Fletcher Jr., and W. W. O. Krueger, "Anterior canal benign paroxysmal positional vertigo: an underappreciated entity," *Otology and Neurotology*, vol. 28, no. 2, pp. 218–222, 2007.

[12] K. D. Heidenreich, K. A. Kerber, W. J. Carender, G. J. Basura, and S. A. Telian, "Persistent positional nystagmus: a case of superior semicircular canal benign paroxysmal positional vertigo?" *Laryngoscope*, vol. 121, no. 8, pp. 1818–1820, 2011.

[13] I. Adamec and M. Habek, "Anterior semicircular canal BPPV with positional downbeat nystagmus without latency, habituation and adaptation," *Neurological Sciences*, vol. 33, no. 4, pp. 955–956, 2012.

[14] P. Vannucchi, R. Pecci, and B. Giannoni, "Posterior semicircular canal benign paroxysmal positional vertigo presenting with torsional downbeating nystagmus: an apogeotropic variant," *International Journal of Otolaryngology*, vol. 2012, Article ID 413603, 9 pages, 2012.

Subglottic Metastatic Rectal Adenocarcinoma: A Specialist Multidisciplinary Airway Team Approach for Optimized Voice and Airway Outcome

Richard Heyes, Ramkishan Balakumar, Krishan Ramdoo, and Taran Tatla

Department of Otolaryngology-Head and Neck Surgery, Northwick Park Hospital,
London North West Healthcare NHS Trust, London, UK

Correspondence should be addressed to Richard Heyes; r.heyes@hotmail.com

Academic Editor: Rong-San Jiang

A 56-year-old female with a background of metastatic rectal adenocarcinoma presented with a subglottic mass causing biphasic stridor. Transoral laser microsurgery and the use of fibrin glue prevented the need for tracheostomy. Six months postoperatively there was no evidence of recurrence. Laryngeal metastasis of colorectal adenocarcinoma, although remarkably rare, is perhaps more prevalent than commonly perceived and the presence of laryngeal symptoms in a patient with colorectal adenocarcinoma should raise concern. This case is presented to aid physicians should they encounter a similar presentation of metastasis to the subglottis.

1. Introduction

An inpatient otolaryngology consult, although often for common and benign conditions, has the potential to recognize rare disease which requires urgent surgical intervention. The presence of a mass in the larynx compromising the airway is such a circumstance. The primary presenting feature of a subglottic mass may be airway obstruction, and differentials for these masses should include primary neoplasms of the laryngeal mucosa such as adenoid cystic carcinoma or squamous cell carcinoma, laryngeal chondrosarcoma, and metastasis from a distant primary tumor. A rare case of metastasis to the subglottis causing airway compromise is presented, and its management including the novel use of a common otolaryngological material is described.

2. Case Report

A 56-year-old female presented with a four-week history of increasing shortness of breath, cough, and mild dysphonia. She had been treated with antibiotics for chest X-ray demonstrated pneumonia during this time but received little benefit. On examination she was found to be "wheezy" on auscultation of the chest and she was admitted under the respiratory service.

A new diagnosis of asthma was suggested for which she was started on salbutamol nebulizers and oral prednisone forty milligrams. She made little progress and suffered sporadic episodes of oxygen desaturation. On day nine of admission, a computed tomography scan of the chest demonstrated known pulmonary metastases and an irregular appearance of the larynx. On the tenth day of admission, an otolaryngology consult was sought.

The patient's medical history was significant for locally advanced, Stage IIIb (T4, N1, M0), adenocarcinoma of the rectum which was diagnosed and treated eight years prior to this episode. Adenocarcinoma treatment involved chemoradiation with Capecitabine as an adjunct for abdominoperineal excision of the rectum with vertical rectus abdominis myocutaneous flap. Four years after her initial treatment she required radio-frequency ablation for lung and liver metastases, she underwent a partial right lung resection five years after initial treatment, and six years after initial treatment she required further radio-frequency ablation of liver and lung metastases. Her metastases proved resistant to radio-frequency ablation and at the time of admission she had

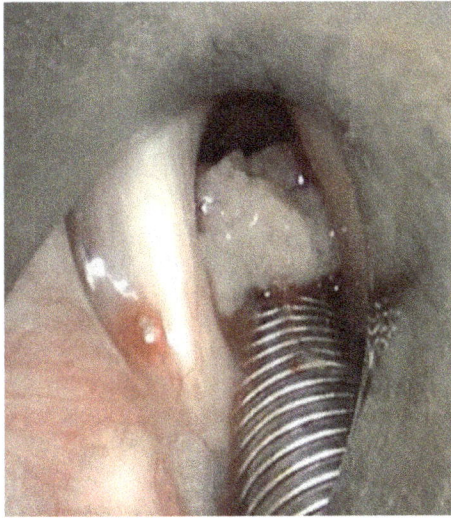

FIGURE 1: Intraoperative telescopic appearance of the subglottic tumor.

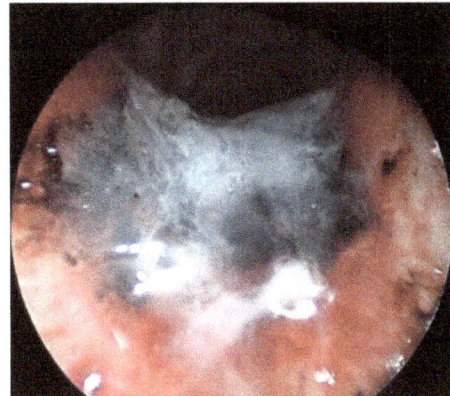

FIGURE 2: Telescopic appearance of the underlying tissues following transoral laser resection of the remnant subglottic tumor.

received four cycles of palliative Capecitabine and Mitomycin chemotherapy. She had suffered two pulmonary emboli, one six years before this episode and one six months prior, for which she took regular prophylactic low molecular weight heparin.

On otolaryngology review, she had biphasic stridor on deep breathing. Flexible nasendoscopy (FNE) was performed at the bedside which visualized a large nodular subglottic mass. Epinephrine nebulizers and intravenous dexamethasone were initiated. On the day of review, a head and neck operative list was taking place. Between cases, a specialist head and neck otolaryngologist and a specialist "difficult airway" anesthesiologist reviewed the patient with repeat FNE. A decision was quickly made to add the patient to their operative list for surgical resection of the mass while securing the airway.

Intubation was performed with the assistance of the Karl Storz C-MAC video laryngoscope and an endotracheal tube was "railroaded" beyond the subglottic mass with an Eschmann tracheal tube introducer. Microlaryngoscopy demonstrated a large sessile subglottic mass arising from the posterior commissure (Figure 1). The bulk of this mass was easily removed en masse by a laryngeal grasper. After a surgical pause to assess for bleeding, the endotracheal tube was replaced with jet ventilation to allow for laser resection of the mass remnant and its underlying mucosa; ten watts of carbon dioxide laser was used on super-pulse mode for the resection. Following laser resection the tissue was extremely friable and bleeding followed any contact (Figure 2). Therefore, in an effort to ensure no further bleeding into the airway, Tisseel fibrin glue (Baxter AG, Vienna, Austria) was applied over the site of laser ablation through a catheter inserted in the operative channel of the bronchoscope with the endoscopic applicator provided by the manufacturer. During Tisseel application, jet ventilation was held for between ninety seconds and two minutes. Two application cycles of Tisseel were employed with five minutes between applications

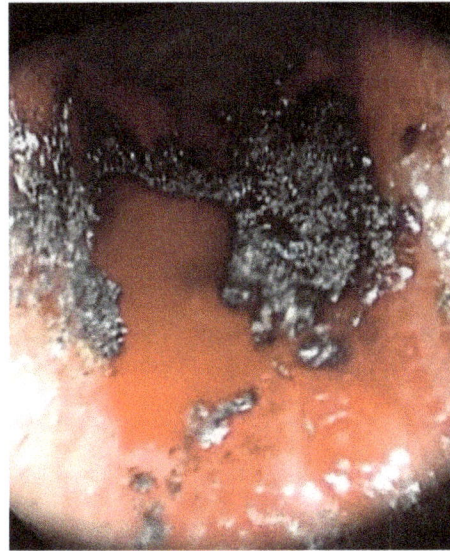

FIGURE 3: Appearance of the subglottis following the first fibrin sealant application.

(Figure 3). Five minutes after the second application of Tisseel cessation of anesthesia was initiated (supplementary video online in Supplementary Material available online at https://doi.org/10.1155/2017/2131068).

The mass measured twelve millimeters in its longest diameter and was histologically described as moderately differentiated adenocarcinoma morphological consistent with metastatic colorectal carcinoma, with positive expression of Cytokeratin 20 and Caudal Type Homeobox 2 without Cluster of Differentiation 7. Immunohistochemical studies for mismatch repair proteins found no evidence to support a diagnosis of Lynch syndrome. Pathological analysis is therefore strongly suggestive of primary tumor origin in the large intestine, confirming this mass as a metastasis of the patient's rectal adenocarcinoma and not a primary laryngeal tumor.

The patient was closely monitored for forty-eight hours on the high dependency unit with clear instructions to intubate if there was evidence of bleed into the airway. Subsequently she was stepped-down to the ward where significant resolution of her shortness of breath and cough were reported, and oxygen saturations above 96% were maintained throughout. Chest auscultation did not elicit any wheeze. Postoperative speech and language therapy evaluation found excellent speech and swallow function, and the patient was discharged from the speech and language therapy service prior to discharge. She was discharged from hospital one week after the procedure having had an uncomplicated postoperative course. Nine months postoperatively she was clinically stable, without evidence of tumor recurrence within the larynx.

3. Discussion

Metastatic disease to the larynx accounts for only 0.09 to 0.40% of all laryngeal tumors, although laryngeal metastasis may be under diagnosed since Friedmann and Osborn reported that 23.9% of patients with metastasis to the head and neck had laryngeal and tracheal diseases on autopsy [1, 2]. Ferlito et al. reported in 1988 that the most common primary sites for these metastases are the skin (melanoma) and the kidney (renal cell carcinoma); a recently published review of the English literature since 1988 proposes that colorectal adenocarcinoma is more common than previously anticipated, accounting for a quarter of 41 published cases [3, 4].

The route for hematogenous spread of colon cancer to the larynx via the systemic circulation is the inferior vena cava, right heart, lungs, left heart, aorta, external carotid artery, superior thyroid artery, and superior laryngeal artery [5]. The vertebral venous plexus has been specifically implicated in retrograde metastatic spread of colorectal carcinoma [6]. Lymphatic metastases spread via the thoracic duct, left supraclavicular lymph nodes, and subglottic lymph nodes [5]. Isolated metastasis to the larynx is extremely rare and patients with a colorectal primary are especially likely to suffer from concurrent metastasis, with lung metastases most common [7].

The location prevalence of metastatic tumors of the larynx is as follows: 39% transglottic, 27% supraglottic, 27% subglottic, and 7% glottic [4]. The site of laryngeal metastasis of colorectal adenocarcinoma is known for 14 patients: 50% were subglottic, 21% transglottic, 14% supraglottic, and 7% glottic [8]. The median age of laryngeal metastasis presentation is 59 years with a male predominance [4]. The symptoms of laryngeal metastases resemble the symptoms of primary laryngeal tumors. Common presenting complaints include dysphonia (66%) and dyspnea on exertion (60%); stridor occurs in approximately 20% of cases [4, 8]. Generally supraglottic masses are symptomatic earlier than subglottic masses, which may remain silent until airway obstruction occurs.

Although due to the rarity of laryngeal metastases treatment guidelines do not exist, symptomatic and palliative treatment is recommended in cases of concurrent distal metastasis. In isolated laryngeal metastases, or when accompanied by a single pulmonary metastasis, curative treatment should be offered following specialist multidisciplinary discussion [4, 8]. Airway protection is paramount to management. In all previous cases of rectal cancer metastasizing to the larynx, tracheostomy or extended laryngectomy has been performed. Our approach prevented significant distress to the patient (as tracheostomy recovery was her primary preoperative concern), in addition to reducing postoperative morbidity.

A successful outcome was achieved by cohesive teamwork. Early expert involvement and the presence of a specialist airway team reduced management discourse and spared the patient radical surgery. Close links with those providing intensive postoperative care and the availability of "24/7" onsite anesthesiologists and otolaryngologists allowed for safe novel intervention.

To our knowledge this is the first description of the use of fibrin glue to cover the site of laser-excised tumor in the larynx in an attempt reduce the risk of postoperative bleeding, which is associated with significant morbidity and mortality. The senior author's involvement in an unpublished case of postoperative bleeding following laser resection of a supraglottic laryngeal tumor was instrumental in the adoption of the described technique. In that case, the patient developed chest pain and ECG signs of myocardial ischemia postoperatively resulting in the administration of anticoagulative therapy and, although the wound bed was dry immediately postoperatively, basal bronchopneumonia, respiratory failure, and death resulted from presumed slow laryngeal bleeding. This experience highlights the risk of an unprotected friable wound in the airway. Fibrin glue (fibrin sealant) is composed of human plasma proteins and mimics the final pathway of the coagulation cascade, yielding a stable and insoluble clot [9]. The role of fibrin sealants throughout surgery is expanding and the use of fibrin has been described to line the repair of cricopharyngeal myotomy and in tracheal lacerations [9, 10]. Our patient suffered no complications associated with the use of fibrin glue and we have demonstrated that Tisseel can be applied to the larynx with the use of jet ventilation provided a pause in ventilation is permitted.

4. Conclusion

Laryngeal metastasis of colorectal adenocarcinoma, although remarkably rare, is perhaps more prevalent than commonly perceived and the presence of laryngeal symptoms in a patient with colorectal adenocarcinoma should raise concern. In this report, a specialist multidisciplinary team managed an unusual otolaryngology consult and prevented tracheostomy with the use of transoral laser microsurgery and fibrin glue. This case is presented to aid physicians should they encounter a similar presentation of metastasis to the subglottis.

Ethical Approval

This study was deemed IRB exempt.

Consent

Informed consent has been obtained.

Disclosure

This case was presented at the American Laryngological Association's 2016 Spring Meeting at COSM in Chicago, Illinois on May 18-19, 2016. This case was presented at Northwick Park Hospital's Grand Rounds June 2016, winning the "Ollie Smith Award."

Competing Interests

The authors declare that there are no competing interests regarding the publication of this paper.

References

[1] P. Nicolai, R. Puxeddu, J. Cappiello et al., "Metastatic neoplasms to the larynx: report of three cases," *Laryngoscope*, vol. 106, no. 7, pp. 851–855, 1996.

[2] I. Friedmann and D. A. Osborn, "Metastatic tumours in the ear, nose and throat region," *The Journal of laryngology and otology*, vol. 79, pp. 576–591, 1965.

[3] A. Ferlito, G. Caruso, and G. Recher, "Secondary laryngeal tumors: report of seven cases with review of the literature," *Archives of Otolaryngology—Head & Neck Surgery*, vol. 114, no. 6, pp. 635–639, 1988.

[4] J. Zenga, M. Mehrad, and J. P. Bradley, "Metastatic cancer to the larynx: a case report and update," *Journal of Voice*, vol. 30, no. 6, pp. 774.e9–774.e12, 2016.

[5] J. G. Batsakis, M. A. Luna, and R. M. Byers, "Metastases to the larynx," *Head and Neck Surgery*, vol. 7, no. 6, pp. 458–460, 1985.

[6] M. Vider, Y. Maruyama, and R. Narvaez, "Significance of the vertebral venous (Batson's) plexus in metastatic spread in colorectal carcinoma," *Cancer*, vol. 40, no. 1, pp. 67–71, 1977.

[7] S. Terashima, S. Watanabe, and M. Shoji, "Long-term survival after resection of metastases in the lungs and larynx originating from sigmoid colon cancer: report of a case," *Fukushima journal of medical science*, vol. 60, no. 1, pp. 82–85, 2014.

[8] J. Q. Ta and J. Y. Kim, "Rectal adenocarcinoma metastatic to the larynx," *Ear, Nose & Throat Journal*, vol. 90, no. 4, article E28, 2011.

[9] M. Mortensen, M. R. Schaberg, E. M. Genden, and P. Woo, "Transoral resection of short segment Zenker's diverticulum and cricopharyngeal myotomy: an alternative minimally invasive approach," *Laryngoscope*, vol. 120, no. 1, pp. 17–22, 2010.

[10] G. Cardillo, L. Carbone, F. Carleo et al., "Tracheal lacerations after endotracheal intubation: a proposed morphological classification to guide non-surgical treatment," *European Journal of Cardio-thoracic Surgery*, vol. 37, no. 3, pp. 581–587, 2010.

Juvenile Nasopharyngeal Angiofibroma Presenting with Acute Airway Obstruction

Chikoti Wheat,[1,2] **Ryan J. Bickley,**[3] **Erik Cohen,**[4] **Danya Wenzler,**[5] **Nancy Hunter,**[6] **and Donna Astiz**[2]

[1]*Department of Dermatology, Johns Hopkins University, Baltimore, MD, USA*
[2]*Department of Internal Medicine, Morristown Medical Center, Morristown, NJ, USA*
[3]*Johns Hopkins University School of Medicine, Baltimore, MD, USA*
[4]*Department of Otolaryngology, Morristown Medical Center, Morristown, NJ, USA*
[5]*Department of Infectious Diseases, Morristown Medical Center, Morristown, NJ, USA*
[6]*Department of Pathology, Morristown Medical Center, Morristown, NJ, USA*

Correspondence should be addressed to Chikoti Wheat; chikotim@gmail.com

Academic Editor: Ho-Sheng Lin

We describe a case of a 24-year-old male presenting urgently with a juvenile nasopharyngeal angiofibroma (JNA) with difficulty breathing, inability to swallow, and respiratory distress following throat swelling. The swelling was reduced with administration of dexamethasone and the JNA was surgically resected within 48 hours. This presentation was atypical given the acuity of presentation and the patient's older age.

1. Introduction

Juvenile nasopharyngeal angiofibromas (JNAs) are benign nasopharyngeal tumors of high vascularity occurring almost always in prepubertal and adolescent males [1]. They typically present as insidious onset nasal obstruction (80–90%), epistaxis (45–60%), headache (25%), and facial swelling (10–18%) and are most often associated with a history of chronic sinusitis [2–4]. There are various genetic etiologies that have been proposed; however, none of these have been directly linked to nasopharyngeal angiofibromas so that a causal link is yet to be established [5]. In this case report, we present an unusual case of a nasopharyngeal angiofibroma causing obstruction acutely in an adult male.

2. Case Report

A 24-year-old male from a local state correctional facility presented to the Morristown Medical Center Emergency Department in Morristown, New Jersey, complaining of throat swelling, difficulty breathing, and inability to swallow beginning four hours prior to presentation. He reported a 6-month history of chronic sinusitis with persistent nasal congestion and clear rhinorrhea for which he had been taking over-the-counter decongestants. He denied any prior symptoms of swelling or obstruction and reported no epistaxis. He denied any recent trauma or exposure to allergenic agents. He admitted to the occasional use of inhaled marijuana but denied any other illicit substance abuse. His only relevant past medical history was latent tuberculosis for which he had been taking moxifloxacin for four months due to exposure to a multidrug resistant strain of tuberculosis prevalent amongst the correctional facility inmates.

On exam, he was moderately dyspneic, with drooling and a muffled voice without adenopathy. Within a few minutes of presentation, he developed progressive respiratory distress and was taken emergently to the operating room where he underwent nasal fiber optic intubation. He was started on combination therapy including dexamethasone, diphenhydramine, fluconazole, and vancomycin for coverage of allergic and infectious etiologies.

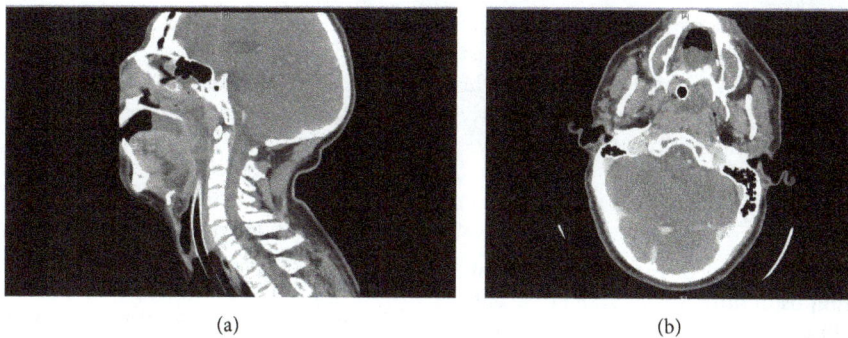

FIGURE 1: Sagittal (a) and axial (b) contrast enhanced CT images of soft tissue of the neck. Sagittal image shows isodense to hypodense central attenuation with a scattered rim of thin peripheral enhancement (a). The axial image shows the mass located in the right frontal sinus with near complete opacification of the anterior and middle ethmoid air cells and maxillary sinuses with thickening of the pharyngeal mucosa consistent with chronic pharyngitis and sinusitis.

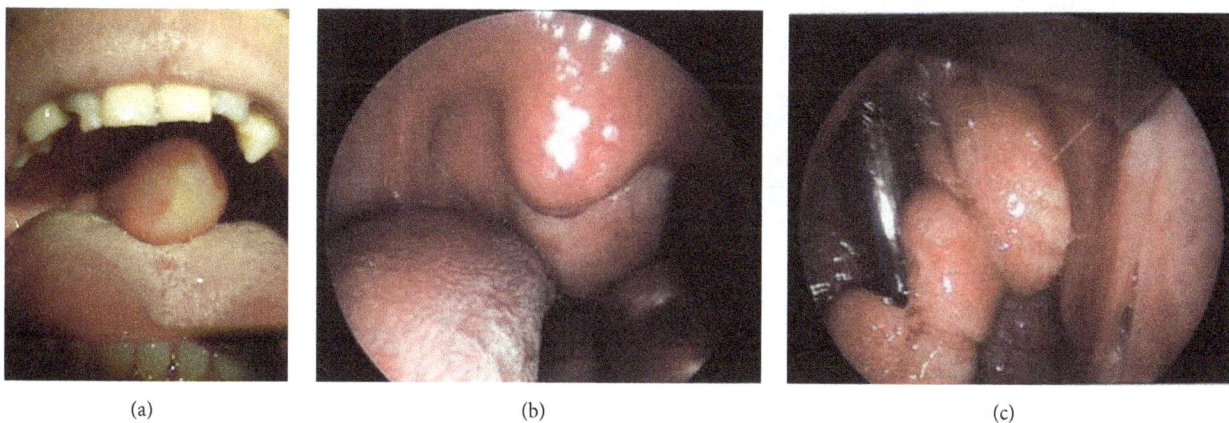

FIGURE 2: Flesh colored polypoid mass attached to the upper posterior nasopharyngeal wall on initial presentation (a), 36 hours after presentation when patient had been treated with steroids and intravenous antibiotics (b) and following transnasal endoscopic and transoral resection (c).

A computed tomography (CT) scan of the neck showed the mass to extend into the oropharynx with surrounding mucosal thickening consistent with chronic sinusitis (Figure 1).

On treatment with dexamethasone, the mass decreased in size, and he underwent transnasal resection 48 hours after presentation. During endoscopic resection, purulent discharge was noted in the middle nasal meatus. Cultures subsequently revealed coagulase negative *Staphylococci* and *Propionibacterium acnes* species.

The resected specimen was a smooth surfaced lobulated mass attached to the upper posterior nasopharyngeal wall (Figure 2). A histologic analysis revealed the mass to be a nasopharyngeal angiofibroma (Figure 3). Microscopic examination of the mass showed high peripheral and reduced central vascularity. The stroma consisted of spindled cells in a sea of randomly arranged collagen with a few scattered vascular channels (Figure 3).

Routine laboratory values appearing on a complete blood count with differential were normal. Additional studies were performed to rule out infectious, allergic, or immunologic etiologies. Both mononucleosis spot test and β-hemolytic

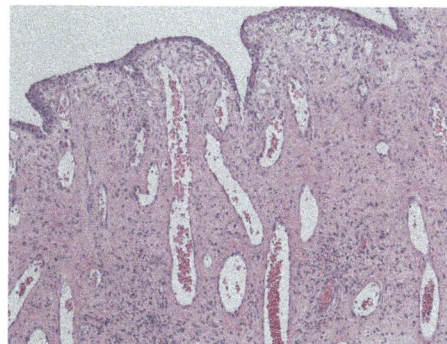

FIGURE 3: Histologic images highlighting the vascular and stromal components characteristic of a nasopharyngeal angiofibroma. Image showing increased peripheral vascularity.

Streptococci blood level test were negative. Lab results were significant for depressed CD4$^+$ and CD8$^+$ counts (178 and 106, resp.) with a CD4$^+$/CD8$^+$ ratio of 1.67. An HIV-1/2 antibody test was negative with an HIV-1 RNA load < 75. C1-INH levels were normal. The patient showed normal immunoglobulin levels except for marginally low IgM. He was noted to have EBV test results consistent with past infection (positive EBV capsid IgG, positive EBV nuclear antigen, negative EBV capsid IgM, and negative EBV early antigen). Fungal and acid-fast bacillus cultures were negative.

3. Discussion

JNAs commonly occur in patients with histories of chronic sinusitis at least a few months in duration, as is the case with our patient. The acuity in presentation makes this presentation atypical. Though literature reports JNAs to be of insidious onset in adolescent males, there have only been a few reports of these masses occurring in adults [4, 6, 7]. The classic presentation is longstanding unilateral nasal obstruction and recurrent epistaxis neither of which were present in this case. Instead, this patient experienced symptoms that manifested acutely over four hours, although the mass certainly did not present in its entirety over this same timeframe.

Coincidentally, the patient had suppressed CD4$^+$ and CD8$^+$ T-lymphocyte counts, suggesting a possible causal relationship. Currently, there has been no suggestion of an association between the immune status of the individual and the susceptibility to developing these tumors.

Given that depressed immune function is a risk factor for chronic sinusitis, it is possible that this may also be a risk factor for developing JNA. As of yet, no reports discuss the immune status of patients except for one case report of an HIV positive individual [8]. While our patient was HIV negative with negative viral load, he did have a depressed CD4$^+$/CD8$^+$ ratio, though not as low a ratio as would be typical for HIV positive patients. Perhaps it is important to consider individual immune status as a risk factor for acute JNAs.

Competing Interests

The authors listed declare that they have no conflict of interests.

Acknowledgments

Special thanks are due to Nimisha Mehta, M.D. (Radiology Resident), and Alexander J. Sikes, M.D. (Emergency Medicine Resident), for providing photographs.

References

[1] R. Rubin, D. S. Strayer, and E. Rubin, *Rubin's Pathology: Clinicopathologic Foundations of Medicine*, Lippincott Williams & Wilkins, 5th edition, 2008.

[2] I. P. Tang, S. Shashinder, G. G. Krishnan, and P. Narayanan, "Juvenile nasopharyngeal angiofibroma in a tertiary centre: ten-year experience," *Singapore Medical Journal*, vol. 50, no. 3, pp. 261–264, 2009.

[3] J. P. Windfuhr and S. Remmert, "Extranasopharyngeal angiofibroma: etiology, incidence and management," *Acta Oto-Laryngologica*, vol. 124, no. 8, pp. 880–889, 2004.

[4] S. L. Mills, E. B. Stelow, and J. L. Hunt, "Tumors of the upper aerodigestive tract and ear," in *AFIP Atlas of Tumor Pathology*, 4th Series, Fascicle 17, Armed Forces Institute of Pathology, 2012.

[5] M. P. Maniglia, M. E. B. Ribeiro, N. M. D. Costa et al., "Molecular pathogenesis of juvenile nasopharyngeal angiofibroma in Brazilian patients," *Pediatric Hematology and Oncology*, vol. 30, no. 7, pp. 616–622, 2013.

[6] R. Madhavan Nirmal, V. Veeravarmal, A. Santha Devy, and C. R. Ramachandran, "Unusual presentation of nasopharyngeal (juvenile) angiofibroma in a 45 year old female," *Indian Journal of Dental Research*, vol. 15, no. 4, pp. 145–148, 2004.

[7] J. A. Patrocínio, L. G. Patrocínio, B. H. C. Borba, B. De Santi Bonatti, and A. H. B. Guimarães, "Nasopharyngeal angiofibroma in an elderly woman," *American Journal of Otolaryngology—Head and Neck Medicine and Surgery*, vol. 26, no. 3, pp. 198–200, 2005.

[8] G. Landonio, A. Nosari, P. Oreste, S. Cantoni, D. Cattaneo, and E. Ghislandi, "Aggressive course of angiofibroma in an HIV-positive patient," *Tumori*, vol. 79, no. 3, pp. 224–226, 1993.

Transnasal, Transethmoidal Endoscopic Removal of a Foreign Body in the Medial Extraconal Orbital Space

Diego Escobar Montatixe,[1] José Miguel Villacampa Aubá,[1] Álvaro Sánchez Barrueco,[1] Beatriz Sobrino Guijarro,[2] and Carlos Cenjor Español[1]

[1]Department of Otolaryngology, Head and Neck Surgery, Hospital Universitario Fundación Jiménez Díaz, Madrid, Spain
[2]Department of Neuroradiology, Hospital Universitario Fundación Jiménez Díaz, Madrid, Spain

Correspondence should be addressed to Diego Escobar Montatixe; diego.escobar@fjd.es

Academic Editor: Nicolas Perez-Fernandez

Intraorbital foreign bodies are located within the orbit but outside the ocular globe. Though not uncommon, removal of these objects poses a challenge for surgeons. External approaches have been the most frequently used but are associated with increased complications and morbidity. An endoscopic endonasal approach can be an appropriate and less complicated technique in these cases. We report a case of a chronic intraorbital foreign body located within the medial extraconal space lateral to the lamina papyracea and behind the lacrimonasal duct, which was successfully removed using a transnasal, transethmoidal endoscopic technique. Neither postoperative complications nor ocular impairment was reported. The patient improved and remains asymptomatic. The transnasal transethmoidal endoscopic approach can be used as a safer and less invasive alternative when removing foreign bodies from the medial orbital compartment.

1. Introduction

Intraorbital foreign bodies are rare and pose a challenge for surgeons. The term "intraorbital" refers to those foreign bodies located within the orbit but outside the ocular globe [1]. Classically, external approaches have been the most widely used; however, these are invasive and associated with several major disadvantages such as postsurgical scarring and considerable morbidity. As technology and the understanding of the anatomy gradually progress, surgeons are using endoscopic techniques for diseases located outside the nasal sinuses.

The medial portion of the orbit shares a boundary with the ethmoid and sphenoid sinuses, and surgeons have exploited this proximity to access the orbit [2]. Foreign bodies located close to the medial wall of the orbit can be safely removed using an endoscopic transnasal approach [3]. This technique is less invasive and, when performed by an experienced surgeon, is associated with fewer complications. We present the case of a female patient with a chronic intraorbital foreign body (a shard of glass) located within the medial extraconal space and successful removal of the body using a transnasal, transethmoidal endoscopic approach.

2. Case Report

A 41-year-old woman presented to our department with a 2-year history of recurrent left orbital edema and erythema which had partially improved with oral antibiotics. The patient also reported mucopurulent rhinorrhea and intermittent bilateral nasal stuffiness not related to the orbital symptomatology. Relevant past history was limited to a road traffic accident approximately 5 years previously; following this accident, a residual foreign body (glass) located medially to the left eye globe was detected on a plain radiograph performed at the time (Figure 1(a)). The patient initially declined to undergo a foreign body removal procedure, although persistence of chronic symptomatology led her to consult with our department on available surgical options.

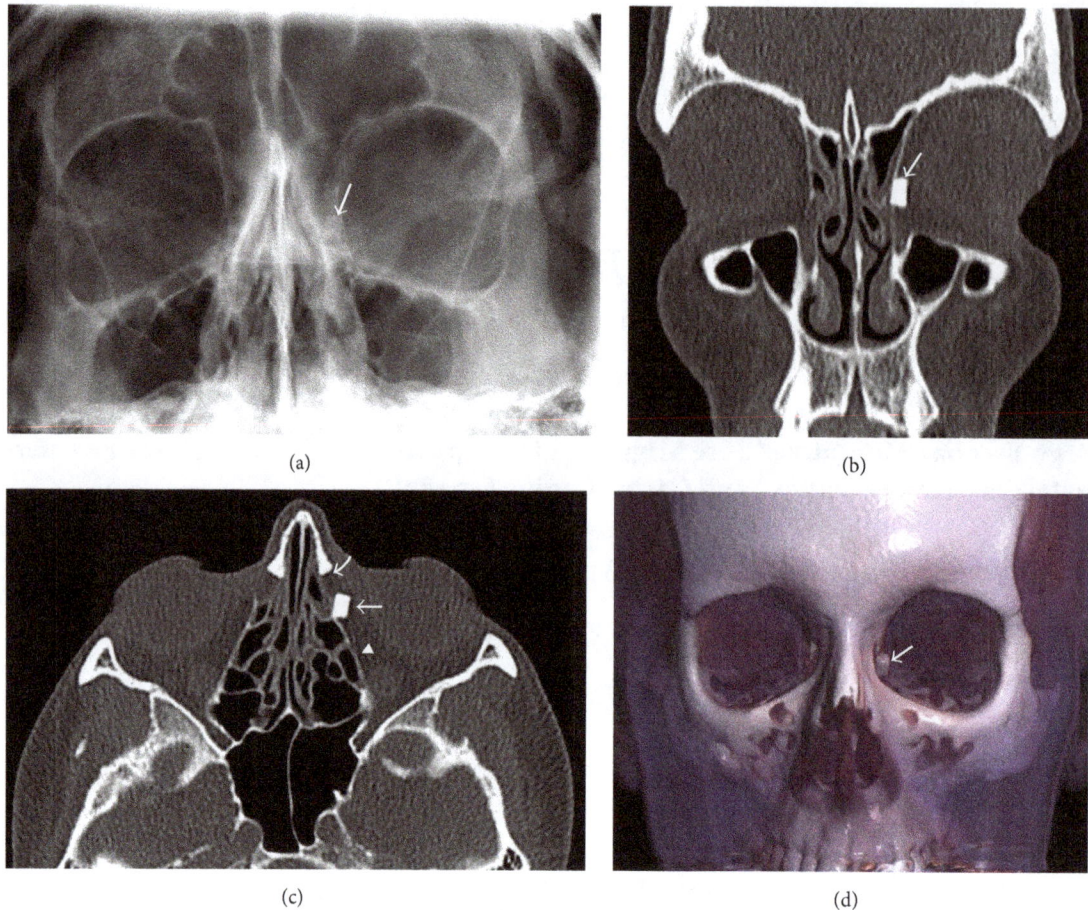

FIGURE 1: (a–d) Frontal plain radiograph revealing (a) a rectangular high-density body (arrow) overlying the left ethmoid cells and in contact with the lamina papyracea. Contrast unenhanced axial (b) and coronal (c) CT scans show a well-delineated hyperdense body (arrow) within the left orbit, adjacent to the lamina papyracea (arrowhead in (c)) and immediately posterior to the lacrimonasal duct (curved arrow in (c)). (d) 3D-CT volume-rendered reconstructed image shows the intraorbital metallic foreign body (arrow).

Nasal endoscopy detected hypertrophy of the left middle turbinate and an accompanying mucopurulent discharge from the middle meatus, without other relevant findings.

A computerized tomography (CT) scan of the facial and paranasal sinuses showed slight middle meatal stenosis due to a bullous left middle turbinate with normal, air-filled sinus cavities and the presence of a hyperdense, well-defined foreign body (a shard of glass) located within the eye orbit in the medial extraconal space, laterally to the lamina papyracea and posteriorly to the nasolacrimal duct (Figures 1(b), 1(c), and 1(d)).

At the request of the patient, we began planning to remove the foreign body endoscopically using a transnasal transethmoidal approach accompanied by a widening of the osteomeatal complex as treatment of her middle meatal stenosis. Partial resections of the bullous middle turbinate, maxillary antrostomy, and anterior ethmoidectomy with aperture of the left lamina papyracea were performed; the foreign body was located within the periorbital fat and was successfully removed without evidence of lesions to the extraocular musculature or the nasolacrimal duct (Figure 2).

No ocular movement anomalies or other immediate postsurgical complications were detected. On follow-up, the patient remains asymptomatic, presenting no additional episodes of left orbital cellulitis to date.

3. Discussion

From an anatomic point of view, the orbit is a highly complex area where critical structures occupy a small space [4]. The cone formed by the extraocular muscles divides the orbit into two compartments: intraconal and extraconal [5]. Intraorbital foreign bodies are located in the orbit and the vast majority are secondary to facial trauma involving penetration of the orbit. The surgical approach employed for extraction depends on the nature of the body, its location (anterior or posterior orbit), and associated complications (infections, optic nerve lesions or compression, and lesions to the extraocular nerve or intraorbital blood vessels) [5].

Complex craniomaxillofacial, transethmoidal, or transcranial approaches have traditionally been used to reach the

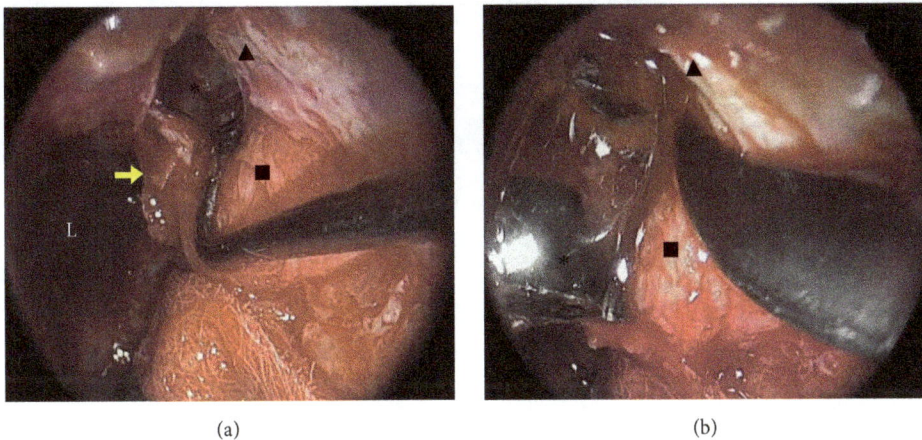

(a)   (b)

Figure 2: (a-b) Left transnasal endoscopic view of a shard of glass (yellow asterisk) following the aperture of the lamina papyracea (yellow arrow) and left periorbital fat (black square) immediately behind the nasolacrimal duct (black arrowhead).

invading material, especially when foreign bodies are located in the medial aspect of the orbit [6, 7]. However, external approaches require skin incisions, osteotomies, and significant displacement of orbital structures, including the globe. The endoscopic endonasal technique can be considered a surgical option to manage the optic nerve and orbital compartments (medial side) for various posttraumatic, inflammatory, infectious, or tumoral diseases; moreover, it minimizes external scarring and preserves cosmesis [8]. From an anatomic viewpoint, this procedure appears to be an excellent surgical approach to access the medial compartment of the orbit and the orbital apex [9]. This alternative should be taken into consideration during surgical planning, especially when dealing with medial extra- and intraconal orbital lesions, including foreign bodies located close to the medial wall of the orbit [3, 8].

Neuronavigation has been shown to be an essential element in endoscopic intervention within the orbit, as it allows for precise location of the target, thereby enabling surgeons to make the smallest possible opening in the bone and periorbita [10–12]; in our patient, however, as the intraorbital foreign body was located in such a concrete and accessible location (beside the lamina papyracea and behind the nasolacrimal duct), we opted not to use this implement. Therefore, we performed a transnasal transethmoidal endoscopic approach to access the lamina papyracea, which preserved our anatomic references (the nasolacrimal duct in this case), thus making this a less invasive approach and a feasible alternative.

4. Conclusion

The transnasal transethmoidal endoscopic approach can be employed as an alternative when removing intraorbital foreign bodies located in the medial extraconal compartment. This is a safe and less invasive approach in comparison with classic surgical techniques.

Competing Interests

There are no financial interests, relationships, and affiliations relevant to the subject of the manuscript. There are no competing interests to declare.

References

[1] T. P. Fulcher, A. A. McNab, and T. J. Sullivan, "Clinical features and management of intraorbital foreign bodies," *Ophthalmology*, vol. 109, no. 3, pp. 494–500, 2002.

[2] V. R. Ramakrishnan, J. D. Suh, A. G. Chiu, and J. N. Palmer, "Addition of a minimally invasive medial orbital approach in the endoscopic management of advanced sino-orbital disease: cadaver study with clinical correlations," *Laryngoscope*, vol. 121, no. 2, pp. 437–441, 2011.

[3] T. Łysoń, A. Sieskiewicz, M. Rogowski, and Z. Mariak, "Transnasal endoscopic removal of intraorbital wooden foreign body," *Journal of Neurological Surgery, Part A: Central European Neurosurgery*, vol. 74, no. 1, pp. e100–e103, 2013.

[4] I. Dallan, V. Seccia, R. Lenzi et al., "Transnasal approach to the medial intraconal space: anatomic study and clinical considerations," *Minimally Invasive Neurosurgery*, vol. 53, no. 4, pp. 164–168, 2010.

[5] D. M. I. Turliuc, V. V. Costan, A. I. Cucu, and C. F. L. Costea, "Intraorbital foreign body," *Revista medico-chirurgicala a Societatii de Medici si Naturalisti din Iasi*, vol. 119, no. 1, pp. 179–184, 2015.

[6] B. D. Edgington, C. E. Geist, and J. Kuo, "Intraorbital organic foreign body in a tree surgeon," *Ophthalmic Plastic and Reconstructive Surgery*, vol. 24, no. 3, pp. 237–238, 2008.

[7] M. Feichtinger, W. Zemann, and H. Kärcher, "Removal of a pellet from the left orbital cavity by image-guided endoscopic navigation," *International Journal of Oral and Maxillofacial Surgery*, vol. 36, no. 4, pp. 358–361, 2007.

[8] P. Castelnuovo, M. Turri-Zanoni, P. Battaglia, D. Locatelli, and I. Dallan, "Endoscopic endonasal management of orbital pathologies," *Neurosurgery Clinics of North America*, vol. 26, no. 3, pp. 463–472, 2015.

[9] S. M. Brown, T. H. Schwartz, and V. K. Anand, "The transethmoidal, transorbital approach to the orbital apex," in *Practical Endoscopic Skull Base Surgery*, pp. 123–133, Plural, San Diego, Calif, USA, 2007.

[10] J. S. Kent, L. H. Allen, and B. W. Rotenberg, "Image-guided transnasal endoscopic techniques in the management of orbital disease," *Orbit*, vol. 29, no. 6, pp. 328–333, 2010.

[11] A. Schramm, M. M. Suarez-Cunqueiro, M. Rücker et al., "Computer-assisted therapy in orbital and mid-facial reconstructions," *The International Journal of Medical Robotics and Computer Assisted Surgery*, vol. 5, no. 2, pp. 111–124, 2009.

[12] A. Sieskiewicz, T. Lyson, Z. Mariak, and M. Rogowski, "Endoscopic trans-nasal approach for biopsy of orbital tumours using image-guided neuro-navigation system," *Acta Neurochirurgica*, vol. 150, no. 5, pp. 441–445, 2008.

Acute Marjolin's Ulcer in a Postauricular Scar after Mastoidectomy

Kholoud A. Alhysoni, Sumaiyah M. Bukhari, and Mutawakel F. Hajjaj

Otolaryngology Department, Ohud Hospital, Medina, Saudi Arabia

Correspondence should be addressed to Kholoud A. Alhysoni; kholoudalhysoni@hotmail.com

Academic Editor: Abrão Rapoport

Background. Marjolin's ulcer is a rare, aggressive cutaneous malignancy that arises primarily in burn scars but can occur in other types of scars. Squamous cell carcinoma is the most common variant, and while malignant degeneration usually takes a long time, it can develop acutely. *Case Report*. a 30-year-old man who developed Marjolin's ulcer acutely in a right postauricular scar after mastoidectomy and the incision and drainage of a mastoid abscess. To the best of our knowledge, this report is the first to describe a Marjolin's ulcer in a postauricular surgical scar. However, it has been reported in others areas in the head and neck. *Conclusion*. Marjolin's ulcer is most commonly observed after postburn scars, but it may be observed after any type of scars, as our patient developed an SCC with a postsurgical scar. Early diagnosis is essential, and a biopsy should be performed on any nonhealing wound or chronic wound that undergoes a sudden change. Tissue samples should be taken from both the centre and the margins of the wound.

1. Introduction

Marjolin's ulcer refers to cancer that most often presents in an area with a chronic burn wound. Marjolin's ulcer is also associated with nonhealing wounds, venous ulcers, lupus vulgaris, vaccination scars, snake bite scars, chronic osteomyelitis fistulae [1], amputation stumps, cystostomy sites, chronic lymphedema, chronic pilonidal sinuses [2], pressure ulcers in spina bifida patients [3], ischial bursitis [4], hidradenitis suppurativa [5], posttraumatic scars [6–9], surgical scars [10], and scars after coronary artery bypass grafting [11].

The most commonly affected sites are the lower extremities, followed by the head and neck region and the trunk [1, 11]. The most commonly involved areas of the head are the scalp [1, 6] and face [1, 10]; in one reported case, the nose was affected [12], and in another, the neck was affected [8].

We report the case of a 30-year-old man who developed Marjolin's ulcer in the right postauricular area only 9 months after the incision and drainage of a right mastoid abscess. There are no other reports of Marjolin's ulcers in this area to date.

2. Case Presentation

A 30-year-old Bangladeshi male presented to the emergency room with a five-day history of right postauricular swelling that had gradually increased in size. There was associated fever and purulent discharge from the right ear.

The patient had a longstanding history of right ear discharge and decreased hearing in the right ear with no tinnitus or vertigo.

The patient had no medical illness and was negative for human immunodeficiency virus.

Examination revealed a right mastoid swelling that was fluctuant, hyperemic, tender, and warm. Needle aspiration revealed 6 cc of purulent fluid. The right external auditory canal (EAC) and right tympanic membrane perforation emitted purulent discharge. The facial nerve was intact on examination, with no palpable lymph nodes.

Pure tone audiometry showed right profound mixed hearing loss.

Axial computerized tomography of the temporal bone showed a mastoid abscess with bone destruction (Figure 1).

(a)

(b)

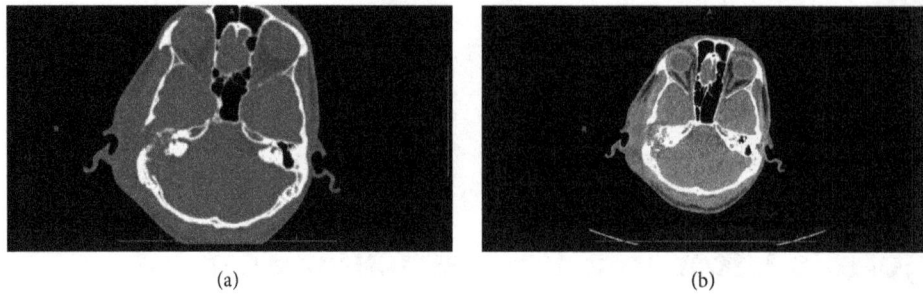

FIGURE 1: Axial CT scan (noncontrast) showing the temporal bone. (a) Bone window and right ill-defined soft tissue density in the right mastoid air cells, middle, and inner ear, associated with bony destruction. Only the basal turn of the cochlea and part of the vestibule are visualized. (b) Soft tissue window and posterior aspect of the tegmentum tympani appear destroyed, thinned, and interrupted, with subcutaneous soft tissue swelling adjacent to the EAC and collection at the superior aspect.

Magnetic resonance imaging of the brain showed enhanced collection in the subcutaneous tissue and auricular region posterior and anterosuperior to the EAC that extended to the mastoid cavity and the middle ear cleft. There was focal area of dural enhancement observed in the right temporal lobe (Figure 2).

A diagnosis of right chronic suppurative otitis media complicated by mastoid abscess was made.

Incision and drainage of the right mastoid abscess with modified radical mastoidectomy were performed and revealed that a large cholesteatoma sac occupied the mastoid cavity and extended to the middle ear cleft. The histopathology results were consistent with cholesteatoma (Figure 3).

Postoperatively, the patient developed right postauricular wound dehiscence. The patient was lost to follow-up for seven months and later presented with 4 cm by 5 cm right postauricular ulcer with raised edges and a necrotic centre (base) (Figure 4).

Computerized axial tomography showed a right periauricular soft tissue mass with an ill-defined border (Figure 5).

Biopsies were taken from the edges and centre of the lesion. The biopsy from the edges showed moderately differentiated squamous cell carcinoma, and those from the centre showed dysplasia with keratinous material (Figure 6).

As the patient after diagnosis chose to return to his home country, no definite treatment was given to him.

3. Discussion

Marjolin's ulcer is a rare and often aggressive cutaneous malignancy that develops in previously traumatized or chronically inflamed skin, particularly after burns [7].

In the first century, Aurelius Cornelius Celsus was the first to report the development of a tumour in old burn scars and chronic nonhealing wounds. In 1828, Jean Nicholas Marjolin, a French surgeon, described a phenomenon that involved the formation of ulcerations within a burn scar and coined the term "ulcere cancroide"; however, the description did not say that the ulcers were malignant [13]. In 1838, Dupuytren observed that de novo malignancy could arise in chronic wounds; he observed this phenomenon in a Belgian man who was treated for a cancer that developed from a scar sustained from a sulphuric acid burn [14]. The name "Marjolin's ulcer" was first used by Da Costa in 1903, when he defined an ulcer arising from burn scars as Marjolin's ulcer [15].

Squamous cell carcinoma is the most common histological type among these wounds, followed by basal cell carcinoma, sarcoma, and melanoma [2, 10, 11, 16]. The male-to-female ratio increases with increasing patient age over 50 years [10, 11, 16].

Various theories have been proposed to explain the pathogenesis of the malignant transformation of these wounds, but none has provided a full explanation. The toxins theory, which proposes that the chronic inflammatory processes that lead to tissue damage produce toxins that may be carcinogenic, was proposed by Treves and Pack [11]. Virchow's theory of chronic irritation explains that, with chronic irritation and repeated tissue injury, the epithelium becomes less stable, loses contact inhibition, and undergoes malignant change. Other proposed theories include epithelial element implantation (Ribet's theory), the cocarcinogenic theory (Friedwald and Rose), and the immunologically privileged site theory. Castillo and Goldsmith suggested that the poor lymphatic flow in scar tissue impairs immunosurveillance, making it difficult for the body to mount an effective antigen-antibody response to protooncogens or tumours within scars. Hereditary theory and the environmental and genetic interaction theory seek to explain the evolution of acute Marjolin's ulcers by suggesting that genetic differences make the individual more susceptible to environmental insults, resulting in a short latency period.

As none of the above theories fully explain the evolution of Marjolin's ulcer, some studies have proposed a multifactorial theory consisting of various combinations of the current theories [3, 17, 18].

Latency has been described as the time between the primary pathology and the confirmation of a pathologic diagnosis of Marjolin's ulcer. The reported latency period for the development of malignancy is between 11 and 75 years [18]. Marjolin's ulcer can be classified as acute or chronic. In acute ulcers, the malignant degeneration occurs within 12 months; in the more common chronic ulcers, the degeneration occurs after 12 months.

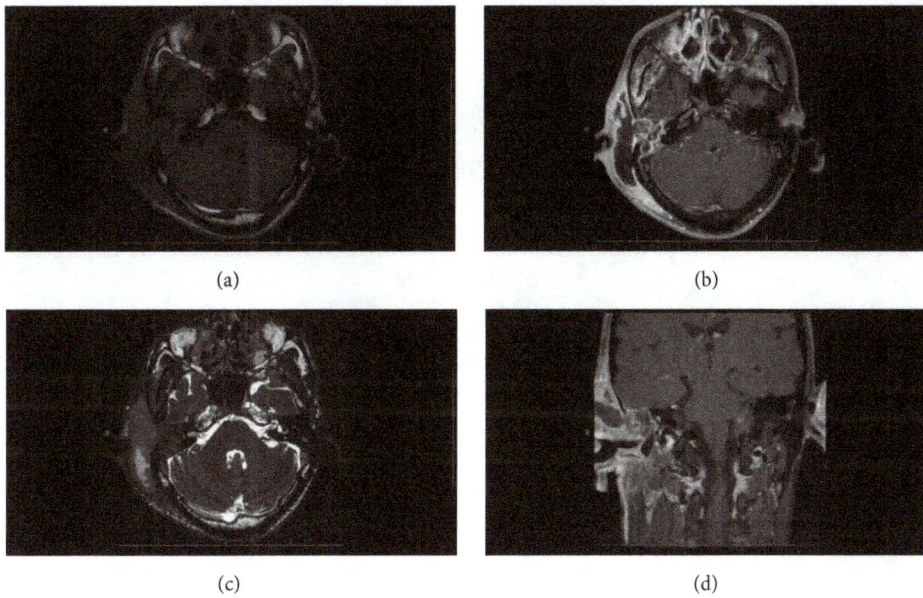

(a)

(b)

(c)

(d)

FIGURE 2: MRI of the brain, IAC, and mastoid with IV contrast. Axial and coronal views show (a) MRI T1 axial view before contrast, (b, c) MRI T1 axial view after contrast, and (d) MRI T1 coronal view after contrast. Right, large, loculated, peripheral enhancing collection is observed in the subcutaneous tissue of the auricular region, posterior and anterosuperior to the external auditory canal and extending to the mastoid air cells and middle ear cavity. The cochlea and semicircular canals are not visualized; only part of the vestibule is observed, and a focal area of dural enhancement is observed in the right temporal lobe.

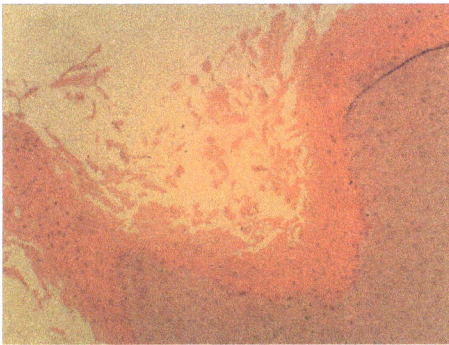

FIGURE 3: Cholesteatoma.

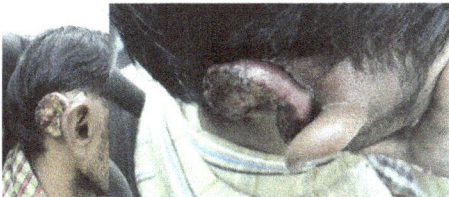

FIGURE 4: A 4 cm by 5 cm right postauricular ulcer with raised edges and a necrotic centre.

When acute, the ulcer is most often basal cell carcinoma and is associated with a more superficial burn scar. However, acute malignant transformations to SCC do occur [5, 10, 19]. Many cases of acute transformation, ranging from weeks [18, 20] to months [7, 14, 21], have been reported in the literature.

Regarding the age of the patient and the burn scar, patient age is inversely proportional to the interval to the formation of cancer. The younger the patient is, the more likely he or she is to have a latency period of less than 1 year; older patients are increasingly likely to have a latency period greater than 1 year [10, 22, 23].

Marjolin's ulcer tends to be more aggressive than other types of skin cancer and has a higher rate of regional metastases [10]. However, head and neck lesions are associated with better survival, as are lesions of the upper extremities. Other factor associated with better survival include a latency to malignancy of less than 5 years, ulcers caused by burns, chronic osteomyelitis, a tumour size less than 2 cm, and ulcers less than 4 mm in thickness [3, 11].

Early diagnosis is essential. A high index of suspicion should be considered in the presence of chronic ulcers persisting longer than 3 months; rolled or everted wound margins; foul-smelling discharge; and an increase in pain, ulcer size, or bleeding [7, 9, 18, 22, 24]. Biopsy of suspicious lesions for histopathology remains the gold standard for diagnosis [24]. Many studies have recommended biopsies of multiple areas, such as the centre and margins [19], at appropriate depths [11].

Treatment of Marjolin's ulcer is quite varied. To prevent wound degeneration into squamous cell carcinoma, it is imperative to provide early and definitive wound coverage after burns and other traumatic injuries. Leaving large wounds to heal by secondary intention creates the potential for a chronic nonhealing ulcer and the ideal conditions for development of a Marjolin's ulcer. Wide local excision and subsequent skin grafting appear to be the standard of care

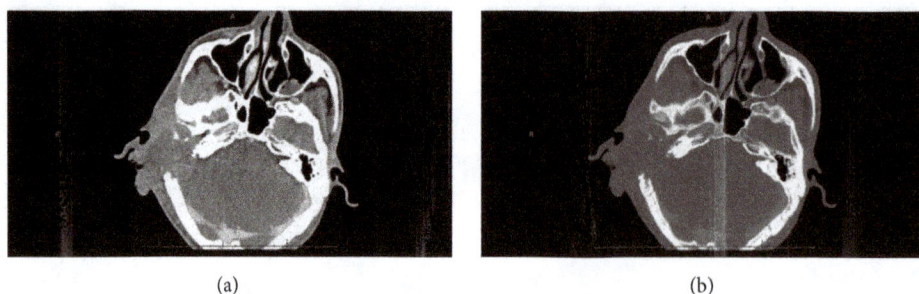

(a)   (b)

FIGURE 5: CT scan of the temporal bone shows that, compared to previous images, the soft tissue component was increased, causing further destruction of the middle and inner ear and a right periauricular soft tissue mass lesion with an ill-defined border.

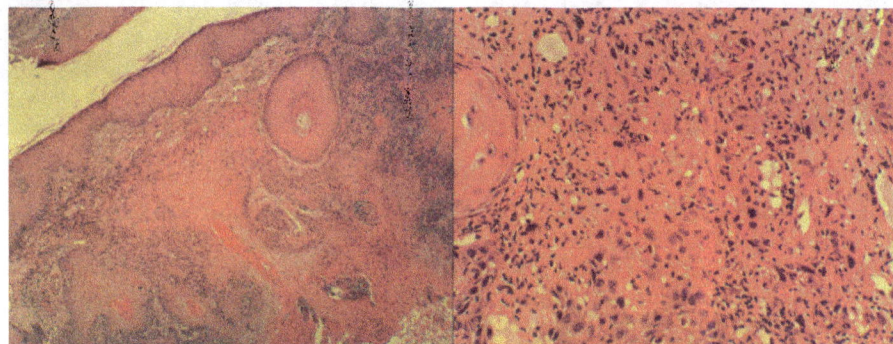

FIGURE 6: Section shows proliferative squamous cells invading the underlying stroma. The cells are hyperchromatic with a high N/C ratio and atypical mitosis.

for most authors [8]. MU is more aggressive than primary skin tumours; therefore nodal assessment and wide surgical excision are recommended [1].

4. Conclusions

Marjolin's ulcer is most commonly observed after postburn scars, but it may be observed after any type of scars, as our patient developed an SCC with a postsurgical scar. Early diagnosis is essential, and a biopsy should be performed on any nonhealing wound or chronic wound that undergoes a sudden change. Tissue samples should be taken from both the centre and the margins of the wound.

Additional Points

Summary. We presented a case of a 30-year-old man who developed Marjolin's ulcer acutely in a right postauricular scar after mastoidectomy and the incision and drainage of a mastoid abscess. To the best of our knowledge, this report is the first to describe a Marjolin's ulcer in a postauricular surgical scar. Early diagnosis is essential, and a biopsy should be performed on any nonhealing wound or chronic wound that undergoes a sudden change.

Competing Interests

The authors declare no competing interests.

Acknowledgments

The authors are grateful to Ahmed Alhujaily, histopathologist at King Fahad Hospital, and Talal Almoghthawey, radiologist at Ohud Hospital.

References

[1] N. Yu, X. Long, J. R. Lujan-Hernandez et al., "Marjolin's ulcer: a preventable malignancy arising from scars," *World Journal of Surgical Oncology*, vol. 11, article 313, 2013.

[2] M. G. Onesti, P. Fino, P. Fioramonti, V. Amorosi, and N. Scuderi, "Ten years of experience in chronic ulcers and malignant transformation," *International Wound Journal*, vol. 12, no. 4, pp. 447–450, 2015.

[3] P. M. Nthumba, "Marjolin's ulcers: theories, prognostic factors and their peculiarities in spina bifida patients," *World Journal of Surgical Oncology*, vol. 8, no. 1, article 108, 2010.

[4] A. H. Cruickshank, E. M. Mcconnell, and D. G. Miller, "Malignancy in scars, chronic ulcers, and sinuses," *Journal of Clinical Pathology*, vol. 16, pp. 573–580, 1963.

[5] J. B. Chang, T. A. Kung, and P. S. Cederna, "Acute marjolin's ulcers: a nebulous diagnosis," *Annals of Plastic Surgery*, vol. 72, no. 5, pp. 515–520, 2014.

[6] C. Ozek, N. Celik, U. Bilkay, T. Akalin, O. Erdem, and A. Cagdas, "Marjolin's ulcer of the scalp: report of 5 cases and review of the literature," *Journal of Burn Care & Rehabilitation*, vol. 22, no. 1, pp. 65–69, 2001.

[7] P. L. Chalya, J. B. Mabula, J. M. Gilyoma, P. Rambau, N. Masalu, and S. Simbila, "Early Marjolin's ulcer developing in a penile

human bite scar of an adult patient presenting at Bugando Medical Centre, Tanzania: a case report," *Tanzania Journal of Health Research*, vol. 14, no. 4, pp. 288–292, 2012.

[8] M. A. Kerr-Valentic, K. Samimi, B. H. Rohlen, J. P. Agarwal, and W. B. Rockwell, "Marjolin's ulcer: modern analysis of an ancient problem," *Plastic and Reconstructive Surgery*, vol. 123, no. 1, pp. 184–191, 2009.

[9] M. E. Asuquo, I. A. Ikpeme, G. Ebughe, and E. E. Bassey, "Marjolin's ulcer: sequelae of mismanaged chronic cutaneous ulcers," *Advances in Skin & Wound Care*, vol. 23, no. 9, pp. 414–416, 2010.

[10] M. S. Fazeli, A. H. Lebaschi, M. Hajirostam, and M. R. Keramati, "Marjolin's ulcer: clinical and pathologic features of 83 cases and review of literature," *Medical Journal of the Islamic Republic of Iran*, vol. 27, no. 4, pp. 215–224, 2013.

[11] V. Challa, V. Deshmane, and M. Ashwatha Reddy, "A retrospective study of Marjolin/s ulcer over an eleven year period," *Journal of Cutaneous and Aesthetic Surgery*, vol. 7, no. 3, p. 155, 2014.

[12] E. Copcu and N. Çulhaci, "Marjolin's ulcer on the nose," *Burns*, vol. 28, no. 7, pp. 701–704, 2002.

[13] T. Wojewoda, W. Wysocki, and J. Mitú, "Marjolin's ulcer—case report and literature review," *Polish Journal of Surgery*, vol. 81, no. 9, pp. 414–418, 2009.

[14] D. Thio, J. H. W. Clarkson, A. Misra, and S. Srivastava, "Malignant change after 18 months in a lower limb ulcer: acute Marjolin's revisited," *British Journal of Plastic Surgery*, vol. 56, no. 8, pp. 825–828, 2003.

[15] J. Da Costa, "III. Carcinomatous changes in an area of chronic ulceration, or Marjolin's ulcer," *Annals of Surgery*, vol. 37, no. 4, pp. 496–502, 1903.

[16] M. Bozkurt, E. Kapi, S. V. Kuvat, and S. Ozekinci, "Current concepts in the management of Marjolin's ulcers: outcomes from a standardized treatment protocol in 16 cases," *Journal of Burn Care & Research*, vol. 31, no. 5, pp. 776–780, 2010.

[17] K. Opara and I. Otene, "Marjolin's ulcers: a review," *The Nigerian Health Journal*, vol. 11, no. 4, pp. 107–111, 2011.

[18] B. Pekarek, S. Buck, and L. Osher, "A comprehensive review on Marjolin's ulcers: diagnosis and treatment," *The Journal of the American College of Certified Wound Specialists*, vol. 3, no. 3, pp. 60–64, 2011.

[19] A. Mohammadi, S. Sayed Jafari, and M. Hosseinzadeh, "Early Marjolin's ulcer after minimal superficial burn," *Iranian Journal of Medical Sciences*, vol. 38, no. 1, pp. 69–70, 2013.

[20] A. N. Wooldridge, M. J. Griesser, T. Scharschmidt, and O. Hans Iwenofu, "Development of Marjolin's ulcer within one month of burn injury with synchronous primary lung squamous cell carcinoma in an elderly patient: report of a case with allelotyping," *Medical Oncology*, vol. 28, no. 1, pp. S586–S592, 2011.

[21] E. Çelik, H. Fýndýk, and A. Uzunismail, "Early arising Marjolin's ulcer: report of three cases," *British Journal of Plastic Surgery*, vol. 58, no. 1, pp. 122–124, 2005.

[22] U. Ochenduszkiewicz, R. Matkowski, B. Szynglarewicz, and J. Kornafel, "Marjolin's ulcer: malignant neoplasm arising in scars," *Reports of Practical Oncology and Radiotherapy*, vol. 11, no. 3, pp. 135–138, 2006.

[23] S. B. Hahn, D. J. Kim, and C. H. Jeon, "Clinical study of Marjolin's ulcer," *Yonsei Medical Journal*, vol. 31, no. 3, pp. 234–241, 1990.

[24] S. Enoch, D. R. Miller, P. E. Price, and K. G. Harding, "Early diagnosis is vital in the management of squamous cell carcinomas associated with chronic non healing ulcers: a case series and review of the literature," *International Wound Journal*, vol. 1, no. 3, pp. 165–175, 2004.

6

Paranasal Rosai-Dorfman Disease with Osseous Destruction

Kevin Hur,[1] Changxing Liu,[1] and Jeffrey A. Koempel[2]

[1]Caruso Department of Otolaryngology, Keck School of Medicine, University of Southern California, Los Angeles, CA 90033, USA
[2]Division of Otolaryngology, Head and Neck Surgery, Children's Hospital Los Angeles, Los Angeles, CA 90027, USA

Correspondence should be addressed to Changxing Liu; changxing.liu@med.usc.edu

Academic Editor: Abrão Rapoport

Rosai-Dorfman disease is a rare histiocytic proliferative disorder of unknown etiology typically characterized by cervical lymphadenopathy. Extranodal involvement often manifests in the head and neck region. We present a 10-year-old male who presented to our hospital with left epiphora from an aggressive paranasal mass invading the left orbit with osseous destruction. The mass was surgically biopsied and debulked with histopathological examination revealing Rosai-Dorfman disease. Although rarely found in the sinuses, Rosai-Dorfman disease should be considered when evaluating sinonasal masses.

1. Introduction

Rosai-Dorfman disease, first described in 1969, is a nonneoplastic histiocytic proliferative disorder of unknown etiology and pathogenesis [1]. The most common presentation is painless bilateral cervical lymphadenopathy accompanied by fever, leukocytosis, increased erythrocyte sedimentation rate, and hypergammaglobulinemia [2]. However, patients with extranodal disease oftentimes lack any constitutional symptoms [2].

Extranodal disease has been reported in up to 43% of cases and commonly involved sites include the skin, central nervous system, orbit and eyelid, upper respiratory tract, and gastrointestinal tract [2–6]. The disease has a variable clinical presentation and requires a pathological review for definitive diagnosis, which is characterized by massive sinusoidal dilation that contains histiocytes, lymphocytes, and plasma cells. Emperipolesis within the histiocyte cytoplasm is a pathognomonic finding [2–4].

Oftentimes patients do not require treatment as the disease has a self-limiting course. Nevertheless, surgical resection is recommended for symptomatic disease. We herein describe a rare case of extranodal sinonasal Rosai-Dorfman disease with osseous destruction of the orbit.

2. Case Report

A 10-year-old Hispanic male presented to the emergency room at Children's Hospital Los Angeles after 6 months of left eye tearing. He was seen by an ophthalmologist a month earlier who found left nasolacrimal duct obstruction on exam. A CT orbit revealed a soft tissue mass involving the medial aspect of the left ethmoid and maxillary sinus with osseous destruction (see Figure 1). The patient denied vision changes, weight loss, fevers, chills, or other symptoms. Laboratory findings were within normal limits with no leukocytosis, increased erythrocyte sedimentation rate, or hypergammaglobulinemia. The mass was not visualized on nasal endoscopy due to a narrow nasal cavity and enlarged middle turbinate. Therefore, an orbital biopsy by ophthalmology was performed, revealing lymphoid tissue with histiocyte proliferation. However, due to the aggressive symptomatic clinical presentation of the sinonasal orbital mass, the patient underwent a left orbitotomy for debulking of the mass. The histopathological examination revealed sheets of histiocytes mixed with few lymphocytes and plasma cells consistent with Rosai-Dorfman disease. There was phagocytic activity identified in the sinus histiocytes characterized as emperipolesis. The histiocytes were CD68(+), S-100(+), C1Da(−), Desmin(−), and EBV(−) (see Figure 2). At 3-month follow-up, the patient reported resolution of left eye tearing and was asymptomatic. Therefore, no further postoperative treatment or imaging was obtained.

3. Discussion

Rosai-Dorfman disease (RDD) presents typically in childhood or early adulthood with a higher incidence in males

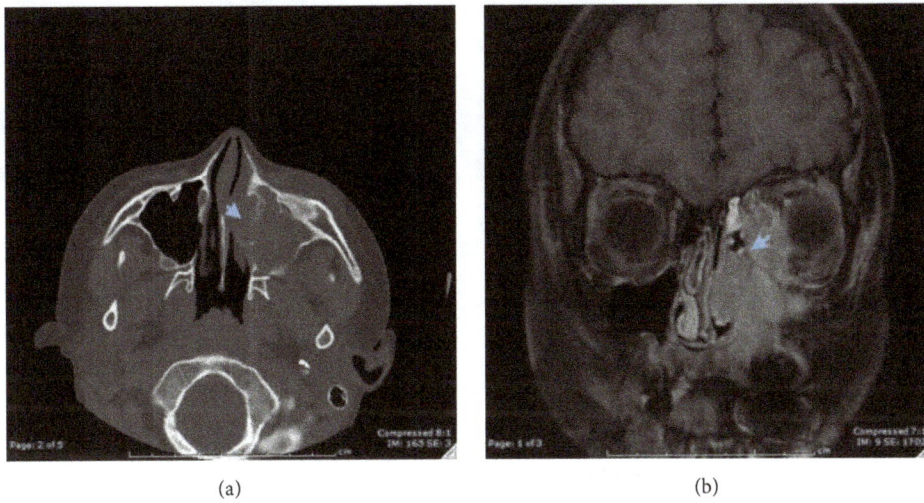

FIGURE 1: Image of mass in left anterior ethmoid cell extending into left medial aspect of orbit on axial sinus CT without contrast (a), and MRI orbit T1 after contrast (b). Blue arrow indicates area of bony destruction.

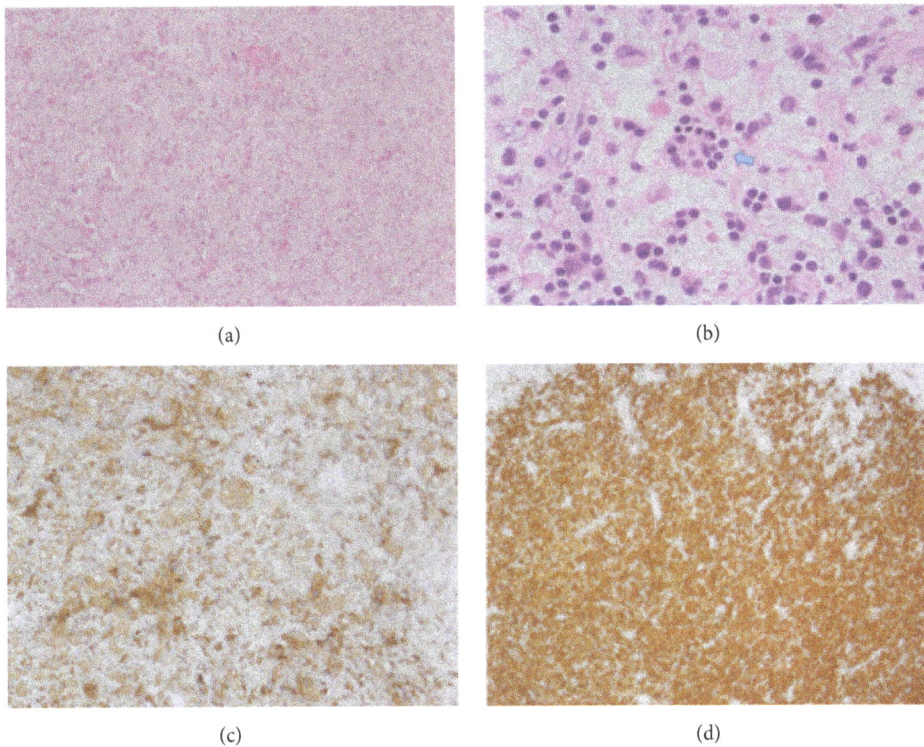

FIGURE 2: Permanent sections showing histology of Rosai-Dorfman disease; low power 100x (a) and high power 400x (b) hematoxylin and eosin stain showing histiocytic infiltrate. Blue arrow indicates emperipolesis. Positive immunostaining for CD68 (c) and S100 (d).

and African-Americans [2]. The etiology of RDD is currently unknown and considered idiopathic. Proposed etiologies include chronic infection or immune dysfunction leading to an exaggerated response to viral agents such as the Epstein-Barr virus, but the overall evidence does not support any one specific theory [2, 4].

When there is an extranodal presentation of RDD, the head and neck region is frequently involved. However, the presentation is variable with case reports of RDD identified in the trachea, nasal septum, dura, orbit, parotid, and so forth [4–14]. The paranasal sinuses are the most common extranodal site of involvement after skin, followed by the orbit, bone, salivary gland, and central nervous system [4]. Patients often present with nasal obstruction, epistaxis, hyposmia, or anosmia [4, 8–11].

A review of RDD imaging manifestations in the head and neck at one institution over a 10-year period found 5 out of 13 head and neck RDD cases had extranodal disease in the paranasal sinuses. None of the paranasal RDD had osseous destruction on imaging [8]. However, there is one case report of sinonasal RDD with osseous destruction of the premaxilla [12]. Also, a pathology quiz case described a young girl with sinonasal RDD extending into the right orbit, but whether the osseous destruction was from her prior surgeries or the disease was unclear [14]. Otherwise, there were no reported cases of osseous destruction of the bony orbit from paranasal RDD identified from our literature search.

The diagnostic workup for RDD relies on histopathologic examination of an incisional or excisional biopsy [2, 11]. The differential diagnosis is extensive and includes other histiocytic proliferative diseases including lymphoma, tuberculosis, granulomatosis with polyangiitis, sarcoidosis, and Langerhans cell histiocytosis. Malignant etiologies such as nasopharyngeal carcinoma and lymphoma should also be considered, especially if aggressive features are seen radiologically as seen in this patient. Identification of emperipolesis within the histiocyte cytoplasm is pathognomonic as originally described by Rosai et al., though histiocytes are less common in extranodal tissue [1–7, 15]. In cases where few histiocytes with emperipolesis are seen, useful immunohistologic markers for RDD include the S100 protein, which is a marker for dendritic cells in lymph nodes and Langerhans cells in skin, and CD68, a pan-macrophage antigen (see Figure 2) [3, 4].

RDD generally has a benign course and does not require treatment. In one review, 82% of untreated patients show spontaneous regression over a period of weeks to years without treatment [16, 17]. However, massive lymphadenopathy, involvement of multiple organs, immunologic abnormalities, and anemia can lead to poor prognosis and in very few cases may be fatal [3, 4]. If patients are symptomatic, the standard treatment is surgical resection. Systemic treatment for extensive disease has not been well established due to rarity of the disease though reported treatment modalities such as steroids, radiation, and chemotherapy have had varying success based on a small case series [2–7]. In patients that require systemic treatment due to symptomatic extensive disease, steroids are typically the first treatment option, having been shown to produce responses in classical and extranodal RDD [2–7]. Radiotherapy can preserve vital organ function in orbital, airway, or CNS involvement but there are no standardized guidelines for treatment in the literature. If steroids and radiotherapy are unsuccessful, chemotherapy can be considered, though data is limited on its effectiveness [2–7].

After diagnosis or treatment, Dalia and colleagues recommend surveillance with clinical and laboratory testing performed every 3–6 months for the first 2 years and then yearly afterwards [2]. Contrast CT scans can be obtained if patients develop symptoms or there is concern for relapse [2].

4. Conclusion

Rosai-Dorfman disease is a rare entity with variable presentations in the head and neck region. Although uncommon, Rosai-Dorfman disease should be considered in the differential diagnosis when evaluating sinonasal masses in children.

Competing Interests

The authors have no financial disclosures and no conflict of interests to report.

References

[1] J. Rosai and R. F. Dorfman, "Sinus histiocytosis with massive lymphadenopathy. A newly recognized benign clinicopathological entity," *Archives of pathology*, vol. 87, no. 1, pp. 64–70, 1969.

[2] S. Dalia, E. Sagatys, L. Sokol, and T. Kubal, "Rosai-Dorfman disease: tumor biology, clinical features, pathology, and treatment," *Cancer Control*, vol. 21, no. 4, pp. 322–327, 2014.

[3] K. Hashimoto, S. Kariya, T. Onoda et al., "Rosai-dorfman disease with extranodal involvement," *Laryngoscope*, vol. 124, no. 3, pp. 701–704, 2014.

[4] S. Gaitonde, "Multifocal, extranodal sinus histiocytosis with massive lymphadenopathy: an overview," *Archives of Pathology and Laboratory Medicine*, vol. 131, no. 7, pp. 1117–1121, 2007.

[5] H.-Y. Li, H.-G. Cui, X.-Y. Zheng, G.-P. Ren, and Y.-S. Gu, "Orbital Rosai-Dorfman disease in a fifty-eight years old woman," *Pakistan Journal of Medical Sciences*, vol. 29, no. 4, pp. 1065–1067, 2013.

[6] A. J. Al-Moosa, R. S. Behbehani, A. E. Hussain, and A. E. Ali, "Orbital rosai-dorfman disease in a five-year-old boy," *Middle East African Journal of Ophthalmology*, vol. 18, no. 4, pp. 323–325, 2011.

[7] G. K. Vemuganti, M. N. Naik, and S. G. Honavar, "Rosai dorfman disease of the orbit," *Journal of Hematology and Oncology*, vol. 1, no. 1, article 7, 2008.

[8] D. V. La Barge III, K. L. Salzman, H. R. Harnsberger et al., "Sinus histiocytosis with massive lymphadenopathy (Rosai-Dorfman disease): imaging manifestations in the head and neck," *American Journal of Roentgenology*, vol. 191, no. 6, pp. W299–W306, 2008.

[9] G. Ottaviano, D. Doro, G. Marioni et al., "Extranodal Rosai-Dorfman disease: involvement of eye, nose and trachea," *Acta Oto-Laryngologica*, vol. 126, no. 6, pp. 657–660, 2006.

[10] L. Gupta, K. Batra, and G. Motwani, "A rare case of Rosai-Dorfman disease of the paranasal sinuses," *Indian Journal of Otolaryngology and Head and Neck Surgery*, vol. 57, no. 4, pp. 352–354, 2005.

[11] A. Akyigit, H. Akyol, O. Sakallioglu, C. Polat, E. Keles, and O. Alatas, "Rosai-Dorfman disease originating from nasal septal mucosa," *Case Reports in Otolaryngology*, vol. 2015, Article ID 232898, 3 pages, 2015.

[12] L. Shemen, M. D'Anton, I. Toth et al., "Rosai-Dorfman disease involving the premaxilla," *Annals of Otology, Rhinology & Laryngology*, vol. 100, no. 10, pp. 845–851, 1991.

[13] R. B. Pradhananga, K. Dangol, A. Shrestha, and D. K. Baskota, "Sinus Histiocytosis with massive lymphadenopathy (Rosai-Dorfman disease): a case report and literature review," *International Archives of Otorhinolaryngology*, vol. 18, no. 4, pp. 406–408, 2014.

[14] X. C. Zhao, J. McHugh, and M. C. Thorne, "Pathology quiz case 2," *JAMA Otolaryngology - Head and Neck Surgery*, vol. 139, no. 5, pp. 529–531, 2013.

[15] E. Foucar, J. Rosai, and R. Dorfman, "Sinus histiocytosis with massive lymphadenopathy (Rosai-Dorfman disease): review of the entity," *Seminars in Diagnostic Pathology*, vol. 7, no. 1, pp. 19–73, 1990.

[16] F. B. Lima, P. S. V. Barcelos, A. P. N. Constâncio, C. D. Nogueira, and A. A. Melo-Filho, "Rosai-Dorfman disease with spontaneous resolution: case report of a child," *Revista Brasileira de Hematologia e Hemoterapia*, vol. 33, no. 4, pp. 312–314, 2011.

[17] E. G. Shaver, S. L. Rebsamen, A. T. Yachnis, and L. N. Sutton, "Isolated extranodal intracranial sinus histiocytosis in a 5-year-old boy. Case report," *Journal of Neurosurgery*, vol. 79, no. 5, pp. 769–773, 1993.

7

Unilateral Head Impulses Training in Uncompensated Vestibular Hypofunction

Ana Carolina Binetti,[1,2] Andrea Ximena Varela,[1,2] Dana Lucila Lucarelli,[1] and Daniel Héctor Verdecchia[1,3]

[1]Vestibular Argentina Institute, Buenos Aires, Argentina
[2]Department of Otolaryngology, British Hospital of Buenos Aires, Buenos Aires, Argentina
[3]Center for Medical Research on Human Movement (CIMMHU), Maimónides University, Buenos Aires, Argentina

Correspondence should be addressed to Daniel Héctor Verdecchia; dhverdecchia@yahoo.com.ar

Academic Editor: Nicolas Perez-Fernandez

The aim of this paper is to report a case of a young woman with unilateral vestibular chronic failure with a poorly compensated vestibuloocular reflex during rapid head rotation. Additionally, she developed migraine symptoms during the treatment with associated chronic dizzy sensations and blurred vision. Her report of blurred vision only improved after she completed a rehabilitation program using fast head impulse rotations towards the affected side for 5 consecutive days. We discuss why we elected this form of treatment and how this method may be useful for different patients.

1. Introduction

The vestibuloocular reflex (VOR) allows us to keep our eyes fixed on an object during head motion. A VOR deficit generates a retinal slip that can be perceived by the patient as a jump or movement of the observed object while turning the head. This same retinal slip also can serve, by means of adaptive mechanisms, to stimulate cerebellar neuroplasticity. VOR plasticity is therefore modulated by vestibulocerebellar-cortical microcircuits that are activated by specific exercises [1].

Following unilateral vestibular lesions, the vestibular compensation process makes it possible for angular VOR responses to low acceleration head rotations to return to normal. However, a marked asymmetry may persist in response to high velocity head rotation [2].

The head impulse test (HIT) was first described by Halmagyi and Curthoys in 1988 [3]. The HIT is a valuable clinical method for detecting a unilateral vestibular hypofunction and for identifying the affected canals [4, 5]. In 2009, Weber et al. [6] presented a video-assisted version of the HIT (vHIT) that enabled a graphic record of the VOR deficit in each of the six semicircular canals and a means to measure their recovery

[7]. This system also enabled the detection of overt saccades, which are a sign of vestibular hypofunction when they appear after head rotation, and covert saccades, which appear during head rotation and cannot be detected by the human eye in a clinical examination but rather can only be identified with this equipment. Recently, Schubert and Migliaccio [8] found that the angular vestibuloocular reflex (aVOR) is stable over repeated test sessions when examined using canal plane head impulses using the scleral search coil technique.

Since the beginning of the 1990s, VOR adaptation has been attempted by repeating head movements on one plane from side to side while the patient fixes his eyes on a letter or a point at a given distance. This exercise, which is known as paradigm $x1$, is repeated for one or two minutes from three to five times per day. In addition, the $x1$ viewing exercises are often performed with vertical head movements [9, 10].

Initially, our female patient suffered from chronic vestibular hypofunction, with minimal and fluctuating changes in dynamic visual acuity and her perception of handicap even after having participated in several months of vestibular rehabilitation. She did not experience an improvement until we changed her treatment by adding a unique VOR exercise

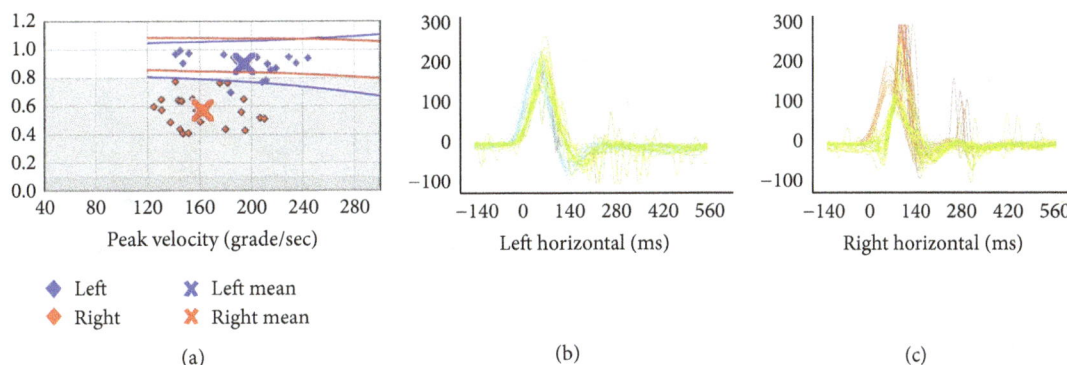

FIGURE 1: Horizontal passive vHIT before unilateral training: left gain: 0.90 ± 0.08; right gain: 0.57 ± 0.11; asymmetry: 37%.

that asked her to make ipsilesional, high frequency, and low amplitude head impulses. The head rotation was only done towards the affected ear, while the patient used the vHIT equipment concurrently. Here we report the changes observed in the results of the vHIT, the dynamic visual acuity clinical test (DVA), and the perception of handicap after unilateral training with vHIT equipment.

2. Case Report

A young female, 30 years old, presented in our clinic suffering a right side unilateral vestibular hypofunction (UVH) due to vestibular neuritis (VN) [11]. At the time of diagnosis, she reported sudden and severe rotatory vertigo with associated autonomic symptoms over the previous 48 hours. Pure tone audiometry (PTA) in both ears was 5 dBHL; she had no tinnitus. The patient denied any previous history of related problems, although her mother was suffering from migraine headache. The patient was hospitalized three days, where she received intravenous steroids and antiemetics. Inner ear and cerebellar magnetic resonance imaging (MRI) were normal. She began vestibular rehabilitation treatment, with a progressive exercise regimen. Initially, she performed gaze stability and balance exercises 3–5 times a day in her home, for a total stimulus time of 20–40 min daily. The gaze stability exercises included the $x1$ and $x2$ paradigms for both near and far target distances. The balance exercises were provided to improve her use of vestibular information to maintain balance. We progressed these exercises by reducing the base of support, altering vision, and proprioceptive input (eyes open or closed; standing on a firm or soft surface). The gait exercises included walking in tandem, with eyes closed, with cephalic movement in the sagittal and horizontal planes. Habituation exercises were indicated based on the result of the 16 movements from the Motion Sensitivity Quotient [12]. The habituation movements included 4 repetitions, 4 times a day, until the exercises did not generate any symptoms for 48 hours, at which time the patient suspended them. Videonystagmography (VNG) showed unilateral weakness of the right ear at 78%. At the time of discharge, her Dizziness Handicap Inventory (DHI) was 66. The patient continued with this rehabilitation treatment for 9 months,

after which the final DHI improved to 36. Although she said that she did all the prescribed exercises, she reported blurred vision and a permanent dizzy sensation. She decided to discontinue treatment but returned to the clinic after three months with the same symptoms. Additionally, she now reported a new onset of periodic headaches that did not fulfill migraine or vestibular migraine criteria [13]. A repeated VNG exam showed spontaneous nystagmus towards the left, with a slow phase velocity (SPV) of 7°/sec. At that moment DHI was 54; the Motion Sensitivity Quotient (MSQ) was 11.81 points; Functional Gait Assessment (FGA) was normal; and modified Clinical Test of Sensory Interaction and Balance (mCTSIB) was 120/120. She restarted vestibular rehabilitation and after 10 sessions her DHI was not better (64 points). Laboratory studies showed normal levels for FAN (Antinuclear Factor), folic acid, Anti-DNA, ionogram, magnesium, calcium, proteinogram, VDRL, and vitamin B12. However, she reported that her headaches had become premenstrual and they now fulfilled the criteria for a migraine diagnosis. She was started on 12.5 mg oral amitriptyline daily and prescribed dietary measures. Subsequently this patient reported less blurred vision and dizziness and no headaches for two months. A new MRI and an angiocerebral MRI were normal. Nevertheless, the patient returned two months later complaining of persistent dizziness, blurred vision, and no benefits from the amitriptyline in spite of the fact that the dosage had been raised to 50 mg daily. We modified her treatment to start vestibular rehabilitation again (her initial DHI was 40) and she was started on 25 mg oral topiramate daily. The patient did not tolerate this medication and discontinued its use. Next, she was prescribed 10 mg of flunarizine daily with good tolerance. Repeated VNG showed spontaneous left nystagmus with a SPV of 3°/sec. Her DHI was now 34, but her clinical dynamic visual acuity was abnormal showing a 6-line difference from static visual acuity. During the next 4 months, the patient did not come to the clinic, after which period of time she came in and was treated with 25 mg of oral venlafaxine daily (provided by another clinic). At this point, we tested with the vHIT (ICS impulse 1085 Otometrics®), which showed a gain of 0.57 in the right horizontal canal with overt and covert saccades (Figure 1). The other semicircular canals had normal gains. Electrocochleography was normal, Brainstem Auditory Evoked Response was normal, a new

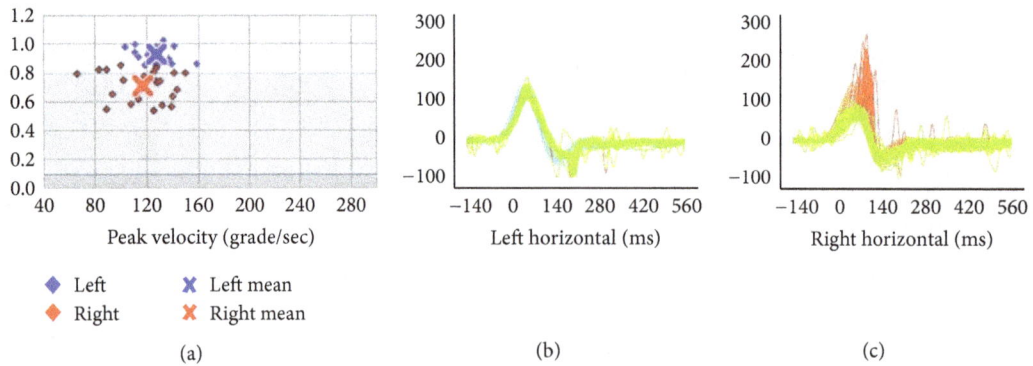

(a)

(b)

(c)

FIGURE 2: Horizontal passive vHIT after unilateral training: left gain: 0.93 ± 0.05; right gain: 0.71 ± 0.10; asymmetry: 24%.

MRI was normal, and PTA was normal. A 4th VNG showed spontaneous horizontal nystagmus to the right, with a SPV of −3°/sec (was interpreted as a recovery nystagmus), and an orthoptic evaluation was normal. Though she said she still suffered from blurred vision and dizziness, she reported fewer headaches. We prescribed 24 mg daily of betahistine (8 mg every 8 hours) to improve compensation. While the patient experienced an improvement, she reported that the dizziness persisted throughout the day. She began working again but had to stop 1 month later due to blurred vision, headaches, and dizziness. Once again, she began vestibular rehabilitation plus psychological therapy. This combination of therapies resulted in some improvement, though her symptoms persisted during head movement, especially in the dark. Her constant blurred vision made it difficult for her to read. Her 5th VNG showed that a spontaneous nystagmus to the left was 1.8°/sec, while the vHIT was the same as before. Based on persistent symptoms and lack of improvement with traditional vestibular rehabilitation, we elected to treat her using passive and predictive, yaw head impulses towards the affected side only. This was done for five consecutive days. Video HIT was used to ensure that the velocity of impulse was correct to stimulate her right horizontal canal in the field of fast movements. When the patient did the head impulse exercises, she sat in front of a solid black circle of 10 mm in diameter on a white background placed at one meter. This circle was positioned at the same level or height as her occipitonasal axis. Stimulation of the affected semicircular canal was done with 10 series of 15 passive head impulses (done by the therapist) with 30 seconds of rest between each series. The initial head position was such that the patient's gaze was centered on the point in front of her with ±2° between the horizontal and vertical planes [14]. The head impulses were small and fast, with a peak amplitude of 15 degrees, a peak velocity of 150°/sec, and peak acceleration of 3000°/sec; the return to the initial position was slow. Video HIT equipment was used to monitor the velocity and amplitude of movements, which were corrected when necessary.

After this treatment, the patient reported resolution of blurred vision and dizziness, with no premenstrual migraines or vertigo. Her final vHIT showed a gain of 0.71 for the right horizontal semicircular canal with covert saccades (Figure 2). The VOR gain remained normal in the vertical canals. Her final DHI was 12. The clinical horizontal dynamic visual acuity test was now within 2 lines of her static visual acuity (normal). After 6 and 12 months, she returned for follow-up to report that she had no more vestibular symptoms. Her premenstrual migraines persisted and she continued to have a spontaneous nystagmus beating towards the left at 1.8°/sec SPV, in the dark (Table 1).

3. Discussion

Today there is moderate to strong evidence that vestibular rehabilitation is a safe and effective treatment for patients with unilateral peripheral vestibular disorders [15, 16]. However, the evidence on frequency, intensity, and time, as well as details on vestibular rehabilitation (for example, in compensation exercises) is still limited, due in part to the heterogeneity of research papers [15]. The objectives of vestibular rehabilitation include a reduction in dizziness and in the risk of falls, increased confidence in equilibrium, and better VOR function [17, 18]. In 2012, Herdman et al. [19] did a study on the possible variables that could affect the results of vestibular rehabilitation and found that patients with greater loss of vestibular function were less likely to return to normal DVA following a course of vestibular exercises, although they still showed significant improvement. In our own clinical practice, we have observed that some patients do not achieve normal DVA in spite of doing the $x1$ paradigm exercises daily. Our observation leads us to think that patients with unilateral vestibular hypofunction who do these exercises at home might not be moving their heads with the appropriate velocity or amplitude in order to avoid the sensation of dizziness and blurred vision caused by the retinal slip. We therefore suspect that the lack of improvement in our patient during the traditional vestibular rehabilitation was due to errors of execution. Asymmetry in vestibular function can cause oscillopsia, which is a sensation of blurred vision during head rotation. In patients with UVH, this can occur during ipsilesional head rotations [20–22]. In one study [23], done on monkeys subjected to a unilateral labyrinthectomy, the

TABLE 1: Evolution of the symptoms, diagnosis, and treatment.

June 2011	2011–2014	July 2014	August 2014	November 2016
Initial symptoms	Evolution	Before treatment with unilateral head impulses	After treatment with unilateral head impulses	Phone communication
Sudden rotational vertigo lasting more than 48 hours, intense autonomic symptoms	Beginning of menses migraine	Migraine, less intensity and frequency	Premenstrual migraine	Sporadic migraine
Unsteadiness +++	Unsteadiness ++	Unsteadiness ++	Unsteadiness +	Unsteadiness +
	Blurred vision with head movements +++	Blurred vision with head movements +++	Blurred vision with head movements +	Blurred vision with head movements ++
Nausea and vomiting		DVA 6 lines (abnormal)	DVA 2 lines (normal)	
	DHI: 66	DHI: 34	DHI: 12	
	Dizziness ++	Dizziness ++	Dizziness +	Dizziness +
	Dizziness in darkness ++	Dizziness in darkness ++	Dizziness in darkness +	Dizziness in darkness ++
Unilateral weakness right ear 78% (VNG)		Unilateral weakness right ear 80% (VNG)		
Diagnosis: vestibular neuritis	Diagnosis: right vestibular hypofunction without compensation. Premenstrual migraine	Diagnosis: right vestibular hypofunction without compensation. Premenstrual migraine	Diagnosis: right vestibular hypofunction with compensation. Premenstrual migraine	Diagnosis: premenstrual migraine. The patient should do new clinical and lab evaluation
Vestibular rehabilitation	Vestibular rehabilitation and migraine prophylaxis	Betahistine plus unilateral head impulses	No treatment	Waiting for new evaluation

+++: severe; ++: moderate; +: mild; DVA: dynamic visual acuity; VNG: videonystagmography; DHI: Dizziness Handicap Inventory.

authors explain that since "in everyday activity the animal moves its head in both directions and never repeatedly in one direction, there may be a conflict in the error signal induced by motion in the contralesional and ipsilesional directions. This error signal could result because the gain is normal for rotations in the contralesional direction. Therefore, an increase in gain would cause an error signal opposite to the error signal resulting from the low gain in the ipsilesional direction. Rotating the animal exclusively in one direction overcomes this limitation because the animal receives only an error signal to increase the gain." The fundamental finding of this study was that asymmetry in the VOR gain after unilateral labyrinthectomy did not improve until the monkeys received ipsilesional adaptation training. The exercises our patient did were different from those performed by the monkeys in that our patient did head only ipsilesional rotation, not whole-body ipsilesional rotation.

We have compared our results with those of other studies done on humans. Schubert et al. [24] have studied unilateral VOR training using an incremental visual stimulus and measured VOR gain with scleral search coil system. Unlike our study, active head impulses only were used in ten series of 15 stimuli towards each side, and the laser was activated only when the head was moved towards the side where adaptation was desired. The laser was gradually adjusted by increments of ten percent of the head movement velocity, until reaching 100 percent in the last series. The range of movement (15°), the velocity (150 m/s), and the acceleration (3000° m/s²) were the same as those we used for our patient. The authors found that adaptation to unilateral stimuli was possible in healthy subjects. Measurements were taken for both active and passive head rotation, even though the subjects were trained using active only head rotation. The gain in the VOR towards the adaptive side after training increased by 22% with active head movements and 11% with passive head movements. In a recent pilot study done by the same authors [25] on ten subjects (six controls and four patients with unilateral and bilateral vestibular hypofunction), active and passive VOR gains were measured during high acceleration stimulation, before and after training for unilateral VOR adaptation, using a helmet with a laser and a gyroscope. VHIT equipment like that used with our patient was used to measure gains in the VOR and it was found that these improved with both active and passive head impulses in patients with unilateral and bilateral hypofunction, though, given the small number of patients, these results were not statistically significant. The exercise variant we had our patient do was different from those used in these studies, in that we used a fixed point as in the x1 paradigm described by Herdman. Additionally, we did not use an incremental stimulus, nor did we use a helmet with an attached laser. Instead, in our study the head impulses were performed by the patient with chronic vestibular hypofunction.

We found it useful to know the VOR gain and presence of saccades as provided by the vHIT software, during our training. We believe that knowing this information was helpful and further believe that vHIT might be useful to assist other clinicians in training the VOR [24, 25].

One limitation of our study is the difference in passive head velocity used to measure VOR gain between the pre- and postmeasures. The lower head velocity for the postmeasure would not be expected to inhibit the contralesional afferents. However, the covert and overt saccades did still change as evidence by their more consistent latency. Another weakness of our study is our lack of a control subject, which limits the ability to make strong conclusions. However, we feel that our results suggest that, after 5 consecutive daily sessions, the VOR gain increased, the covert saccades were reprogrammed, and vHIT asymmetry was reduced. Additionally, gaze instability as measured by DVA and her perception of handicap both improved.

The vHIT and the caloric test of the VNG are known to present with different responses of the VOR, presumably due to stimulating the VOR at different frequencies. Redondo-Martínez et al. [26] found no correlation between the VHIT, the caloric test, and the DHI test in patients with vestibular neuritis, none of which were indicative of the subjective clinical status of the patient at any given time. In line with recent scientific literature [26–28], our patient showed improved DHI and DVA without significant changes in her vHIT. One study [29] has demonstrated that persistent dizziness after VN is not significantly associated with sustained vestibular impairment as assessed by the quantitative search coil head impulse testing (qHIT); more specifically, severe vestibular deficit in the chronic patient group did not imply a high score on the shortened version of the Vertigo Symptom Scale (sVSS), assessing dizziness, vertigo, and imbalance during the past 12 months. Similar findings were reported in a study [30] on patients who suffered from vestibular neuritis; the high velocity VOR was not different between patients who felt they had recovered and patients who felt they had not and suggests that chronic symptoms of dizziness following VN are not associated with the high velocity VOR of the single or combined ipsilesional horizontal and anterior or posterior semicircular canals.

To better understand the possible benefits of these exercises, other studies should be done in patients with unilateral and bilateral vestibular hypofunction to compare the x1 paradigm exercises with our novel, ipsi-rotational exercises. A recent review [31] concluded that investigations would be required to determine the evolution of the VOR gain with the progression of the vestibular disease. We also recommend further evaluation of the use of active or passive head movements and the relation between these exercises and different variations of them as well as evaluation of the possibility of performing this exercise at patients' homes without expensive equipment.

4. Conclusion

Passive unilateral head impulses applied to the affected side appear to be a useful method for stimulating recovery of gaze stabilization in our subject with unilateral vestibular hypofunction and abnormal DVA. Larger studies are needed to evaluate the efficacy of this exercise.

Competing Interests

The authors declare that there is no conflict of interests regarding the publication of this paper.

Acknowledgments

The authors are grateful to Dr. Michael Schubert for his assistance in editing.

References

[1] M. Ito, "Cerebellar long-term depression: characterization, signal transduction, and functional roles," *Physiological Reviews*, vol. 81, no. 3, pp. 1143–1195, 2001.

[2] M. Lacour, C. Helmchen, and P.-P. Vidal, "Vestibular compensation: the neuro-otologist's best friend," *Journal of Neurology*, vol. 263, supplement 1, pp. S54–S64, 2016.

[3] G. M. Halmagyi and I. S. Curthoys, "A clinical sign of canal paresis," *Archives of Neurology*, vol. 45, no. 7, pp. 737–739, 1988.

[4] L. B. Minor and D. M. Lasker, "Tonic and phasic contributions to the pathways mediating compensation and adaptation of the vestibulo-ocular reflex," *Journal of Vestibular Research: Equilibrium and Orientation*, vol. 19, no. 5-6, pp. 159–170, 2009.

[5] P. C. Carriel and O. M. Rojas, "Prueba de impulso cefálico: bases fisiológicas y métodos de registro del reflejo vestíbulo oculomotor," *Revista de Otorrinolaringología y Cirugía de Cabeza y Cuello*, vol. 73, no. 2, pp. 206–212, 2013.

[6] K. P. Weber, H. G. MacDougall, G. M. Halmagyi, and I. S. Curthoys, "Impulsive testing of semicircular-canal function using video-oculography," *Annals of the New York Academy of Sciences*, vol. 1164, pp. 486–491, 2009.

[7] H. G. MacDougall, K. P. Weber, L. A. McGarvie, G. M. Halmagyi, and I. S. Curthoys, "The video head impulse test: diagnostic accuracy in peripheral vestibulopathy," *Neurology*, vol. 73, no. 14, pp. 1134–1141, 2009.

[8] M. C. Schubert and A. A. Migliaccio, "Stability of the aVOR to repeat head impulse testing," *Otology & Neurotology*, vol. 37, no. 6, pp. 781–786, 2016.

[9] S. J. Herdman, R. A. Clendaniel, D. E. Mattox, M. J. Holliday, and J. K. Niparko, "Vestibular adaptation exercises and recovery: acute stage after acoustic neuroma resection," *Otolaryngology—Head and Neck Surgery*, vol. 113, no. 1, pp. 77–87, 1995.

[10] S. Herdman and R. Clendaniel, *Vestibular Rehabilitation*, F. A. Davis Company, 2014.

[11] S.-H. Jeong, H.-J. Kim, and J.-S. Kim, "Vestibular neuritis," *Seminars in Neurology*, vol. 33, no. 3, pp. 185–194, 2013.

[12] N. T. Shepard, S. A. Telian, and M. Smith-Wheelock, "Habituation and balance retraining therapy. A retrospective review," *Neurologic Clinics*, vol. 8, no. 2, pp. 459–475, 1990.

[13] T. Lempert, J. Olesen, J. Furman et al., "Vestibular migraine: diagnostic criteria," *Journal of Vestibular Research*, vol. 22, no. 4, pp. 167–172, 2012.

[14] N. Pérez-Fernández, V. Gallegos-Constantino, L. Barona-Lleo, and R. Manrique-Huarte, "Clinical and video-assisted examination of the vestibulo-ocular reflex: a comparative study," *Acta Otorrinolaringologica Espanola*, vol. 63, no. 6, pp. 429–435, 2012.

[15] M. N. McDonnell and S. L. Hillier, "Vestibular rehabilitation for unilateral peripheral vestibular dysfunction," *Cochrane database of systematic reviews*, vol. 1, Article ID CD005397, 2011.

[16] C. D. Hall, S. J. Herdman, S. L. Whitney et al., "Vestibular rehabilitation for peripheral vestibular hypofunction: an evidence-based clinical practice guideline: from the American physical therapy association neurology section," *Journal of Neurologic Physical Therapy*, vol. 40, no. 2, pp. 124–155, 2016.

[17] A. H. Alghadir, Z. A. Iqbal, and S. L. Whitney, "An update on vestibular physical therapy," *Journal of the Chinese Medical Association*, vol. 76, no. 1, pp. 1–8, 2013.

[18] S. Whitney, A. Alghwiri, and A. Alghadir, "An overview of vestibular rehabilitation," in *Handbook of Clinical Neurology*, vol. 137, pp. 187–205, Elsevier, Amsterdam, Netherlands, 2016.

[19] S. J. Herdman, C. D. Hall, and W. Delaune, "Variables associated with outcome in patients with unilateral vestibular hypofunction," *Neurorehabilitation and Neural Repair*, vol. 26, no. 2, pp. 151–162, 2012.

[20] S. J. Herdman, M. C. Schubert, and R. J. Tusa, "Role of central preprogramming in dynamic visual acuity with vestibular loss," *Archives of Otolaryngology—Head & Neck Surgery*, vol. 127, no. 10, pp. 1205–1210, 2001.

[21] S. J. Herdman, M. C. Schubert, V. E. Das, and R. J. Tusa, "Recovery of dynamic visual acuity in unilateral vestibular hypofunction," *Archives of Otolaryngology—Head and Neck Surgery*, vol. 129, no. 8, pp. 819–824, 2003.

[22] M. C. Schubert, A. A. Migliaccio, R. A. Clendaniel, A. Allak, and J. P. Carey, "Mechanism of dynamic visual acuity recovery with vestibular rehabilitation," *Archives of Physical Medicine and Rehabilitation*, vol. 89, no. 3, pp. 500–507, 2008.

[23] M. Ushio, L. B. Minor, C. C. Della Santina, and D. M. Lasker, "Unidirectional rotations produce asymmetric changes in horizontal VOR gain before and after unilateral labyrinthectomy in macaques," *Experimental Brain Research*, vol. 210, no. 3-4, pp. 651–660, 2011.

[24] M. C. Schubert, C. C. Della Santina, and M. Shelhamer, "Incremental angular vestibulo-ocular reflex adaptation to active head rotation," *Experimental Brain Research*, vol. 191, no. 4, pp. 435–446, 2008.

[25] A. A. Migliaccio and M. C. Schubert, "Unilateral adaptation of the human angular vestibulo-ocular reflex," *Journal of the Association for Research in Otolaryngology*, vol. 14, no. 1, pp. 29–36, 2013.

[26] J. Redondo-Martínez, C. Bécares-Martínez, M. Orts-Alborch, F. J. García-Callejo, T. Pérez-Carbonell, and J. Marco-Algarra, "Relationship between video head impulse test (vHIT) and caloric test in patients with vestibular neuritis," *Acta Otorrinolaringologica Espanola*, vol. 67, no. 3, pp. 156–161, 2016.

[27] S. Zellhuber, A. Mahringer, and H. A. Rambold, "Relation of video-head-impulse test and caloric irrigation: a study on the recovery in unilateral vestibular neuritis," *European Archives of Oto-Rhino-Laryngology*, vol. 271, no. 9, pp. 2375–2383, 2014.

[28] D. L. McCaslin, G. P. Jacobson, M. L. Bennett, J. M. Gruenwald, and A. P. Green, "Predictive properties of the video head impulse test: measures of caloric symmetry and self-report dizziness handicap," *Ear and Hearing*, vol. 35, no. 5, pp. e185–e191, 2014.

[29] A. Palla, D. Straumann, and A. M. Bronstein, "Vestibular neuritis: vertigo and the high-acceleration vestibulo-ocular reflex," *Journal of Neurology*, vol. 255, no. 10, pp. 1479–1482, 2008.

[30] M. Patel, Q. Arshad, R. E. Roberts, H. Ahmad, and A. M. Bronstein, "Chronic symptoms after vestibular neuritis and the high-velocity vestibulo-ocular reflex," *Otology and Neurotology*, vol. 37, no. 2, pp. 179–184, 2016.

[31] S. F. Alhabib and I. Saliba, "Video head impulse test: a review of the literature," *European Archives of Oto-Rhino-Laryngology*, pp. 1–8, 2016.

8

Tortuous Common Carotid Artery: A Report of Four Cases Observed in Cadaveric Dissections

Joe Iwanaga, Koichi Watanabe, Saga Tsuyoshi, Yoko Tabira, and Koh-ichi Yamaki

Department of Anatomy, Kurume University School of Medicine, Kurume, Fukuoka 830-0011, Japan

Correspondence should be addressed to Joe Iwanaga; iwanaga_jyou@med.kurume-u.ac.jp

Academic Editor: Augusto Casani

A tortuous common carotid artery poses a high risk of injury during tracheotomy. Preoperative diagnosis is therefore important to avoid serious complications. We found four cases of tortuous common carotid artery during an anatomical dissection course for students. The first case was a 91-year-old woman who had bilateral tortuous common carotid arteries without arteriosclerosis. Case 2 was a 78-year-old woman who had bilateral tortuous common carotid arteries without arteriosclerosis. Case 3 was an 86-year-old woman who died from bladder cancer and who also had a right tortuous common carotid artery without arteriosclerosis. Case 4 was an 89-year-old woman who had bilateral tortuous common carotid arteries and a tortuous brachiocephalic artery with severe arteriosclerosis. Case 4 was also examined using computed tomography to evaluate the arteriosclerosis. Computed tomography revealed severe calcification of the vascular wall, which was confirmed in the aortic arch and origins of its branches. In all four cases, the tortuosity was located below the level of the thyroid gland. Based on prior study results indicating that fusion between the carotid sheath and visceral fascia was often evident at the level of the thyroid gland, we speculated that the major region in which tortuosity occurs is at the same level or inferior to the level of the thyroid gland.

1. Introduction

Tortuous common carotid artery (CCA) is associated with a risk of injury during surgical procedures in the anterior cervical region, such as tracheotomy [1, 2]. Therefore, the preoperative examination is important. Computed tomographic angiography (CTA) can provide an accurate diagnosis [3]. For patients with a tortuous CCA who require tracheotomy, evaluation of the three-dimensional relation between the CCA and the thyroid gland is of great interest. There have been few reports, however, that included an accurate description of those structures.

We describe four cases of tortuous CCA that were found among 32 cadavers during a gross anatomical dissection course for students in 2015 to explore the cause of tortuous CCA and its relation with the thyroid gland. To clarify the appearance of the tortuous CCA more definitively, one of the four cases (with bilateral severe tortuous CCA and arteriosclerosis) underwent radiological examination as well.

This study was performed in keeping with the requirements of the Declaration of Helsinki.

2. Case Reports

Case 1 was a 91-year-old woman who died from lung cancer and who also had bilateral tortuous CCAs (Figure 1(a)). The position of the right tortuosity was at the mid-thyroid level and posterior to the gland. The position of the left tortuosity was slightly lower than and lateral to the inferior border of the thyroid gland. The left CCA was more tortuous than that on the right. There was no evidence of arteriosclerosis.

Case 2 was a 78-year-old woman who died from multiple organ failure. She was also found to have bilateral tortuous CCAs (Figure 1(b)). The position of the right tortuosity was at the mid-thyroid level and lateral to the gland. The position of the left tortuosity was lower than the inferior border of the thyroid gland. The right CCA was more tortuous than that on the left. There was no evidence of arteriosclerosis.

(a) (b) (c) (d)

(e) (f)

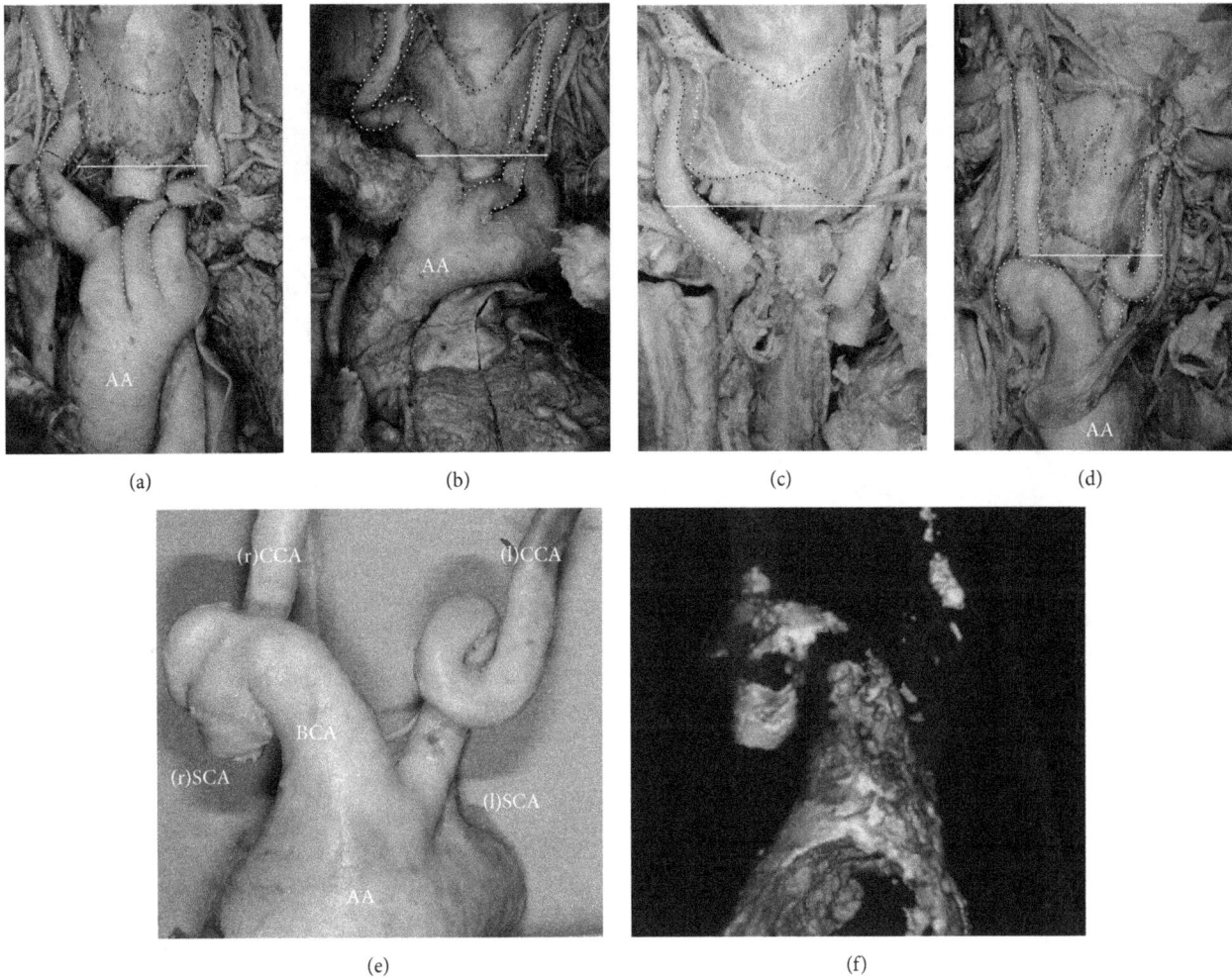

FIGURE 1: Four cases of tortuous common carotid artery (CCA) reported in the present study. Black dotted lines indicate the thyroid glands. White dotted lines indicate the common carotid arteries. White lines show the inferior border of the thyroid glands. (a) Case 1. Bilateral tortuous CCAs ascend posterior to the thyroid gland. The left side is especially tortuous. (b) Case 2. Bilateral tortuous CCAs ascend posterior to the thyroid gland. The right side is especially tortuous. (c) Case 3. Tortuous CCA on the right side ascends posterior to the thyroid gland. The aortic arch had been removed during dissection. (d) Case 4. Bilateral tortuous CCAs ascend posterior to the thyroid gland with a $360°$ turn. The brachiocephalic trunk is also tortuous and hypertrophied. (e) Case 4. Aortic arch and its branches after removal from the body. The vascular wall is highly calcified and has lost its elasticity. (f) Case 4. Computed tomography (CT) image shows the calcified part of the aortic arch and its branches. White parts, which had high CT values, are suspected to be calcified. AA: aortic arch; BCA: brachiocephalic artery; CCA: common carotid artery; SCA: subclavian artery.

Case 3 was an 86-year-old woman who died from bladder cancer and who had a right tortuous CCA (Figure 1(c)). The position of the tortuosity was at the level of the inferior border of, and posterior to, the thyroid gland. There was no evidence of arteriosclerosis.

Case 4 was an 89-year-old woman who died of old age. At postmortem evaluation, she was found to have bilateral tortuous CCAs and a tortuous brachiocephalic artery (BCA; Figure 1(d)). The right and left tortuosities were both located below the level of the inferior border of the thyroid gland. The BCA protruded and was positioned anterior to the thyroid gland. Palpation of the aortic arch and its branches led to a suspicion of severe arteriosclerosis, so CT was performed after resection. The CT images indicated arteriosclerotic changes in the aortic arch, BCA, and both CCAs (Figures 1(e) and 1(f)).

3. Discussion

Tortuous CCA is generally asymptomatic, although occasionally a patient becomes aware of a pulsating mass in the neck region, indicating tortuous CCA. Tortuous CCA is also sometimes found incidentally during imaging. An arterial vascular lesion due to a tortuous CCA aneurysm could affect blood flow to the brain and may result in cerebrovascular disease [4]. Rare cases of a tortuous CCA causing dysphagia [5] and a tortuous CCA presenting as a pediatric submandibular mass lesion [6] have been reported.

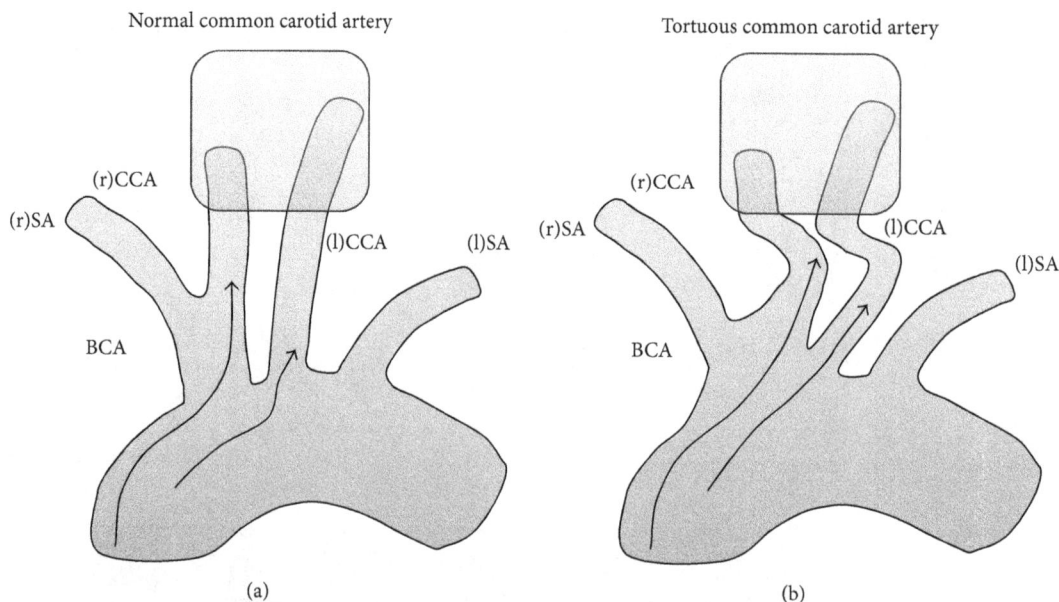

FIGURE 2: Relations among the carotid sheath, visceral fascia, and tortuosity. The square indicates the region of tight fusion between the carotid sheath and cervical visceral fascia. (a) Ejection power of the heart (black arrow) directly affects the brachiocephalic artery and right and left carotid arteries. (b) Ejection power of the heart (black arrow) results in tortuosity of the brachiocephalic artery and the right and left carotid arteries. BCA: brachiocephalic artery; (l)CCA: left common carotid artery; (l)SA: left subclavian artery; (r)SA: right subclavian artery; (r)CCA: right common carotid artery.

Tortuous CCA is sometimes found in the clinical setting, more often in women than men. It appears more frequently on the right side than on the left. Risk factors are old age, obesity, arteriosclerosis, hypertension, and heart enlargement [7]. The ages of the present four cases were 78–91 years, and all were women. Three cases showed tortuous CCA without arteriosclerosis, and one case had severe tortuous CCA and arteriosclerosis. Calcification of the vascular wall in case 4 was found especially in the aortic arch and at the origins of its branches, not in the middle of the tortuosity.

Our findings led us to presume that arteriosclerosis was not an immediate trigger of tortuosity of the CCA, but a complication of it. We presumed that the cardiac pumping and the strength of the connection between the cervical visceral fascia and carotid sheath comprise the potential cause of tortuous CCA. Originally, cardiac pumping is stronger in patients with hypertension and cardiac hypertrophy than in healthy people. The BCA and left CCA are the vessels most commonly affected by the force of the cardiac pumping (Figure 2). The farther the vessels are from the heart, the less the pumping influences them.

Hayashi [8] reported that fusion between the carotid sheath and visceral fascia was often evident at the level of the thyroid gland. We therefore speculated that a fixed CCA does not curve at the level of the thyroid gland. In fact, the tortuous CCAs in our four cases were found at the same level as the thyroid gland or inferior to it (Figures 1(a)–1(d)). In addition, the length and direction of the ascending aorta (which were not investigated in this study) could affect the tortuosity. Hence, surgical procedures in the anterior neck region (e.g., tracheotomy) should be modified in patients

who have a tortuous CCA that protrudes or is positioned higher than the normal CCA [9, 10]. Because tracheotomy in a patient with a tortuous CCA puts the patient at high risk of injury to a major artery, a three-dimensional analysis, such as CTA [3], is required when the situation allows. The consensus is that a procedure that can evaluate the relations between the tortuous CCA and cervical organs, not only morphology, is needed.

Competing Interests

The authors have no competing interests to declare.

Acknowledgments

The authors thank the individuals who donated their bodies for the advancement of education and research.

References

[1] G. Choi, S. H. Han, and J. O. Choi, "Tortuous common carotid artery encountered during neck dissection," *European Archives of Oto-Rhino-Laryngology*, vol. 255, no. 5, pp. 269–270, 1998.

[2] J. K. Muhammad, E. Major, A. Wood, and D. W. Patton, "Percutaneous dilatational tracheostomy: haemorrhagic complications and the vascular anatomy of the anterior neck. A review based on 497 cases," *International Journal of Oral and Maxillofacial Surgery*, vol. 29, no. 3, pp. 217–222, 2000.

[3] M. J. W. Koelemay, P. J. Nederkoorn, J. B. Reitsma, and C. B. Majoie, "Systematic review of computed tomographic

angiography for assessment of carotid artery disease," *Stroke*, vol. 35, no. 10, pp. 2306–2312, 2004.

[4] T. J. Leipzig and G. J. Dohrmann, "The tortuous or kinked carotid artery: pathogenesis and clinical considerations. A historical review," *Surgical Neurology*, vol. 25, no. 5, pp. 478–486, 1986.

[5] A. Gupta and M. C. Winslet, "Tortuous common carotid artery as a cause of dysphagia," *Journal of the Royal Society of Medicine*, vol. 98, no. 6, pp. 275–276, 2005.

[6] C. C. Xu and T. C. Uwiera, "Tortuous common carotid artery presenting as a pediatric submandibular neck mass," *International Journal of Pediatric Otorhinolaryngology Extra*, vol. 5, no. 2, pp. 53–56, 2010.

[7] R. A. Deterling, "Tortuous right common carotid artery simulating aneurysm," *Angiology*, vol. 3, no. 6, pp. 483–492, 1952.

[8] S. Hayashi, "Histology of the human carotid sheath revisited," *Okajimas Folia Anatomica Japonica*, vol. 84, no. 2, pp. 49–60, 2007.

[9] A. Comert, E. Comert, S. Ozlugedik, S. Kendir, and I. Tekdemir, "High-located aberrant innominate artery: an unusual cause of serious hemorrhage of percutaneous tracheotomy," *American Journal of Otolaryngology—Head and Neck Medicine and Surgery*, vol. 25, no. 5, pp. 368–369, 2004.

[10] N. Shankar, V. Raveendranath, R. Ravindranath, and K. Y. Manjunath, "Anatomical variations associated with the carotid arterial system in the neck," *European Journal of Anatomy*, vol. 12, no. 3, pp. 175–178, 2008.

9

Eosinophilic Angiocentric Fibrosis as a Stenosing Lesion in the Subglottis

Ivan Keogh,[1] Rohana O'Connell,[1] Sean Hynes,[2] and John Lang[1]

[1]Otorhinolaryngology Department, University College Hospital Galway and Academic Department of Otorhinolaryngology, National University of Ireland Galway, Newcastle Road, Galway, Ireland
[2]Department of Pathology, University College Hospital Galway, Newcastle Road, Galway, Ireland

Correspondence should be addressed to Rohana O'Connell; rohana.oconnell@gmail.com

Academic Editor: Hsing-Won Wang

Subglottic Eosinophilic Angiocentric Fibrosis (EAF) is an extremely rare disease of an elusive aetiology. It is chronically progressive benign condition that causes narrowing of the subglottic region leading to dysphonia and airway compromise. The diagnosis is historical and imaging is nonspecific. We report a case xc of 56-year-old lady referred to our institution with globus sensation, hoarseness, and mild stridor. Incidental subglottic mass was found at time of diagnostic microlaryngoscopy and biopsy confirmed subglottic EAF. All laboratory investigations were unremarkable. Lesion was removed with laryngeal microdebrider and three courses of intravenous dexamethasone were administered. Patient's postoperative period was uneventful and had remained disease free for 1 year. To date, no consensus has been reached on the optimal treatment of subglottic EAF. We recommend regular follow-up to detect early recurrence.

1. Introduction

Eosinophilic Angiocentric Fibrosis (EAF) had been described as rare submucosal fibrosing vasculitis, believed by some to be the mucosal counterpart of granuloma faciale [1]. Numerous cases have been reported to date, mainly involving the upper airway, and are particularly common at the nasal septum [2, 3].

To date, 51 cases have been reported in the English literature and majority of reported occurrences of this benign condition are in the nasal cavity [4]. Only three cases have been identified in the subglottic region.

Holmes and Panje were the first to describe this condition in 1983 followed by Roberts and McCann two years later, who reported two cases of female patients with rare stenosing lesion involving the upper airway and coined the descriptive diagnosis of *Eosinophilic Angiocentric Fibrosis* [1, 5]. Roberts and McCann also believed that it might be allergies associated with an environmental agent [1]. Recently, EAF has been classified as an IgG4-related disease (IgG4-RD) [2].

EAF typically presents in young to middle aged females, as slowly progressive upper airway obstruction. Although rare, involvement of other anatomic regions such as the orbits, larynx, and trachea has also been reported with patients presenting with diplopia, epiphora, and stridor [6–9].

We report a rare case of subglottic EAF and review of patient's clinical course, her radiological findings, historical diagnosis, and treatment.

2. Case Report

A 58-year-old lady was referred to us with 2 years' history of hoarseness and globus sensation in her throat. She had no dysphagia or odynophagia but reported slowly progressive noisy breathing. She had no previous history of any surgery requiring intubation and no allergies or atopy or aspirin sensitivity. Mild audible biphasic stridor was noted. Oropharyngeal examination was normal. Fibreoptic nasoendoscopy revealed asymmetry of the glottis and limited view of the subglottis. Chest X-ray was normal.

On the basis of these findings and to further evaluate her airway, microlaryngoscopy was arranged. Difficulties were encountered during anaesthesia with poor visualisation

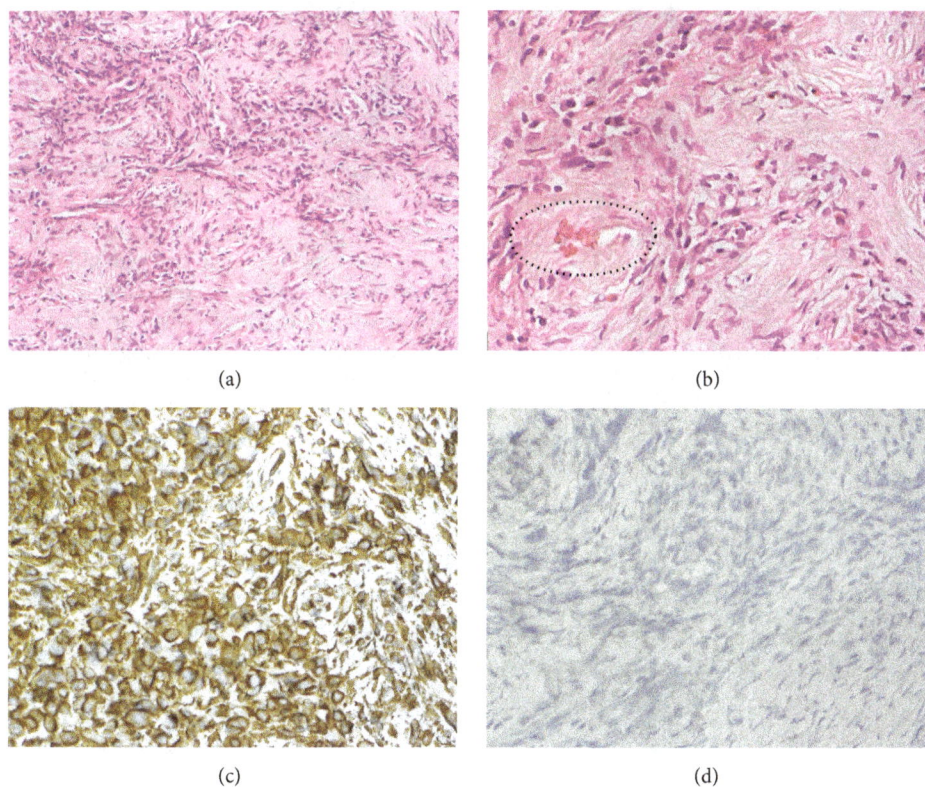

FIGURE 1: (a) Histology of the dense collagenous sclerosing lesion with acute and chronic inflammatory cells (10x objective). (b) Histology demonstrating significant numbers of eosinophils in the inflammatory infiltrate which surrounds a vessel (circled) (40x objective). (c) Positive staining of the lesion's cells for vimentin with immunohistochemistry (40x objective). (d) Negative staining for S100 and AE1/AE3 (40x objective).

during intubation leading to trauma to an incidental lesion in the subglottic region. After successful intubation with microlaryngeal tube, the subglottic mass was thoroughly assessed by the senior author. Biopsies were taken and haemostasis was ensured. Intraoperative intravenous dexamethasone was administered and patient was extubated safely. The rest of her postoperative course was uneventful.

Histology of the lesion under low power view (20x objective) revealed dense collagenous sclerosing lesion with acute and chronic inflammatory cells and examination under high power (40x objective) revealed significant numbers of eosinophil in the inflammatory infiltrate which surrounds vessels (see Figure 1). Lesion also showed positive staining for vimentin and negative for S100 and AE1/AE3 (see Figure 1).

Imaging with CT scan that was carried out two weeks after biopsy confirmed laryngeal asymmetry; the lesion appeared homogenous with no surrounding cartilaginous or bony invasion (see Figure 2). MRI confirmed soft tissue mass approximately 1 cm in diameter confined to the subglottic region (see Figure 3).

Laboratory investigations, including routine blood examinations, blood biochemistry, and erythrocyte sedimentation rate (ESR), and coagulation parameters were all within the normal ranges. Antinuclear antibody (ANA), anti-PR3 antibody (c-ANCA), and anti-MPO antibody (p-ANCA) were also within the normal range.

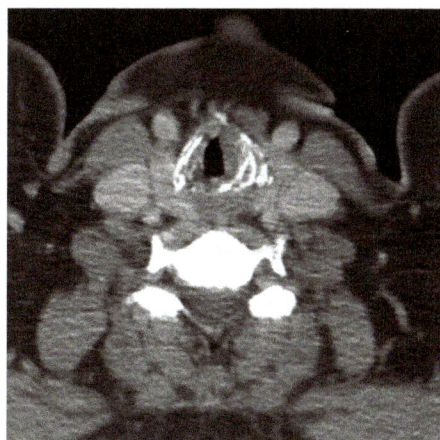

FIGURE 2: Axial section of CT scan showing left-sided laryngeal asymmetry and homogenous soft tissue mass in the subglottic region.

This case was discussed in the multidisciplinary meeting. Diagnosis of EAF was confirmed and the need for definitive management was acknowledged. Patient was booked in for definitive surgery 6 weeks after biopsy. This time precautions were taken not to traumatise the lesion and vocal cords during intubation with microlaryngeal tube (see Figure 4).

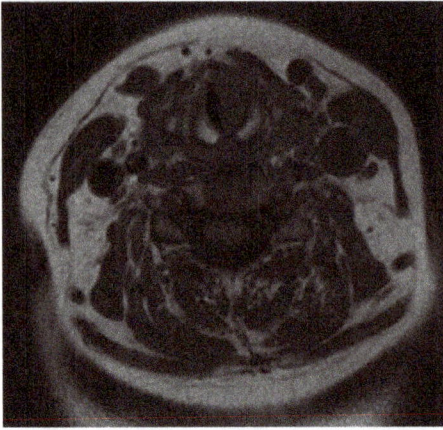

FIGURE 3: T1-weighted MRI scan showing homogenous soft tissue mass in the left subglottic region.

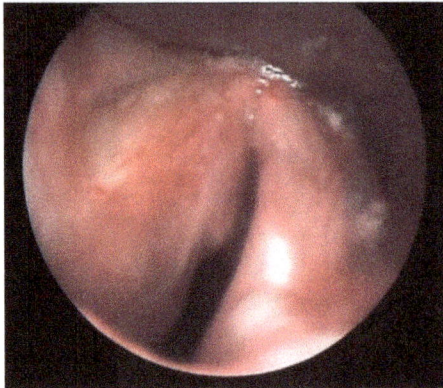

FIGURE 4: View of the glottis and superior aspect of the subglottic mass.

Initially submucosal flap was elevated and laryngeal microdebrider was used to remove the tumour. Minimal bleeding was encountered and all macroscopic tumours were removed successfully.

Patient received dexamethasone intraoperatively and two further doses 8 hours apart. Her postoperative period was uneventful and was discharged home the following day. She was seen subsequently in the outpatient clinic, with improvement in her breathing and resolution of her stridor.

We recommend long term clinical follow-up, based on patient's symptoms and clinical examination with fibreoptic nasoendoscopy. So far, one year after surgery, there has been no sign or symptoms of local recurrence.

3. Discussion

Subglottic EAF is an exceedingly rare condition with no definitive aetiology. Three cases of subglottic EAF had been reported previously. The first case was reported by Roberts and McCann, of a 33-year-old female with asymptomatic subglottic stenosis noted at intubation [1]. This patient was successfully treated with cricotracheal resection [1]. Fageeh et al.

reported the case of a 25-year-old female with history of progressive dyspnea [9]. Imaging revealed subglottic narrowing [9]. This patient had negative serological (CBC, ESR, and ANCA) studies [9]. She was initially treated with tracheotomy and dilatation and was given Tamoxifen [9]. Ultimately, she underwent cricotracheal resection for definite management [9]. The third case of subglottic EAF was reported by Nogueira et al. in 2011 [10]. The patient in this case report was a 68-year-old female who presented with nasal plaques, hoarseness, and dyspnea. Serological test revealed eosinophilia (6.7%) and mildly elevated ESR. CT scan revealed a concentric subglottic narrowing. This patient underwent wide local excision of the subglottic lesion.

EAF shares similar histological features to granuloma faciale of the skin and sometimes can occur concurrently in association with this benign skin condition, as reported by Nogueira et al. [10]. The histology of EAF is pathognomonic and is characterised by progression from an early eosinophil-rich perivascular fibrosing inflammatory lesion to a late dense perivascular "onion-skin" fibrosis formation with decreased inflammatory infiltration [11, 12]. Eosinophils are the predominant inflammatory cells [11, 12]. The main histological differential diagnosis includes granuloma faciale, Wegener's granulomatosis, Churg-Strauss syndrome, and Kimura's disease [13]. All these lesions have prominent eosinophil infiltrates. Negative blood test for c-ANCA and p-ANCA excludes Wegener's granulomatosis and Churg-Strauss syndrome while absence of dense lymphoid aggregates with prominent germinal centres exclude Kimura's disease [13].

Based on most literature, the average duration of clinical symptoms ranged from 3 to 6 years, with majority experiencing symptoms for more than 4 years [1, 9, 14]. Our patient suffered for almost 2 years with globus sensation, hoarseness, and stridor. The long history of the symptoms suggests chronically progressive upper airway obstructive disease resulting in substantial narrowing of the subglottic region. Therefore, it is crucial for subglottic EAF to be evaluated and confirmed historically.

The radiological findings of subglottic EAF in our case were nonspecific and included soft tissue mass in the subglottic region. There was no evidence of focal bony or cartilaginous erosion. On nonenhanced CT scan, the subglottic lesion appeared homogenous and similar finding was also noted on T1-weighted MRI scan. The characteristic whorled "onion-skin" collagenous tissue that is usually observed in the late stage on T2-weighted MRI scan was not seen.

To date, no consensus has been reached on the treatment strategy of EAF, let alone on subglottic EAF. It has been generally accepted that EAF lacks malignant degeneration with no potential for distant metastasis. But it still has the ability to cause focal destruction leading to organ malfunction. Slowly progressive EAF in the subglottic region has the potential to cause dysphonia, dysphagia, and life threatening airway obstruction. The most common treatment modality of EAF in most case reports is surgical resection [4, 6, 7, 11, 14]. The recurrence rate reported is extremely high with approximately 70% of patients experiencing persistence disease following treatment [4].

In most instances, medical treatment has not been effective, although few reported symptomatic relief. Fageeh et al. reported good results with intralesional injection of subglottic EAF [9]. Surgical resections of EAF located elsewhere have resulted in disease-free follow-up in approximately 30% of patients [15]. Majority of patients with recurrences still require multiple resections. Nogueira et al. combined both surgical and medical therapies in treatment of concurrent granuloma faciale on the face and subglottic EAF [10]. He reported excellent response to an intralesional corticosteroid on the GF lesion, CO_2 laser on the EAF lesion, and oral dapsone treatment [10].

Regular and longer follow-ups are necessary to confirm surgical completeness. Our patient has remained disease free for almost 1 year now with no evidence of disease recurrence and is completely asymptomatic.

In conclusion, subglottic EAF is an exceedingly rare and chronically progressive disease with an elusive aetiology. Though benign, subglottic EAF has the potential to cause dysphonia, dysphagia, and airway obstruction. It has historical diagnosis and radiological findings are often nonspecific. Treatment remains a challenge, necessitating regular follow-up after surgery to confirm surgical completeness.

Disclosure

This study was presented at Royal Academy of Medicine-Otolaryngology session, 24/12/2012.

Competing Interests

The authors declare that they have no competing interests.

References

[1] P. F. Roberts and B. G. McCann, "Eosinophilic angiocentric fibrosis of the upper respiratory tract: a mucosal variant of granuloma faciale? A report of three cases," *Histopathology*, vol. 9, no. 11, pp. 1217–1225, 1985.

[2] V. Deshpande, A. Khosroshahi, G. P. Nielsen, D. L. Hamilos, and J. H. Stone, "Eosinophilic angiocentric fibrosis is a form of IgG4-related systemic disease," *American Journal of Surgical Pathology*, vol. 35, no. 5, pp. 701–706, 2011.

[3] B. T. Yang, Y. Z. Wang, X. Y. Wang, and Z. C. Wang, "Nasal cavity eosinophilic angiocentric fibrosis: CT and MR imaging findings," *American Journal of Neuroradiology*, vol. 32, no. 11, pp. 2149–2153, 2011.

[4] Y. Li, H. Liu, D. Han, H. Zang, T. Wang, and B. Hu, "Eosinophilic angiocentric fibrosis of the nasal septum," *Case Reports in Otolaryngology*, vol. 2013, Article ID 267285, 6 pages, 2013.

[5] D. K. Holmes and W. R. Panje, "Intranasal granuloma faciale," *American Journal of Otolaryngology—Head and Neck Medicine and Surgery*, vol. 4, no. 3, pp. 184–186, 1983.

[6] H. Kiratli, S. Önder, S. Yıldız, and H. Özşeker, "Eosinophilic angiocentric fibrosis of the orbit," *Clinical and Experimental Ophthalmology*, vol. 36, no. 3, pp. 274–276, 2008.

[7] O. Kosarac, M. A. Luna, J. Y. Ro, and A. G. Ayala, "Eosinophilic angiocentric fibrosis of the sinonasal tract," *Annals of Diagnostic Pathology*, vol. 12, no. 4, pp. 267–270, 2008.

[8] A. Valenzuela, K. Whitehead, I. Brown, and T. J. Sullivan, "Eosinophilic angiogentric fibrosis: an unusual entity producing complete lacrimal duct obstruction," *Orbit*, vol. 25, no. 2, pp. 159–161, 2006.

[9] N. A. Fageeh, K. T. Mai, and P. F. Odell, "Eosinophilic angiocentric fibrosis of the subglottic region of the larynx and upper trachea," *Journal of Otolaryngology*, vol. 25, no. 4, pp. 276–278, 1996.

[10] A. Nogueira, C. Lisboa, A. F. Duarte et al., "Granuloma faciale with subglottic eosinophilic angiocentric fibrosis: case report and review of the literature," *Cutis*, vol. 88, no. 2, pp. 77–82, 2011.

[11] D. B. Nguyen, J. C. Alex, and B. Calhoun, "Eosinophilic angiocentric fibrosis in a patient with nasal obstruction," *Ear, Nose and Throat Journal*, vol. 83, no. 3, pp. 183–186, 2004.

[12] S. Önder and A. Sungur, "Eosinophilic angiocentric fibrosis: an unusual entity of the sinonasal tract," *Archives of Pathology and Laboratory Medicine*, vol. 128, no. 1, pp. 90–91, 2004.

[13] R. Jain, J. V. Robblee, E. O'Sullivan-Mejia et al., "Sinonasal eosinophilic angiocentric fibrosis: a report of four cases and review of literature," *Head and Neck Pathology*, vol. 2, no. 4, pp. 309–315, 2008.

[14] L. D. R. Thompson and D. K. Heffner, "Sinonasal tract eosinophilic angiocentric fibrosis: a report of three cases," *American Journal of Clinical Pathology*, vol. 115, no. 2, pp. 243–248, 2001.

[15] J. Sunde, K. A. Alexander, V. V. B. Reddy, and B. A. Woodworth, "Intranasal eosinophilic angiocentric fibrosis: a case report and review," *Head and Neck Pathology*, vol. 4, no. 3, pp. 246–248, 2010.

10

Two Cases of Ectopic Hamartomatous Thymoma Masquerading as Sarcoma

Takahito Kondo,[1] Yukiko Sato,[2] Hiroko Tanaka,[3] Toru Sasaki,[1] Kazuyoshi Kawabata,[1] Hiroki Mitani,[1] Hiroyuki Yonekawa,[1] Hirofumi Fukushima,[1] and Wataru Shimbashi[1]

[1]*Department of Head and Neck Oncology, Cancer Institute Hospital of Japanese Foundation for Cancer Research, 3-8-31 Ariake, Koutou-ku, Tokyo 135-8550, Japan*
[2]*Department of Pathology, Cancer Institute Hospital of Japanese Foundation for Cancer Research, 3-8-31 Ariake, Koutou-ku, Tokyo 135-8550, Japan*
[3]*Department of Diagnostic Imaging, Cancer Institute Hospital of Japanese Foundation for Cancer Research, 3-8-31 Ariake, Koutou-ku, Tokyo 135-8550, Japan*

Correspondence should be addressed to Takahito Kondo; takajinkun25@yahoo.co.jp

Academic Editor: Abrão Rapoport

Ectopic hamartomatous thymoma (EHT) is an extremely rare benign tumor. EHTs are difficult to differentiate from sarcomas, especially synovial sarcomas. We encountered two cases of EHT that were referred from other hospitals because sarcoma was suspected. In these cases, fusion gene detection via polymerase chain reaction or fluorescence in situ hybridization was useful for differentiating EHT from synovial sarcoma. EHT requires accurate diagnosis before surgery to avoid excessive treatment. Both tumor location and the presence of fat inside the tumor are important imaging findings for EHT, and confirmation of spindle cells, epithelial cells, and mature adipose cells in the tumor is an important pathological finding. It is important to exclude synovial sarcoma from the differential diagnosis via fusion gene analysis.

1. Introduction

Ectopic hamartomatous thymoma (EHT) is a benign tumor that occurs with extreme rarity in the lower neck. Although EHT disease is referred to as a thymoma, there is no evidence of thymic origin or differentiation [1]. Because EHT is an extremely rare tumor, it is often difficult to diagnose. Additionally, EHT is difficult to differentiate from synovial sarcoma (SS) or other malignant tumors. If EHT is diagnosed incorrectly, treatment leads to unnecessary resection.

Here, we report two cases of EHT in whom the differentiation of EHT from SS was assisted by fusion gene detection using polymerase chain reaction (PCR) or fluorescence in situ hybridization (FISH), as genetic diagnostic techniques [2].

2. Case Presentation

2.1. Case 1. A 60-year-old woman had been aware of a mass in her left lower neck for 5 months. She underwent an open biopsy of the left neck by a previous physician. The findings of the histopathological examination indicated spindle cell sarcoma. On physical examination, an extremely soft mass was palpated in the left lower neck. Computed tomography (CT) scans (Figure 1(a)) revealed a $60 \times 26 \times 42$ mm well-marginated soft tissue mass in the left lower anterior neck. The sternocleidomastoid muscle was markedly displaced anteriorly. The mass presented with heterogeneous enhancement and low-density areas, suggesting the presence of intralesional fat. On magnetic resonance imaging (MRI), the tumor exhibited soft tissue intensity with scattered high intensity that was suggestive of fat in T1-weighted images (WI) (Figure 1(b)) and T2WI (Figure 1(c)). In fat-suppressed gadolinium-enhanced T1WI (Figure 1(d)), the mass showed marked enhancement, and high-intensity areas were suppressed. On ^{18}fluorodeoxyglucose positron emission tomography/CT (FDG-PET/CT) imaging, the maximum standard uptake volume in the tumor was 2.1. Histopathological examination of the previous open biopsy revealed spindle

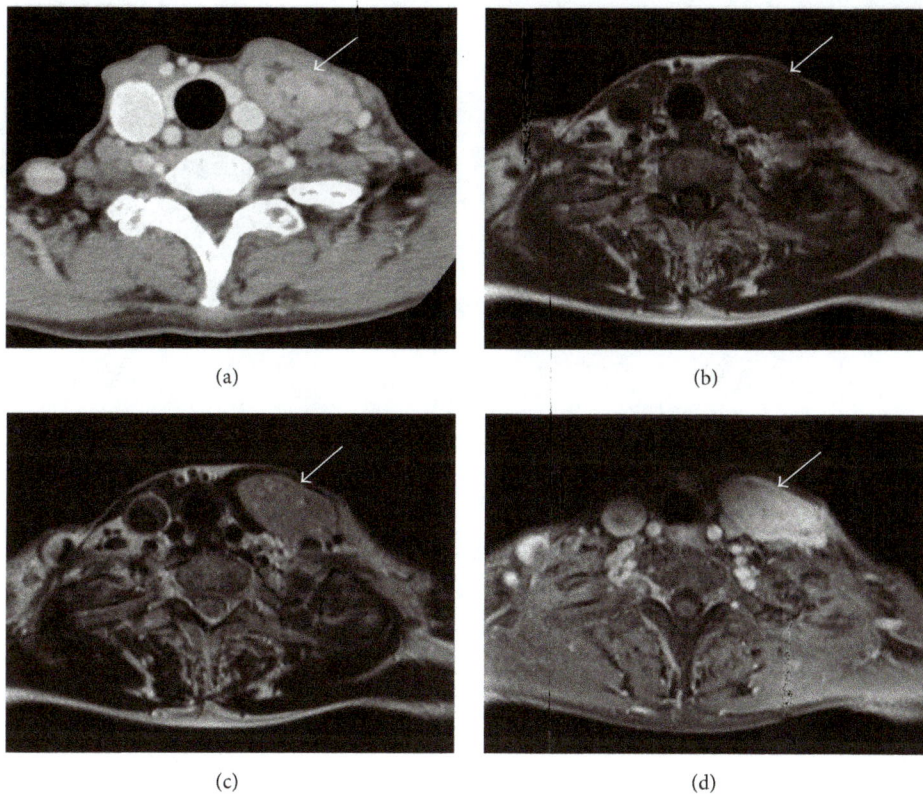

FIGURE 1: Preoperative imaging findings for Case 1. (a) Contrast-enhanced computed tomography image. T1-weighted axial (b), T2-weighted axial (c), and fat-suppressed gadolinium-enhanced T1-weighted axial (d) magnetic resonance images. Computed tomography and magnetic resonance images show a soft tissue tumor with adipose tissue between the sternocleidomastoid muscle and the anterior strap muscle.

cells with epithelioid differentiation. On immunohistochemical examination, the spindle cells and epithelial cells were cytokeratin (CK) AE1/3 (+). The spindle cells were alpha-smooth muscle actin (α-SMA) (+), S100 (−), desmin (−), Bcl2 (+), and terminal deoxynucleotidyl transferase (TdT) (−). SS and spindle cell carcinoma were suspected.

The tumor was resected from the left neck under general anesthesia. The scar created by the previous open biopsy was also resected. The sternocleidomastoid muscle around the tumor was also resected. Resection progressed along the deep cervical fascia with attaching adipose tissue surrounding the tumor. A phrenic nerve running to the deep portions of the tumor was resected. The tumor was detached from the surrounding tissue. Intraoperative frozen section examination results indicated the presence of a spindle cell tumor.

We used frozen samples to assess SYT-SSX fusion gene expression by PCR. cDNA was prepared from total RNA extracted from the excised specimen. We used the SYT51 (5′-cagggaccacctccacaacag-3′) and SSX124-31 (5′-cctctgctggcttct-tgggc-3′) primers, which recognize SSX1/2/4, to perform the 35-cycle PCR. The SYT-SSX fusion gene was not expressed, and thus SS was eliminated from the differential diagnosis. On histopathological examination of the resected tumor, the tumor consisted of plump to thin spindle cells growing in a bundle shape (Figure 2(a)), epithelial cells that formed

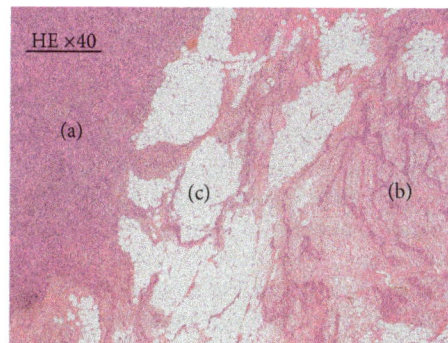

FIGURE 2: Hematoxylin and eosin (HE) staining findings in Case 1 (×40). (a) Plump to thin spindle cells with a low degree of cellular atypia can be observed. (b) Epithelial cells form anastomosing cords. (c) Intermingled adipose cells are present in the tumor.

anastomosing cords (Figure 2(b)), and epithelial islands with solid or microcystic extension areas. In addition, mature adipose cells (Figure 2(c)) and lymphocytes were observed between spindle cells and epithelial cells. Upon evaluation of the overall lesion, we diagnosed the tumor as EHT. The patient has had no recurrence for 56 months after surgery.

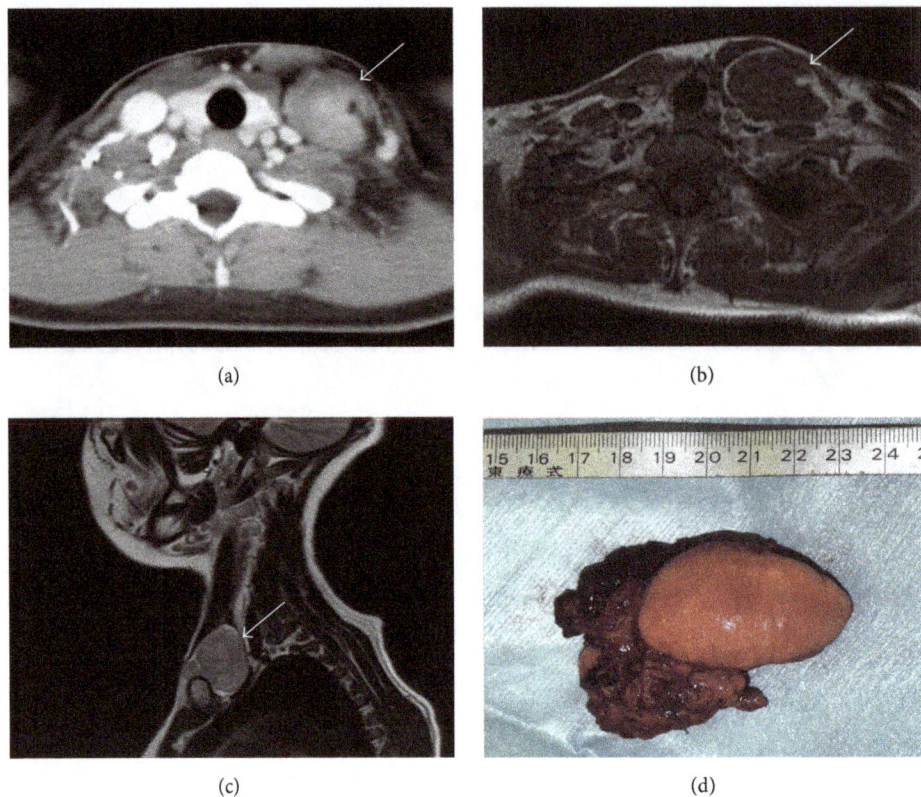

(a)

(b)

(c)

(d)

FIGURE 3: Preoperative imaging findings for Case 2. (a) Contrast-enhanced computed tomography image. T1-weighted axial (b) and T2-weighted sagittal (c) magnetic resonance images. Computed tomography and magnetic resonance images show a tumor with a clear margin and intralesional adipose tissue in the left lower neck. (d) Gross findings of the tumor. The tumor was encapsulated and had a smooth external surface.

The patient provided written informed consent for all medical procedures and for the publication of this case report.

2.2. Case 2. A 24-year-old woman had been aware of a lower left neck swelling for several days. She underwent an open biopsy of the left neck by a previous physician. The histopathological examination suggested SS. The previous physician planned to perform surgery after chemotherapy or chemoradiotherapy. The patient was referred to our department to obtain more detailed examinations before surgery. On physical examination, a soft mass was palpated in the lower left neck. CT scans (Figure 3(a)) revealed a 42 × 35 × 48 mm well-circumscribed mass with nonhomogeneous enhancement between the sternocleidomastoid muscle and internal jugular vein. The mass had low signal intensity similar to muscle on T1WI (Figure 3(b)) and higher intensity than muscle on T2WI (Figure 3(c)). Densities and intensities resembling those of intralesional and marginal fat were observed. On FDG-PET/CT, there was no accumulation in the tumor. Upon histopathological examination of the open biopsy performed by the previous physician, the tumor consisted of comparatively even spindle cells and adipose-like cells. According to the immunohistochemical examination, the spindle cells were CK AE1/3 (+), α-SMA (+), S100 (−), desmin (−), Bcl2 (+), and TdT (−). The tumor was suspected

of being SS. We used the Vysis SS18 Break-Apart FISH Probe Kit (Abbott Laboratories, Abbott Park, Illinois, USA). The gene was not disrupted in the sample, and SS was excluded from the differential diagnosis.

On the basis of the findings in Case 1, we suspected EHT, but a definitive diagnosis could not be obtained from the biopsy. Tumor resection from the left neck was performed under general anesthesia. The scar created by the previous open biopsy was also resected. Part of the sternocleidomastoid muscle between the skin scar and the tumor was also resected. The tumor (Figure 3(d)) was encapsulated with a smooth surface, and there was no adhesion to the surroundings. The surrounding organs were preserved, aside from the partial resection of the sternocleidomastoid muscle between the tumor and the scar, which was performed because the possibility of malignancy could not be excluded.

On intraoperative frozen section examination, spindle cells with no pleomorphism and adipose tissue were seen inside the lesion. Necrosis and mitotic figures were absent. These findings were compatible with a diagnosis of EHT. On histopathological examination of the resected tumor, the tumor consisted of plump to thin spindle cells growing in a bundle shape (Figure 4(a)) and adipose cells (Figure 4(b)). Based on immunohistochemical examination and fusion gene examination, we diagnosed the tumor as EHT. The

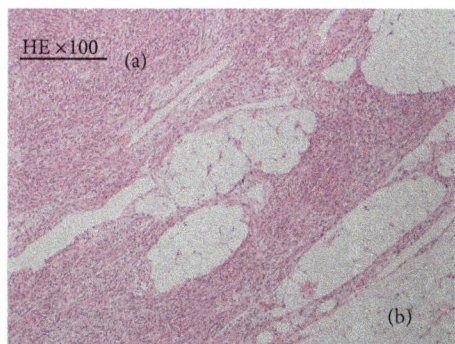

FIGURE 4: Hematoxylin and eosin (HE) staining findings in Case 2 (×100). (a) Plump to thin spindle cells with a low degree of cellular atypia and low mitotic activity can be observed. (b) Adipose cells can be observed within the tumor.

patient has had no recurrence for 29 months after surgery. The patient provided written informed consent for all medical procedures and for the publication of this case report.

3. Discussion

EHT is a disease that has characteristics of both hamartomas and tumors. It was first described in 1982 by Smith and McClure [3] and Rosai et al. [4]. Chan and Rosal [5] defined EHT as a benign "tumor of the neck showing thymic or related branchial pouch differentiation." There was no evidence that this tumor had any relationship with the thymus. Fetsch et al. [6] proposed that "branchial anlage mixed tumor" might be a better name for this disease.

EHT has a markedly higher incidence in men, with a male-to-female ratio of >10 to 1. The tumor most commonly affects adults, with a median age at diagnosis of 42.5 years. It occurs exclusively in the superficial or deep soft tissues of the supraclavicular, suprasternal, or presternal regions. Tumor development is slow, and the clinical course is long. Recurrence after complete surgical excision or metastasis is extremely rare, and most patients experience a benign clinical course [1].

Histopathologically, EHT consists of spindle cells, epithelial cells, and mature adipose cells. Immunohistochemically, both spindle cells and epithelial cells are CK AE1/3 (+), and the spindle cells are α-SMA (+). EHT lacks any population of immature T-cells, and TdT is negative in this tumor. In the histopathological differential diagnosis, SS is the most important tumor to exclude [1, 7]. Although the spindle cell arrays are similar in EHT and SS, SS has larger spindle cells and cellular atypia. In our cases, differentiating between SS and EHT was difficult, and the elimination of SS required fusion gene analysis using PCR or FISH. SS is characterized by the t(X;18)(p11;q11) translocation. This translocation or complex variants are present in more than 95% of all cases. Through this translocation, the SS18 gene (also known as SYT) localized on chromosome 18 and the SSX genes (SSX1, SSX2, or SSX4) localized on the X chromosome become fused, and a SYT-SSX chimeric gene is created. PCR and Break-Apart FISH for assessing fusion transcript expression have been employed widely for accurate diagnoses of SS [2]. We used frozen samples to test for SYT-SSX fusion gene expression via PCR in Case 1. We acquired the Vysis SS18 Break-Apart FISH Probe Kit between the times at which we encountered Case 1 and Case 2. Therefore, we were able to analyze a paraffin-embedded section and perform SS18 Break-Apart FISH for Case 2.

EHT has no specific radiological characteristics. In our cases, however, CT and MRI images showed well-marginated masses in the lower anterior neck with scattered fat density or intensity. Iida et al. [8] also reported the radiological differential diagnosis of fat-containing tumors. Mature adipose cells are pathological components of EHT. Therefore, we concluded that well-circumscribed masses with fat in the lower anterior neck were specific imaging features of EHT.

The treatment for EHT is usually simple resection [7]. Although EHT is a disease that should be differentiated as a lower anterior neck tumor, it may be misdiagnosed as a malignant tumor, such as a sarcoma, because it is so rare. If EHT is not properly diagnosed, it leads to potentially excessive treatment. On the other hand, if a malignant tumor cannot be excluded, we must avoid giving the patient too little treatment. Since a definitive diagnosis of EHT before surgery was impossible in Case 1, the resection included some of the surrounding organs. We strongly suspected EHT before surgery in Case 2 and, therefore, we were able to preserve the surrounding organs, except for the sternocleidomastoid muscle.

The ideal strategy for EHT is definitive diagnosis before surgery and simple resection to avoid excessive surgery. Regarding imaging findings, both tumor location (supraclavicular, suprasternal, or presternal region) and the presence of adipose inside the tumor are important. Regarding histopathological findings, spindle cells, epithelial cells, and mature adipose cells within the tumor are important, as is the exclusion of SS by fusion gene analysis using PCR or FISH.

In conclusion, EHT should be included in the differential diagnosis of lower anterior neck tumors. Fusion gene assessment using PCR or FISH is useful for differentiating between EHT and SS.

Competing Interests

The authors report that there are no competing interests to disclose.

Acknowledgments

The authors would like to thank Dr. Takurou Nakamura from the Division of Carcinogenesis at the Cancer Institute of the Japanese Foundation for Cancer Research and Dr. Noriko Motoi from the Department of Pathology and Clinical Laboratories at the National Cancer Center Hospital.

References

[1] J. K. C. Chan, "Ectopic hamartomatous thymoma," in WHO Classification of Tumours of Soft Tissue and Bone, C. D. M. Fletcher, J. A. Bridge, P. C. W. Hogendoorn, and F. Mertens,

Eds., pp. 201–202, International Agency for Research on Cancer Press, Lyon, France, 4th edition, 2013.

[2] A. J. H. Suurmeijer, D. de Bruijn, A. G. van Kessel, and M. M. Miettinen, "Synovial sarcoma," in *WHO Classification of Tumours of Soft Tissue and Bone*, C. D. M. Fletcher, J. A. Bridge, P. C. W. Hogendoorn, and F. Mertens, Eds., pp. 213–215, International Agency for Research on Cancer Press, Lyon, France, 4th edition, 2013.

[3] P. S. Smith and J. McClure, "Unusual subcutaneous mixed tumour exhibiting adipose, fibroblastic, and epithelial components," *Journal of Clinical Pathology*, vol. 35, no. 10, pp. 1074–1077, 1982.

[4] J. Rosai, G. D. Levine, and C. Limas, "Spindle cell thymic anlage tumor: four cases of a previously undescribed benign neoplasm of the lower neck," *Laboratory Investigation*, vol. 46, p. 70, 1982.

[5] J. K. C. Chan and J. Rosal, "Tumors of the neck showing thymic or related branchial pouch differentiation: a unifying concept," *Human Pathology*, vol. 22, no. 4, pp. 349–367, 1991.

[6] J. F. Fetsch, W. B. Laskin, M. Michal et al., "Ectopic hamartomatous thymoma: a clinicopathologic and immunohistochemical analysis of 21 cases with data supporting reclassification as a branchial anlage mixed tumor," *The American Journal of Surgical Pathology*, vol. 28, no. 10, pp. 1360–1370, 2004.

[7] D. R. Gnepp, "Ectopic hamartomatous thymoma," in *Diagnostic Surgical Pathology of the Head and Neck*, pp. 863–864, Saunders Press, Philadelphia, Pa, USA, 2nd edition, 2009.

[8] E. Iida, M. Okazaki, S. Sarukawa, T. Motoi, and Y. Kikuchi, "Ectopic hamartomatous thymoma growing in the sternocleidomastoid muscle masquerading as sarcoma," *Scandinavian Journal of Plastic and Reconstructive Surgery and Hand Surgery*, vol. 40, no. 4, pp. 249–252, 2006.

11

Case of Superficial Cancer Located at the Pharyngoesophageal Junction Which Was Dissected by Endoscopic Laryngopharyngeal Surgery Combined with Endoscopic Submucosal Dissection

**Kenro Kawada,[1] Tatsuyuki Kawano,[1] Taro Sugimoto,[2] Kazuya Yamaguchi,[1]
Yuudai Kawamura,[1] Toshihiro Matsui,[1] Masafumi Okuda,[1] Taichi Ogo,[1]
Yuuichiro Kume,[1] Yutaka Nakajima,[1] Andres Mora,[1] Takuya Okada,[1] Akihiro Hoshino,[1]
Yutaka Tokairin,[1] Yasuaki Nakajima,[1] Ryuhei Okada,[2] Yusuke Kiyokawa,[2]
Fuminori Nomura,[3] Takahiro Asakage,[2] Ryo Shimoda,[4] and Takashi Ito[5]**

[1]*Department of Gastrointestinal Surgery, Tokyo Medical and Dental University, Tokyo, Japan*
[2]*Department of Head and Neck Surgery, Tokyo Medical and Dental University, Tokyo, Japan*
[3]*Department of Otorhinolaryngology, Tokyo Medical and Dental University, Tokyo, Japan*
[4]*Department of Internal Medicine and Gastrointestinal Endoscopy, Saga Medical School, Saga, Japan*
[5]*Department of Human Pathology, Tokyo Medical and Dental University, Tokyo, Japan*

Correspondence should be addressed to Kenro Kawada; kawada.srg1@tmd.ac.jp

Academic Editor: Guangwei Zhou

Aims. In order to determine the indications of transoral surgery for a tumor located at the pharyngoesophageal junction, the trumpet maneuver with transnasal endoscopy was used. Its efficacy is reported here. *Material and Methods.* An 88-year-old woman complaining of dysphagia, diagnosed with cervical esophageal cancer, and hoping to preserve her voice and swallowing function was admitted to our hospital. Conventional endoscopy showed that the tumor had invaded the hypopharynx. When inspecting the hypopharynx and the orifice of the esophagus, we asked the patient to blow hard and puff her cheeks with her mouth closed (trumpet maneuver). After the trumpet maneuver, the pharyngeal mucosa was stretched out. The pedicle of the tumor arose from the left-anterior wall of the pharyngoesophageal junction, so we decided to perform endoscopic resection. *Result.* Under general anesthesia, the curved laryngoscope made it possible to view the whole hypopharynx, including the apex of the piriform sinus and the orifice of the esophagus. The cervical esophageal cancer was pulled up to the hypopharynx. Under collaboration between a head and neck surgeon and an endoscopist, the tumor was resected en bloc by endoscopic laryngopharyngeal surgery combined with endoscopic submucosal dissection. *Conclusion.* Transnasal endoscopy using the trumpet maneuver is useful for a precise diagnosis of the pharyngoesophageal junction. Close collaboration between head and neck surgeons and endoscopists can provide good results in treating tumors of the pharyngoesophageal junction.

1. Introduction

With increasing progress in endoscopy, superficial cancers in the head and neck regions are being identified with greater incidence [1–3]. Several methods have been reported as low-invasive transoral surgical approaches, including transoral laser microsurgery (TLM) [4], transoral robotic surgery (TORS) [5], endoscopic laryngopharyngeal surgery (ELPS) [6], and transoral videolaryngoscopic surgery (TOVS) [7]. Endoscopic submucosal dissection (ESD), which was developed as a treatment for gastrointestinal mucosal neoplasia, is now widespread in Japan, and its indications have been expanded to the treatment of pharyngeal lesions [8, 9]. ESD is recognized as an organ preservation strategy, especially

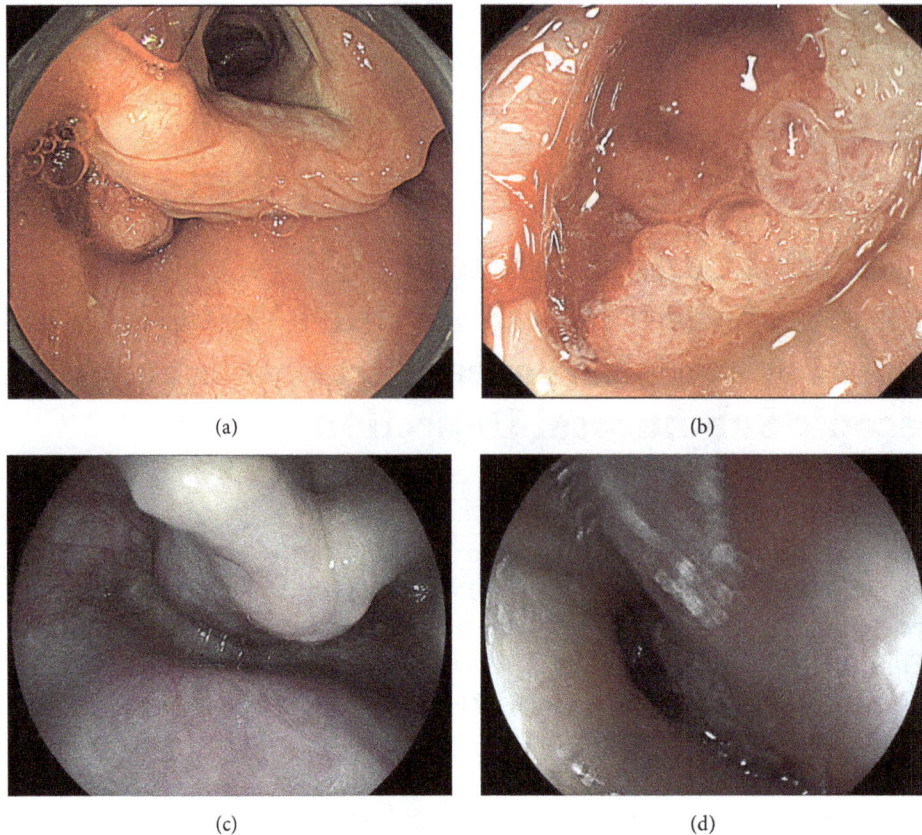

FIGURE 1: (a) Conventional endoscopy showed that the protruded mass was located at the left piriform sinus. (b) The tumor was very movable and was diagnosed as cervical esophageal cancer. (c) Transnasal endoscopy using the trumpet maneuver showed that the tumor had not widely invaded the hypopharynx. (d) The pedicle of the tumor was located at the left-anterior wall of the pharyngoesophageal junction.

with respect to functional outcomes such as swallowing and use of the voice. It is very important to determine the indication, so we must estimate the depth of tumor invasion precisely at the preoperative examination. However, circumferential observation of the hypopharyngeal mucosa is difficult during conventional endoscopy due to its anatomically closed nature. We previously reported the utility of transnasal endoscopy using the trumpet maneuver for precise inspection before treatment [10]. We herein report a case of a tumor located at the pharyngoesophageal junction treated by ELPS combined with ESD.

2. Case Presentation

An 88-year-old woman had suffered from a cough for the past 2 years and had recently felt dysphagia. The dysphagia progressed to the extent that she was unable to tolerate solid foods. She also reported an episode of regurgitation of a mass into her mouth. Three months before, she was diagnosed with cervical esophageal cancer at the clinic near her home, at which point she was admitted to a local tertiary medical center. On the further examination, she was diagnosed with cervical esophageal cancer invading the hypopharynx (Figures 1(a) and 1(b)). A histopathological examination revealed squamous cell carcinoma. Computed tomography

and positron emission tomography (PET) revealed no lymph nodal metastasis or distant metastasis. She was recommended to undergo total pharyngolaryngoesophagectomy or chemoradiotherapy. However, she was elderly; she refused these invasive treatments and hoped to preserve her voice and swallowing function. She was therefore referred to our hospital for a second opinion. The present patient received a transnasal endoscopic examination. We have routinely performed the trumpet maneuver using transnasal endoscopy for patients with esophageal cancer since 2009, using the following procedure. First, the patient is asked to bow the head deeply in the left lateral position. We then place a hand on the back of the patient's head and push it forward. To examine the hypopharynx and the orifice of the esophagus, the patient is asked to blow hard and puff the cheeks while the mouth remains closed (trumpet maneuver). The image of the pharynx using the trumpet maneuver with transnasal endoscopy in the present patient is shown in Figure 1(c). The postcricoid was difficult to visualize during esophagogastroduodenoscopy; however, the view could be improved by using trumpet maneuver. We therefore concluded that the tumor of the cervical esophagus had not invaded the hypopharynx. The pedicle of the tumor was located at the left-anterior wall of the pharyngoesophageal junction (Figure 1(d)). We therefore planned to observe it under

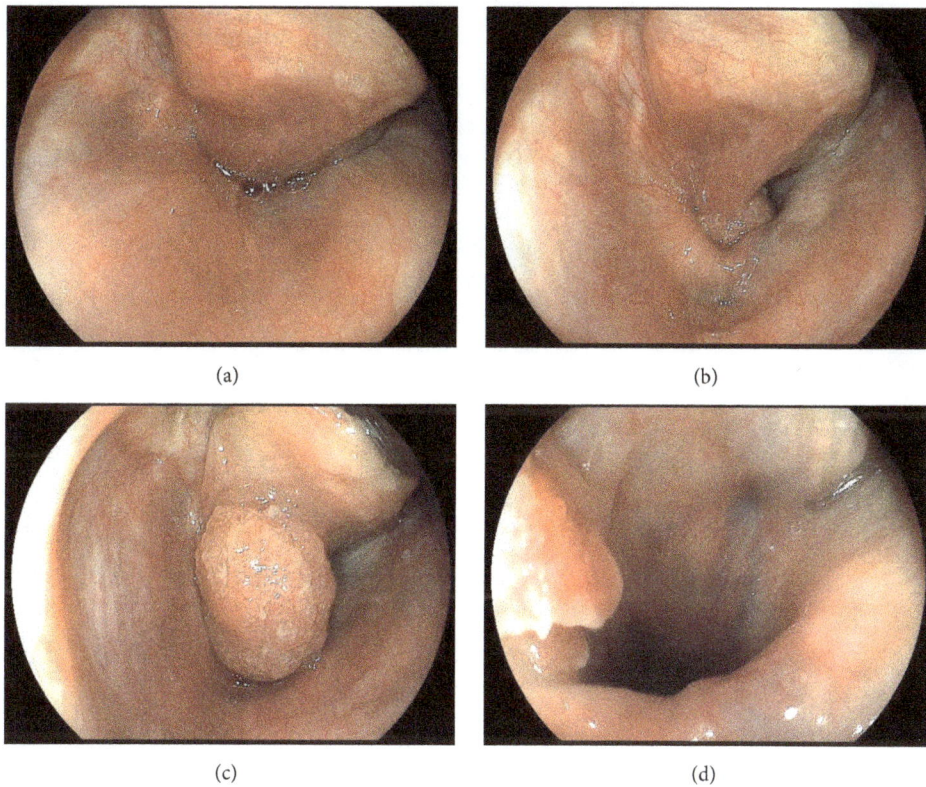

FIGURE 2: (a) The curved laryngoscope enabled a view of the whole hypopharynx, including the apex of the piriform sinus and the orifice of the esophagus. The tumor was invisible from the hypopharynx. (b) The tumor was pulled up from the cervical esophagus to the hypopharynx. (c) The pedicle of the tumor was mainly located at the postcricoid area. (d) The flat, superficial part and the anal side of the tumor had spread to the cervical esophagus.

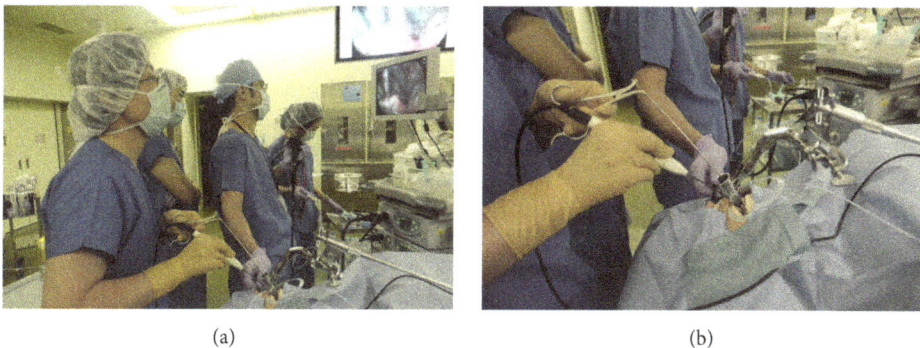

FIGURE 3: (a) ELPS is a video-assisted surgery performed by two physicians: a head and neck surgeon acting as the operator and an endoscopic specialist acting as the endoscopist. They observe the same TV monitor in the operation room. (b) The operator uses the curved forceps and the electric needle knife, while the endoscopist inserts the transnasal endoscope through the nose.

general anesthesia. A specially designed curved laryngoscope was inserted into the anesthetized patient to create a working space in the pharyngoesophageal lumen. Initially, the tumor was invisible from the hypopharynx (Figure 2(a)), as most of it was located in the cervical esophagus. Using the forceps, the tumor was pulled up from the cervical esophagus to the hypopharynx (Figure 2(b)). The pedicle of the tumor was mainly located at the postcricoid area (Figure 2(c)). The flat superficial part and anal side of the tumor had spread to the cervical esophagus (Figure 2(b)). It was easy to grasp the

pedicle with the forceps inserted transorally, and the lesion was moving well, so we concluded that the tumor had not invaded the muscle layer.

3. Therapeutic Procedure

Endoscopic laryngopharyngeal surgery is a video-assisted surgery performed by two physicians (Figure 3(a)): an operator and endoscopist who is an endoscopic specialist [7]. The endoscopist inserts the esophagogastroduodenoscope

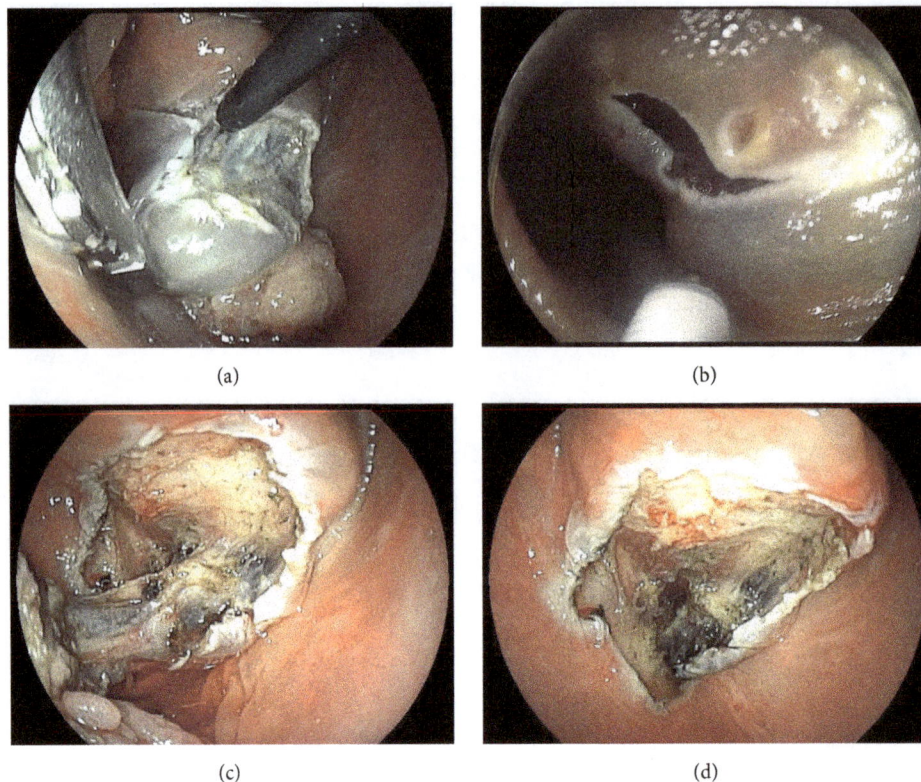

(a)

(b)

(c)

(d)

FIGURE 4: (a) After saline was injected into the subepithelial layer, the head and neck surgeon dissected the lesion using the orally inserted curved grasping forceps with one hand and the orally inserted curved electric needle knife with the other. (b) The esophageal portion was resected by ESD. (c) The pharyngeal portion was resected by ELPS. (d) After tumor removal, the tumor was resected en bloc.

and obtains images of the lesion on a monitor. The operator uses the curved forceps and the electric needle knife, while the endoscopist inserts the transnasal endoscope through the nose (Figure 3(b)).

In the present patient, the endoscope first identified and demarcated the lesion margins using iodine dye, which was then marked by endoscopist. Next, a solution of epinephrine (0.02 mg/mL) and saline was then injected into the subepithelial layer to separate the mucosa from the muscle layer proper. Then a head and neck surgeon performed the circumferential mucosal incision using an electric needle knife (KD-600, Olympus Medical Systems, Tokyo, Japan) and forceps inserted transorally (Figure 4(a)). At the esophageal portion, the needle knife could not reach the lesion, inserted transorally as it was, so it was difficult for the head and neck surgeon to perform the operation alone. An endoscopist was therefore called in to help the operator dissect the anal margin using the electric knife inserted through a flexible endoscope (Figure 4(b), ESD procedure). After the circumferential incision, dissection was performed using the orally inserted curved grasping forceps with an electric knife in combination (Figure 4(c) with video https://www.youtube.com/watch?v=2FCFVLQtAN8). The tumor was resected en bloc (Figure 4(d)). Finally, triamcinolone was injected endoscopically to prevent the posttreatment formation of stricture.

The operation time was 62 minutes. The patient was extubated immediately after surgery. The fasting period was two days after surgery, and the postoperative hospital stay was five days. There were no complications and no hoarseness or swallowing discomfort.

The histopathological findings were squamous cell carcinoma, $25 \times 18 \times 10$ mm, subepithelial invasion, no microvascular permeation, and a negative vertical margin (Figure 5). On the anal side of the specimen, the muscularis mucosa was examined (Figure 6), and the tumor was confirmed to have spread to the cervical esophagus. According to the TNM classification, the final stage was Stage III (T3N0M0). The follow-up examinations after treatment included cervical ultrasound and the measurement of her tumor marker levels every three months and computed tomography every six months. Balloon dilation was not required. The patient is currently alive with no recurrence at 8 months after the surgery (Figure 7(a)), and there is no stricture at the cervical esophagus (Figure 7(b)).

4. Discussion

With increasing progress in esophagogastroduodenoscopy, superficial cancers in the head and neck regions are being identified with greater incidence. Transoral surgery is becoming a major strategy in the treatment of laryngopharyngeal

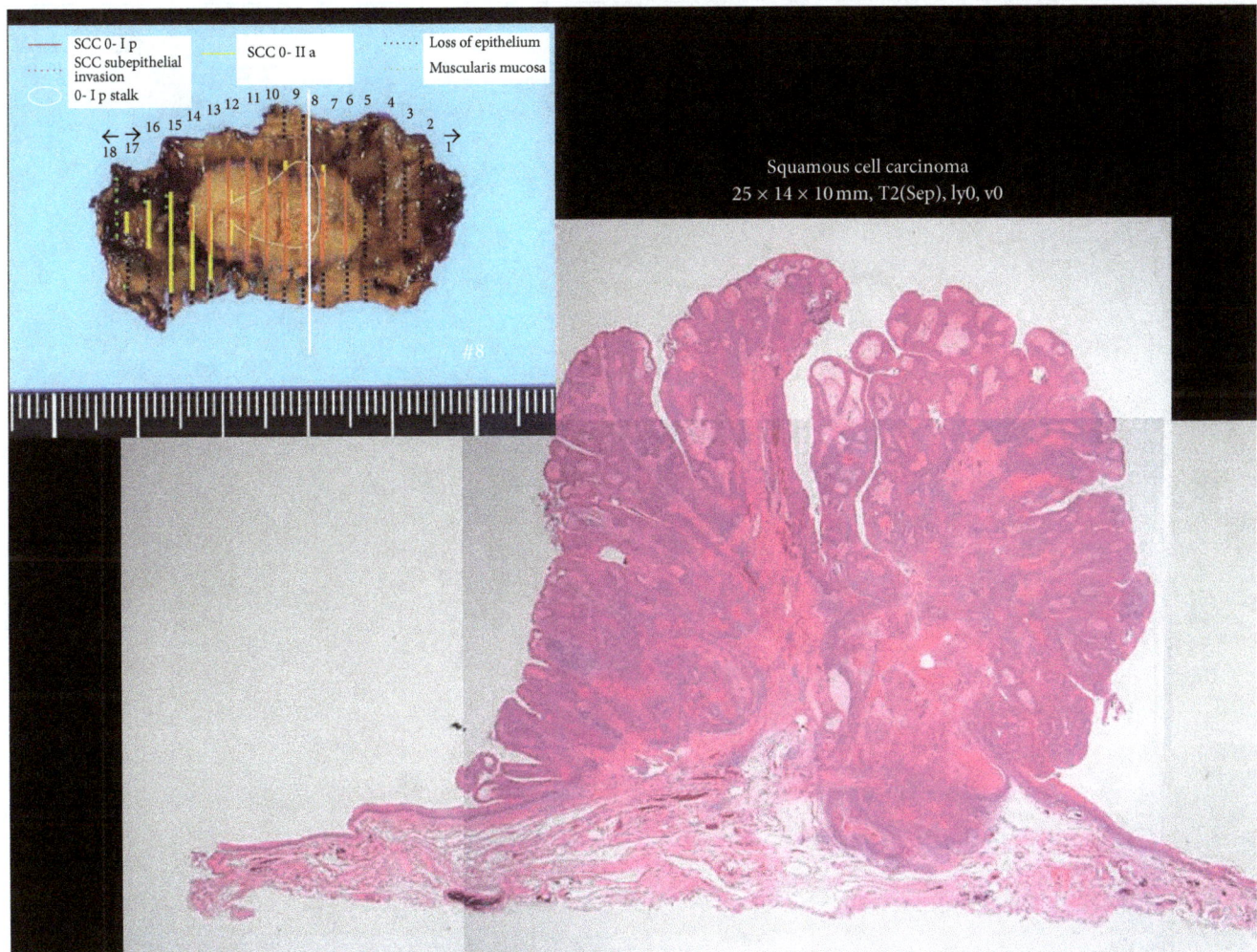

FIGURE 5: A histopathological examination revealed a diagnosis of invasive squamous cell carcinoma. A 25 × 18 × 10 mm superficial lesion was removed by en bloc resection.

cancer [11]. However, the choice of an adequate therapeutic strategy for treating neoplasms located at the pharyngoesophageal junction is not clearly defined and therefore difficult. Chemoradiotherapy is widely performed at present but is associated with a high frequency of complications during and after treatment [12]. Total pharyngolaryngoesophagectomy is considered the most complicated and most invasive surgery for the gastrointestinal tract [13]. In determining the treatment strategy, the stage and location of the tumor and the general status of the patient should be considered. The indications of voice-preserving surgery can be examined using transoral endoscopy or esophagogram, but it can sometimes be difficult to observe the pharyngoesophageal junction. However, determining the precise location of tumor is important in determining the optimum method of treatment. We previously reported the utility of transnasal endoscopy using the trumpet maneuver for observing the pharyngoesophageal junction [14]. This method is also useful for determining the oral surgical margin of cervical esophageal cancer preoperatively [15].

We first diagnosed the patient with cervical esophageal cancer that had not widely invaded the hypopharynx and the pedicle was located only in the junction. However, the tumor was actually mainly located at the postcricoid, and a curved laryngoscope under general anesthesia was very effective in obtaining a wide space to examine the hypopharynx. This preoperative study using transnasal endoscopy was also important for determining whether or not her larynx could be preserved.

Kawano et al. [16] previously reported a case of superficial carcinoma located at the pharyngoesophageal junction treated with endoscopic mucosal resection (EMR). In EMR, a small-diameter snare (SD-7P, Olympus, Tokyo, Japan) is used for resection. A weak point of EMR is that endoscopists cannot confirm an accurate cutting line until resection is performed, occasionally requiring multiple instances of resection [17]. ESD is now a standard procedure in the gastrointestinal tract in Japan, with a gastroenterologist easily resecting the mucosa containing the lesion at the submucosal

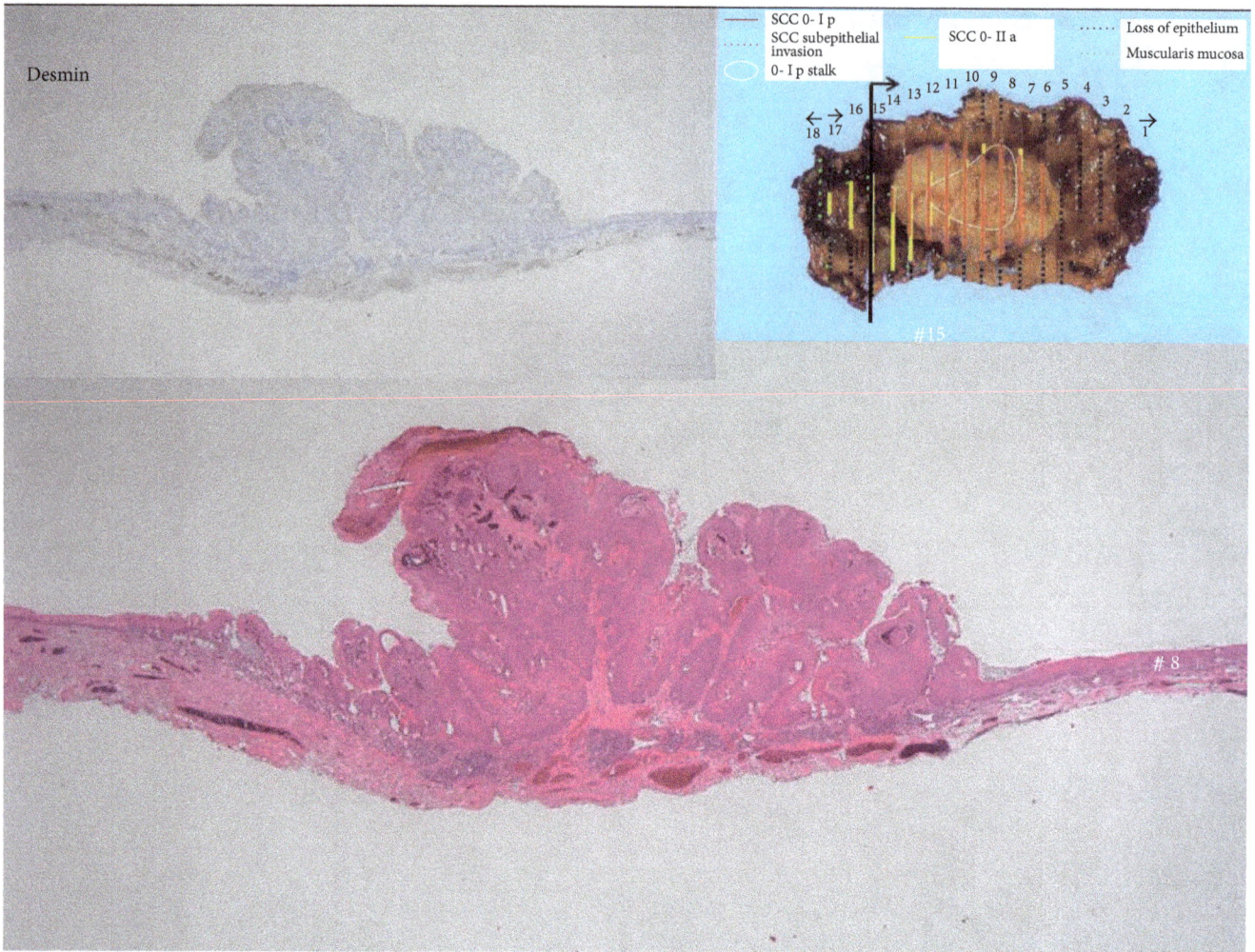

FIGURE 6: At the anal side of the specimen, the muscularis mucosa was examined, and the tumor was confirmed to have spread to the cervical esophagus.

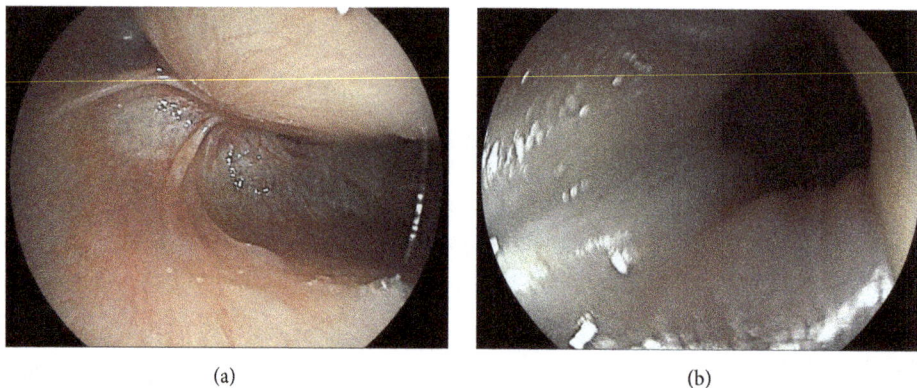

(a)   (b)

FIGURE 7: (a) At 8 months after treatment, no local recurrence was observed. (b) No stricture was observed at the cervical esophagus.

level of the esophageal region. We performed ELPS combining with ESD in the present patient.

In Japan, most cases of superficial squamous cell carcinoma located at the cervical esophagus are treated endoscopically. To avoid the perforation of esophageal wall, saline is first injected into the subepithelial layer to separate the mucosa from the muscle layer proper. It was reported that the endoscopic injection of steroid is useful for preventing stricture after esophageal ESD [18]. In this case, we could easily perform surgery without any complications. Collaboration between a head and neck surgeon and a gastroenterologist on ELPS combined with ESD has been reported useful for treating even the hypopharyngeal lesions that have spread to the cervical esophagus which is difficult with TLM, TOVS, and TORS [19]. Although we do not have any robotic surgery systems in our institution, we were able to perform the treatment with human power alone.

More cases and longer follow-up periods will be required to obtain conclusive findings, and future studies will need to determine the indications of this treatment.

5. Conclusion

Transnasal endoscopy using the trumpet maneuver is useful for diagnosing the pharyngoesophageal junction. Collaboration between head and neck surgeon and an endoscopist can provide a good result in treating tumors of the pharyngoesophageal junction. ELPS combined with ESD for treating superficial neoplasm of the pharyngoesophageal junction is a promising therapeutic option for elderly patients.

Competing Interests

The authors declare that there is no conflict of interests regarding the publication of this paper.

References

[1] M. Muto, M. Nakane, C. Katada et al., "Squamous cell carcinoma in situ at oropharyngeal and hypopharyngeal mucosal sites," *Cancer*, vol. 101, no. 6, pp. 1375–1381, 2004.

[2] M. Muto, K. Minashi, T. Yano et al., "Early detection of superficial squamous cell carcinoma in the head and neck region and esophagus by narrow band imaging: a multicenter randomized controlled trial," *Journal of Clinical Oncology*, vol. 28, no. 9, pp. 1566–1572, 2010.

[3] A. Watanabe, H. Tsujie, M. Taniguchi, M. Hosokawa, M. Fujita, and S. Sasaki, "Laryngoscopic detection of pharyngeal carcinoma in situ with narrowband imaging," *The Laryngoscope*, vol. 116, no. 4, pp. 650–654, 2006.

[4] W. Steiner, "Experience in endoscopic laser surgery of malignant tumours of the upper aero-digestive tract," *Advances in Oto-rhino-laryngology*, vol. 39, pp. 135–144, 1988.

[5] B. W. O'Malley Jr., G. S. Wienstein, and N. G. Hockstein, "Transoral robotic surgery for base of tongue neoplasms," *The Laryngoscope*, vol. 116, pp. 1465–1472, 2006.

[6] Y. Sato, T. Omori, and M. Tagawa, "Surgical treatment for hypopharyngeal superficial cancer: endoscopic laryngo-pharyngeal surgery," *Nihon Jibiinkouka Gakkai Kaiho*, vol. 109, pp. 581–586, 2006.

[7] A. Shiotani, "Transoral surgery for laryngeal and hypopharyngeal cancer," *Practica Oto-Rhino-Laryngologica Journal*, vol. 101, no. 1, pp. 68–69, 2008.

[8] Y. Shimizu, J. Yamamoto, M. Kato et al., "Endoscopic submucosal dissection for treatment of early stage hypopharyngeal carcinoma," *Gastrointestinal Endoscopy*, vol. 64, no. 2, pp. 255–259, 2006.

[9] T. Iizuka, D. Kikuchi, S. Hoteya, N. Yahagi, and H. Takeda, "Endoscopic submucosal dissection for treatment of mesopharyngeal and hypopharyngeal carcinomas," *Endoscopy*, vol. 41, no. 2, pp. 113–117, 2009.

[10] K. Kawada, T. Kawano, T. Sugimoto et al., "Case of a superficial hypopharyngeal cancer at the pharyngoesophageal junction which is detected by transnasal endoscopy using trumpet maneuver," *Open Journal of Gastroenterology*, vol. 5, no. 1, pp. 1–6, 2015.

[11] I. Tateya, A. Shiotani, Y. Satou et al., "Transoral surgery for laryngo-pharyngeal cancer—the paradigm shift of the head and cancer treatment," *Auris Nasus Larynx*, vol. 43, no. 1, pp. 21–32, 2016.

[12] A. Nakajima, K. Nishiyama, M. Morimoto et al., "Definitive radiotherapy for T1-2 hypopharyngeal cancer: a single-institution experience," *International Journal of Radiation Oncology Biology Physics*, vol. 82, no. 2, pp. e129–e135, 2012.

[13] N. Sagawa, S. Okushiba, K. Ono et al., "Reconstruction after total pharyngolaryngoesophagectomy: comparison of elongated stomach roll with microvascular anastomosis with gastric pull up reconstruction or something like that," *Langenbeck's Archives of Surgery*, vol. 385, no. 1, pp. 34–38, 2000.

[14] K. Kawada, T. Kawano, T. Sugimoto et al., "Observation of the pharynx to the cervical esophagus using transnasal endoscopy with blue laser imaging," in *Endoscopy—Innovative Uses and Emerging Technologies*, S. Amornyotin, Ed., chapter 10, InTech, 2015.

[15] Y. Nakajima, K. Kawada, Y. Tokairin et al., "Larynx-preserving surgery for cervical esophageal carcinoma," *Journal of the Japan Bronchoesophageal Society*, vol. 65, pp. 447–456, 2014 (Japanese).

[16] T. Kawano, K. Nagai, and T. Iwai, "A case of cancer on the pharyngoesophageal junction treated by ambulatory endoscopic mucosectomy," *Surgical Endoscopy*, vol. 16, no. 5, pp. 871–872, 2002.

[17] K. Nagai, K. Kawada, T. Nishikage et al., "Endoscopic treatment for superficial hypopharyngeal carcinoma," *Stomach and Intestine*, vol. 38, pp. 331–338, 2003 (Japanese).

[18] S. Hashimoto, M. Kobayashi, M. Takeuchi, Y. Sato, R. Narisawa, and Y. Aoyagi, "The efficacy of endoscopic triamcinolone injection for the prevention of esophageal stricture after endoscopic submucosal dissection," *Gastrointestinal Endoscopy*, vol. 74, no. 6, pp. 1389–1393, 2011.

[19] I. Tateya, M. Muto, S. Morita et al., "Endoscopic laryngo-pharyngeal surgery for superficial laryngo-pharyngeal cancer," *Surgical Endoscopy*, vol. 30, no. 1, pp. 323–329, 2016.

12

Intra-Attack Vestibuloocular Reflex Changes in Ménière's Disease

Dario A. Yacovino[1,2] and John B. Finlay[1,3]

[1]Department of Neurology, Cesar Milstein Hospital, Buenos Aires, Argentina
[2]Memory and Balance Clinic, Buenos Aires, Argentina
[3]Princeton University, Princeton, NJ, USA

Correspondence should be addressed to Dario A. Yacovino; yac@intramed.net

Academic Editor: Augusto Casani

Ménière's attack has been shown to temporarily alter the vestibuloocular reflex (VOR). A patient with unilateral Ménière's disease was serially evaluated with the video Head Impulse Test during single, untreated episodes of acute vertigo. Spontaneous nystagmus activity was concurrently recorded in order to establish the three typical phases of Ménière's attack (irritative, paralytic, and recovery) and correlate them with VOR performance. The onset of attack was associated with a quick change in VOR gain on the side of the affected ear. While a rapidly progressive reduction of the VOR was evident at the paralytic nystagmus phase, in the recovery phase the VOR gain returned to normal and the direction of the previous nystagmus reversed. The membrane rupture potassium intoxication theory provides a good foundation with which to explain these dynamic VOR changes and the observed triphasic direction behavior of the spontaneous nystagmus. We additionally postulated that endolymphatic fluid displacement could have a synergic effect during the earliest phase of attack.

1. Introduction

Ménière's disease (MD) is a fluctuating audiovestibular disorder. The recurrent vertigo attacks, among others, are the most stressful symptoms. According to the temporal direction of spontaneous nystagmus, three classic phases of the attack have been recognized: an initial "irritative" phase beating toward the affected ear, the contralateral "paralytic" phase, and the final "recovery" phase beating again toward the affected side. However, to date, few studies have considered vestibular function measurements during the progression of the attack, and the exact VOR performance in each of the three phases is unknown [1].

The new video Head Impulse Test (vHIT) provides an objective way to measure the dynamic vestibuloocular reflex (VOR) and can be used even in acute vestibular episodes [2]. This procedure is a very valuable, brief test to assess online VOR function, which is particularly helpful for studying short-lived vestibular phenomenon such as Ménière's attack.

The aim of this work is to report the VOR changes measured with vHIT throughout a single Ménière's attack in the following patient.

2. Case Report

An 82-year-old male with right-sided MD for the last 10 years suffered spontaneous attacks of vertigo ranging in frequency from 2 to 4 times per year. He had also occasionally suffered from right posterior canal benign paroxysmal positional vertigo (PC-BPPV) in the quiescent period of the MD. He came to the clinic with typical positional brief upbeating and torsional nystagmus of right PC-BPPV on the Dix-Hallpike maneuver. As a practical routine in our clinic, a vHIT was performed prior to a Semont maneuver. Ten minutes after the maneuver, while he was in a seated position, the vertigo started again. Reexamination showed right beating horizontal nystagmus lasting 3 to 5 minutes (irritative nystagmus). After this, a change of direction was evident:

progressive build-up of left beating horizontal nystagmus (paralytic nystagmus) reached a peak intensity about 10 to 15 minutes from the beginning (12°/sec of SPV with vision), accompanied by severe vertigo, nausea, sweating, and gait disequilibrium. The duration of the vertigo attack was about 1 hour. VHIT ("Eye see cam," Interacoustics, Inc.) and spontaneous nystagmus (binocular 105 Hz Videonystagmography, VNG/V0425, Interacoustics, Inc.) measurements were taken at regular intervals throughout the episode, interchanging the goggles and recalibrating both devices at each interval (Figure 1). In order to minimize patient intolerance during the vHIT procedure, no more than twenty-five horizontal head impulses were passively and randomly applied toward each side. The horizontal VOR gains were automatically measured by the vHIT software in two forms: the instantaneous 40, 60, and 80 ms velocity gain-VOR (head and eye velocity at 40, 60, and 80 ms head movement), and the slope of the linear regression of head on eye velocity variables (*regression gain*) [3]. Since the latter measurement is a mathematically more robust value in an otherwise unstable vHIT baseline trace (i.e., generated by compensatory eye movements or spontaneous nystagmus), this method was ultimately used to document the VOR changes (Figure 1).

When the vertigo started to decrease, a recovery nystagmus (right beating) was recognized after a short quiescent period without any nystagmus. Screening tests to rule out similar conditions were done beforehand, all with normal results, including blood syphilis antibody, anti-cochlear antibody (68 KD), immunological panel, inner ear MRI, and CT Scan. New controls at 2, 7, and 30 days with BPPV still present showed normal gains on the vHIT and no spontaneous nystagmus (SN). An informed consent for the academic use of patient clinical data was obtained.

3. Discussion

3.1. Pathophysiological Discussion. Supported by the membrane rupture potassium intoxication theory, the mechanism of Ménière's attack is a dynamic, triphasic biological process (irritative, paralytic, and recovery), and the exact time frame regarding how early into the attack the VOR recordings are made is critical.

The severe reduction of the VOR during Ménière's attack has been suspected in the clinical setting. However, to the best of our knowledge, the instantaneous VOR changes over a single episode have never been well-documented.

In the intercrisis period (1 week before and 1 and 4 weeks after attack), the vHIT showed normal gain and symmetry on the 6 semicircular canals, and no corrective saccades were identified. We were unable to detect higher than normal VOR gain during the quiescent phase, as was reported in some MD patients [4]. However, there were severe reductions in VOR gain on the affected side during the attack.

Pertinent histopathologic findings in Ménière's Disease include endolymphatic hydrops and associated rupture in almost every part of the membranous labyrinth (excluding the nonampullated portions of the semicircular canals) [5]. According to this theory, the rupture of the distended membranous labyrinth would release neurotoxic potassium-rich endolymph into the perilymph. Irritative acute (depolarization phase) nystagmus, which later becomes paretic (ATPase pump blocking phase), was thought to result from a complete depolarization of either first-order vestibular afferent nerve fibers passing through the perilymph space, or of sensory cells on their synaptic area directly by the escaping endolymph, which increases perilymphatic potassium concentration [6]. This idea is supported by the observation that the direction of the spontaneous nystagmus documented during the attacks was congruent with both phases in the present case.

A group of patients in nonserial HIT studies during Ménière's attack showed variable VOR gains (from normal to reduced) [7]. Since the nystagmus during the irritative and recovery phases had the same direction (beating toward the affected ear), the authors reasoned that it was impossible to determine the phase of the attack that was studied. As shown in the present case, the attack is a dynamic process.

We detected an irritative nystagmus that was short-lived [8]. Unfortunately, we were unable to perform a vHIT at this phase since it lasted only a few minutes. It has been theorized that the presence of irritative nystagmus depends on the size of the perilymph leak into the endolymph system. A sudden and rapid increase in the potassium concentration in the perilymphatic space on the affected side would induce a paretic nystagmus without a visible irritative phase [9]. Contrarily, a smaller progressive filtration of the endolymph should induce a longer (when present) irritative phase followed by a paretic phase, which was the pattern of this case.

Using the distended membrane theory (hydrops) as a base, we postulated that the location of the membrane rupture (leaking) with respect to the ampullary cupula could induce a sudden endolymphatic fluid displacement with either ampullofugal or ampullopetal endolymphatic flow direction. In the horizontal canal, the ampullopetal is excitatory, so the irritative nystagmus should be evidently brief. On the other hand, in the case of ampullofugal flow, which is inhibitory, the induced nystagmus would have the same direction as the paralytic phase, so the initial phase should not be evident. Finally, once the paralytic phase (nerve blocking) starts the cupula deflection, no clinically visible effects should be produced.

In the case of study, the paralytic phase was associated with severe reduction of the VOR, which could not be explained by either the central adaptation or the baseline SN effect. It was recently reported that when induced in postrotatory conditions, an intense baseline SN (SPV greater than 30°/sec) could affect the VOR absolute gain value in the vHIT [10]. However, these baseline conditions were not obtained in the present case (max SPV of 12°/sec).

In the recovery nystagmus phase, the VOR returned to normal gain, compatible with central mediate adaptation nystagmus without peripheral involvement. According to the floating bias toward the side of less active vestibular input [1], when the side with the less active vestibular input recovers to levels analogous with the contralateral side, the bias becomes unmasked in the form of nystagmus toward the formerly less active side. Vestibular adaptation provides a good conceptual framework for the phenomenon observed here *in vivo* and in other similar conditions (p.e. post caloric reversal nystagmus).

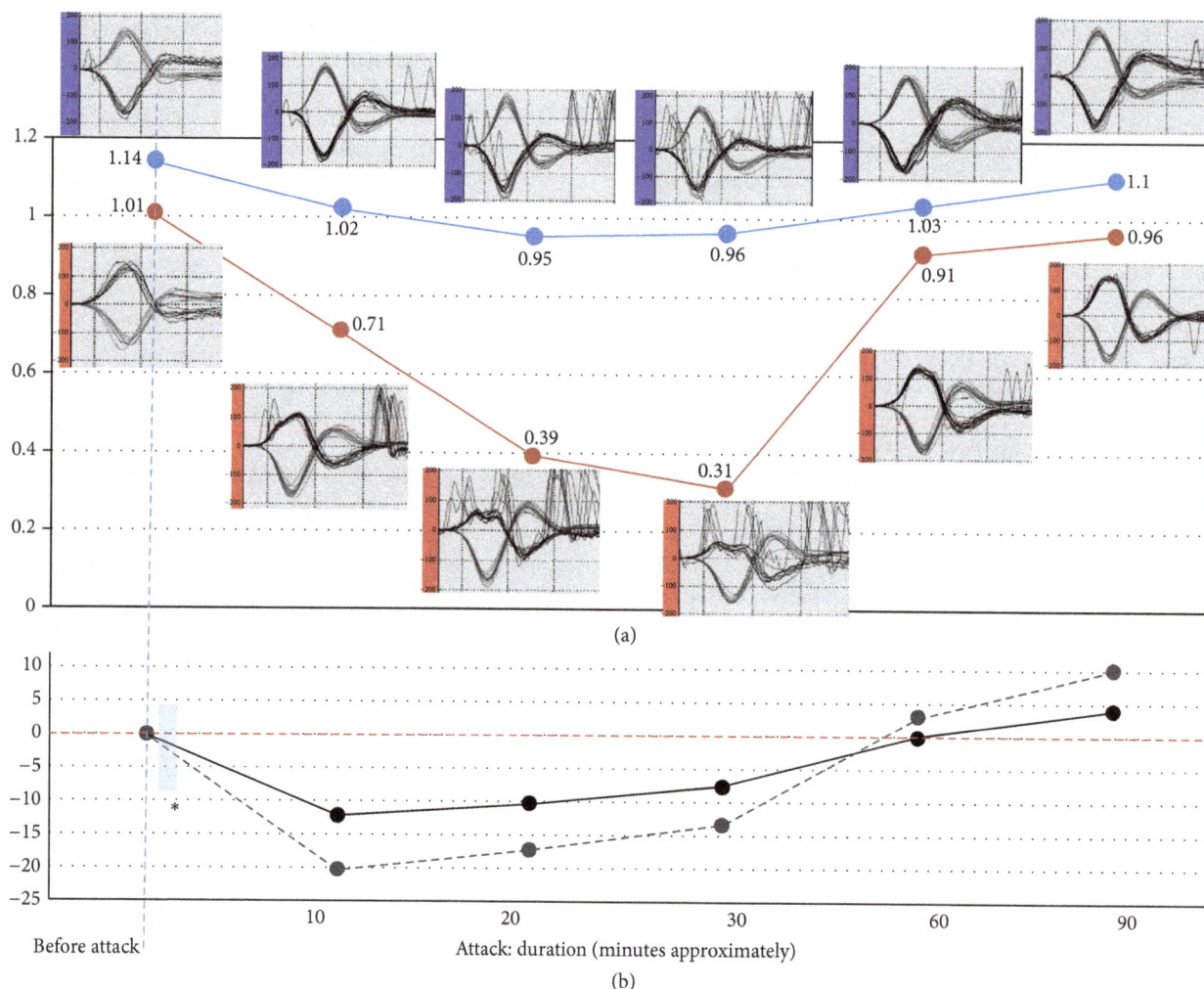

FIGURE 1: (a) The VOR regression gain values on the *y*-axis shows evolution of the right affected side (red line) and left side (blue line) during a vertigo attack from the beginning (0 minutes before attack) to the symptomatic end (90 minutes). The small plots show the video Head Impulse Test (vHIT) recordings; the velocity trajectories (°/s) of the eye (dark grey lines) and head (light grey lines) are depicted during right and left impulses. There are short time mismatches between the vHIT records and the VNG records (spontaneous nystagmus), which can be attributed to the changes and calibration of each instrument. On the right HIT, note the saturated profile of the eye velocity curve and the low VOR gain (from 1.01 to 0.31) as well as the grouped, same direction corrective saccades (at 0.71 right gain). Note also that, with the progression of the attack (at 0.39 and 0.31 right gain), the untidy saccadic movements observed on the ocular velocity baseline trace are due to the interference effect at the onset of the fast phase of the spontaneous nystagmus. At the end of the acute stage (about 60 minutes), the horizontal nystagmus changes direction, and the eye velocity curve regains its normal trajectory, although the VOR gain still shows a slight asymmetry. A week later, the gain was normal (1.09 right and 1.1 left), and no corrective saccades or spontaneous nystagmus were recorded. Technical conditions of the vHIT: number of head impulses technically accepted for analysis: from 10 to 25. Head velocity: from 140 to 190 (°/sec). (b) Spontaneous nystagmus. Velocity SPV °/sec on the *y*-axis is shown with fixation (black line) and without fixation (grey line). At 60 minutes, the nystagmus reversed to the right. *The irritative period was not recorded.

3.2. *Clinical Discussion.* A causal relationship between BPPV and its subsequent development of Ménière's attack has been proposed. Studies of Ménière's disease after physical trauma have described a hypothetical mechanism in which free-floating otoliths could induce hydrops by mechanically obstructing the longitudinal flow and absorption of endolymph [11]. The particle could conceivably provoke the obstruction and accumulation of endolymphatic fluid, which would lead to membrane rupture. In our case, however, the very short period (minutes) between the Semont maneuver performed and the presented Ménière's attack makes this theoretical mechanism less plausible. As further evidence against this hypothesis, the canal reposition maneuver (CRM) was ineffective due to the fact that the Dix-Hallpike test at the follow-up remained positive. There were also various attacks of BPPV without Ménière's attack and vice versa. Another condition that could mimic the VOR features described in the presented case is the plugging of the horizontal canal due to a jamming of particles after the CRM. However, the three observed instances of direction change of the spontaneous horizontal nystagmus, the self-limited evolution, and the progressive reduction of VOR could not be explained by a single canal plugging mechanism [12]

Martinez-Lopez and coauthors reported a similar case and presented additional discussion [13]. However, there were some remarkable clinical differences. First, the ear studied had previously been submitted to a partial chemical ablation procedure (transtympanic gentamicin). Second, the nystagmus found was monophasic (same direction throughout the episode) on the horizontal axis with a vertical component soon added. However, by definition, only one of the typical three stages of attack was documented. Third, although the affected side superior canal did show a gain in VOR reduction, the horizontal did not, even when a significant horizontal component of the SN was observed. The authors hypothesized that the horizontal component could actually be of utricular origin. On the other hand, in our case the spontaneous direction-changing horizontal nystagmus throughout the single attack was associated with a rapid and severe reduction of the VOR on the same horizontal axis. Because of the severity of the vertigo attack, we attempted to minimize stimuli by only performing horizontal impulses in the vHIT. This brief study protocol allowed us to achieve a higher number of VOG and vHIT in an hour-long episode and assess the online VOR behavior during Ménière's attack. Contrary to the cochlear component (progressive hearing reduction), in this case the high VOR changes were rapid and reversible. According to other similar cases [4, 7], in the presence of a fluctuating unilateral gain in the vHIT in a recurrent vertigo case, endolymphatic hydrops should also be considered as a diagnosis.

4. Conclusions

This case showed a severe rapid fluctuation of the high velocity VOR during Ménière's attack. The membrane rupture, fluid displacement, and perilymphatic intoxication theories, postulated *in vitro*, properly explain the dynamic neurophysiological changes presented here, in a human case.

Competing Interests

The authors declare no potential conflicts of interest.

References

[1] M. Bance, M. Mai, D. Tomlinson, and J. Rutka, "The changing direction of nystagmus in acute Meniere's disease: pathophysiological implications," *Laryngoscope*, vol. 101, no. 2, pp. 197–201, 1991.

[2] H. G. MacDougall, K. P. Weber, L. A. McGarvie, G. M. Halmagyi, and I. S. Curthoys, "The video head impulse test: diagnostic accuracy in peripheral vestibulopathy," *Neurology*, vol. 73, no. 14, pp. 1134–1141, 2009.

[3] S. T. Aw, T. Haslwanter, G. M. Halmagyi, I. S. Curthoys, R. A. Yavor, and M. J. Todd, "Three-dimensional vector analysis of the human vestibuloocular reflex in response to high-acceleration head rotations: I. Responses in normal subjects," *Journal of Neurophysiology*, vol. 76, no. 6, pp. 4009–4020, 1996.

[4] L. Manzari, A. M. Burgess, H. G. MacDougall, A. P. Bradshaw, and I. S. Curthoys, "Rapid fluctuations in dynamic semicircular canal function in early Ménière's disease," *European Archives of Oto-Rhino-Laryngology*, vol. 268, no. 4, pp. 637–639, 2011.

[5] H. F. Schuknecht and A. E. Seifi, "Experimental observations on the fluid physiology of the inner ear," *The Annals of Otology, Rhinology, and Laryngology*, vol. 72, pp. 687–712, 1963.

[6] G. F. Dohlman, "Experiments on the mechanism of Ménière attacks," *Journal of Otolaryngology*, vol. 6, no. 2, pp. 135–156, 1977.

[7] S. Lee, H. Kim, J. Koo, and J. Kim, "Comparison of caloric and head-impulse tests during the attacks of Meniere's disease," *The Laryngoscope*, 2016.

[8] J. Hozawa, K. Fukuoka, S. Usami et al., "The mechanism of irritative nystagmus and paralytic nystagmus. A histochemical study of the guinea pig's vestibular organ and an autoradiographic study of the vestibular nuclei," *Acta Oto-Laryngologica. Supplementum*, vol. 481, pp. 73–76, 1991.

[9] G. Dohlman and W. H. Johnson, "Experiments on the mechanism of the Ménière attack," *Proc Can Otolaryngol*, vol. 19, p. 73, 1965.

[10] G. Mantokoudis, A. S. S. Tehrani, L. Xie et al., "The video head impulse test during post-rotatory nystagmus: physiology and clinical implications," *Experimental Brain Research*, vol. 234, no. 1, pp. 277–286, 2016.

[11] M. M. Paparella and F. Mancini, "Trauma and Ménière's syndrome," *Laryngoscope*, vol. 93, no. 8, pp. 1004–1012, 1983.

[12] L. Luis, J. Costa, F. V. Garcia, J. Valls-Solé, T. Brandt, and E. Schneider, "Spontaneous plugging of the horizontal semicircular canal with reversible canal dysfunction and recovery of vestibular evoked myogenic potentials," *Otology and Neurotology*, vol. 34, no. 4, pp. 743–747, 2013.

[13] M. Martinez-Lopez, R. Manrique-Huarte, and N. Perez-Fernandez, "A puzzle of vestibular physiology in a Meniere's disease acute attack," *Case Reports in Otolaryngology*, vol. 2015, Article ID 460757, 5 pages, 2015.

13

Acoustic Neuroma Mimicking Orofacial Pain: A Unique Case Report

Praveenkumar Ramdurg,[1] **Naveen Srinivas,**[1]
Vijaylaxmi Mendigeri,[2] **and Surekha R. Puranik**[3]

[1]*Department of Oral Medicine and Radiology, PMNM Dental College and Hospital, Bagalkot, Karnataka, India*
[2]*Department of Orthodontics, PMNM Dental College and Hospital, Bagalkot, Karnataka, India*
[3]*Department of Oral Medicine and Radiology, PMNM Dental College and Hospital, Bagalkot, Bagalkot District, India*

Correspondence should be addressed to Praveenkumar Ramdurg; praveenod@gmail.com

Academic Editor: Manish Gupta

Acoustic neuroma (AN), also called vestibular schwannoma, is a tumor composed of Schwann cells that most frequently involve the vestibular division of the VII cranial nerve. The most common symptoms include orofacial pain, facial paralysis, trigeminal neuralgia, tinnitus, hearing loss, and imbalance that result from compression of cranial nerves V–IX. Symptoms of acoustic neuromas can mimic and present as temporomandibular disorder. Therefore, a thorough medical and dental history, radiographic evaluation, and properly conducted diagnostic testing are essential in differentiating odontogenic pain from pain that is nonodontogenic in nature. This article reports a rare case of a young pregnant female patient diagnosed with an acoustic neuroma located in the cerebellopontine angle that was originally treated for musculoskeletal temporomandibular joint disorder.

1. Introduction

Orofacial pain is the most common problem encountered by the patient that leads to frequent visits to the dental office, as it mimics vast array of disorders arising from orofacial structures, diseases due to generalized musculoskeletal, peripheral, or central nervous system, and psychological abnormality [1]. In some rare instances, the pain may also arise from neurogenic sources involving cranial nerves V [2, 3], VII [4], VIII [5], and IX [2].

Several reports showed that otologic [6] and ophthalmological [7] clinical manifestations mimic orofacial pain. Thus, well-trained dentists should be capable of diagnosing the source of these complaints before starting any dental treatment in order to avoid unnecessary interventions. One rare cause of orofacial pain is intracranial tumors [8]. According to Bullitt et al., about 1% of patients with orofacial pain will have intracranial tumors as the underlying cause [9]. These patients may undergo unnecessary dental interventions before the correct diagnosis is made.

Tumors of the VIII cranial nerve or acoustic neuroma (AN) is a relatively uncommon, benign, usually slow-growing tumor that develops from the vestibulocochlear nerve supplying the inner ear [10–12].

The Schwann cell sheath from which these tumors develop lies distal to the Glial-Schwann cell junction, which is usually located close to the point where the eighth nerve enters the internal auditory meatus. Consequently, AN arise almost invariably within the meatus itself but expand in a medial direction through the orifice of the meatus and into the potential space formed by the cerebellopontine angle. Here, their close proximity to the roots or proximal portions of various cranial nerves ultimately leads to the development of signs and symptoms due to the pressure on these nerves [13].

Compression of these structures may result in a series of complications with the most common symptoms being tinnitus, hearing loss, and postural imbalance [14]. Despite this, these tumors can also present with other symptoms like temporomandibular disorders (TMD), orofacial pain, numbness or tingling in the face, headache, dizziness, facial paresis, and trigeminal nerve disturbances [15].

To date, there are very few case reports in the dental literature of AN mimicking orofacial pain of nonodontogenic origin; hence, the purpose of this article was to report one such rare case of AN impersonating nonodontogenic orofacial pain.

2. Case Report

A 30-year-old female patient in her third trimester visited a dentist with a chief complaint of pain in the right side of maxilla and preauricular region in the month of April 2014. Pain was gradual in onset, moderate in intensity, and continuous in nature. The pain radiated to the temporal and auricular region of the same side. Examination of the patient revealed tenderness of the TMJ and muscles of mastication on the right side and bilateral attrition of maxillary and mandibular first molars. The intensity of pain was measured using visual analogue scale which was at 8. Correlating the history and clinical findings, a diagnosis of temporomandibular joint disorder secondary to bruxism was considered. Patient was recalled after 15 days with instructions to use night guard, restricted mouth opening, soft diet, and physiotherapy.

Patient reported reduced pain with VAS score of 4 after 20 days; hence, she was was advised to continue with the same instructions and constant follow-up.

Patient reported back to the clinic with aggravated symptoms in December 2015. The pain presented as shock-like that aggravated on brushing and washing face with added symptoms of tinnitus, hearing impairment in right ear, and intermittent loss of balance. Radiographic examination revealed no abnormality with TMJ and surrounding structures. Hence, patient was referred to ENT specialist and audiometry was performed and 48 dB of hearing loss was noted in audiometry test. A more serious pathology was suspected and computed tomography (CT) and magnetic resonance imaging (MRI) were requested. Since the patient was in pain at the time of the examination and the pain had a neuropathic quality and presentation, carbamazepine was initially prescribed for her, which decreased her intensity of pain.

Contrast CT (Figure 1) report showed that an approximately 38 × 27 mm ovoid homogeneous enhancing extra axial mass lesion involving right cerebellopontine cistern was observed. Further contrast MRI revealed 25 × 37 × 31 mm well-defined heterogeneously enhancing T1 hypo and T2 predominantly hyperintense space occupying mass lesion in the right cerebellopontine angle cistern causing mild mass effect on the brain stem with extension to right internal auditory canal with subtle canal widening suggestive of acoustic neuroma (Figures 2 and 3). The extension of the tumor into the internal auditory canal represented "shark fin" appearance (Figure 4). Immediately, the patient was referred to a neurosurgeon to evaluate the lesion. Right retromastoid suboccipital craniotomy and total excision of lesion were performed leading to damage of cranial nerves VII and VIII resulting in hearing loss and facial paralysis with loss of taste sensation on the affected side (Figures 5 and 6).

Histological analysis of the lesion revealed two microscopic patterns in varying amounts. Few areas showed streaming fascicles of spindle shaped Schwann cells (Antoni-A areas). These spindle shaped cells were arranged in a palisaded manner around acellular, eosinophilic areas (Verocay

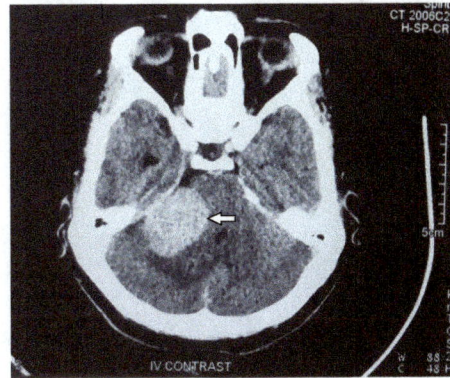

FIGURE 1: Contrast axial CT shows an ovoid homogeneous enhancing lesion (38 mm × 27 mm) involving right cerebellopontine cistern (white arrow).

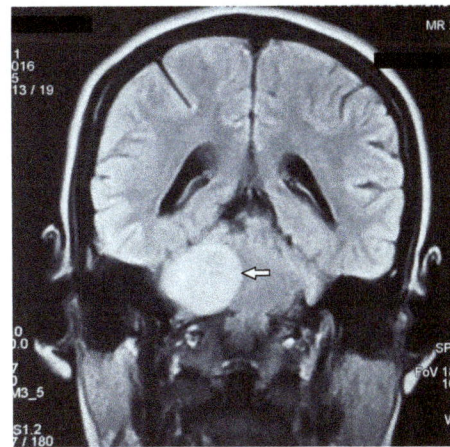

FIGURE 2: Contrast coronal MRI shows well-defined heterogeneously enhancing T1 hypo and T2 predominantly hyperintense lesion in the right cerebellopontine angle (white arrow).

bodies). In other areas, the spindle shaped cells revealed relatively less cellular and less organized areas within a myxomatous stroma (Antoni-B areas). Few blood vessels showed hemorrhage and fibrin within the lumen. Immunohistochemical analysis revealed that the lesion was positive for S-100 protein (Figures 7 and 8).

3. Discussion

A complete history, clinical examination, and through diagnostic work-up ruled out an odontogenic cause for the patient's pain. The absence of work, family, and personal conflicts excluded psychological pain. Initially, the clinical signs of bruxism that is attrition of posterior molars in maxilla and mandible along with the tenderness of the right TMJ tilted the diagnosis towards musculoskeletal-TMD. Bite guard, physiotherapy, and other instructions reduced the pain but the patient did not return for follow-up and further treatment because of pregnancy. After one and half years,

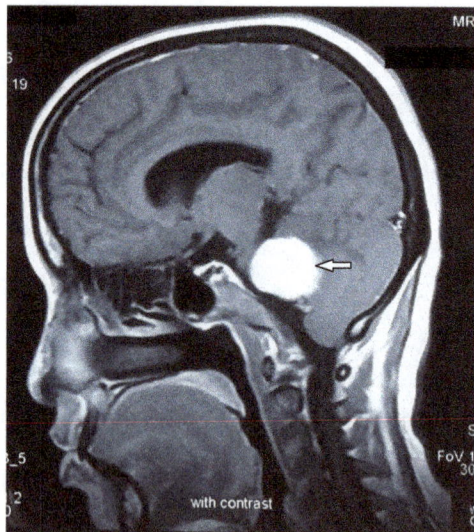

FIGURE 3: Contrast sagittal MRI shows well-defined heterogeneously enhancing T1 hypo and T2 hyperintense mass in the right cerebellopontine angle causing mild mass effect on the brain stem (white arrow).

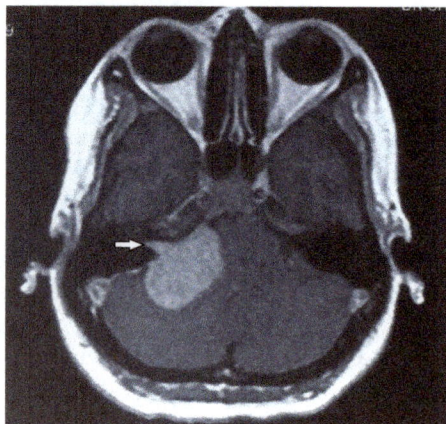

FIGURE 5: Postoperative image shows paralysis of face on right side.

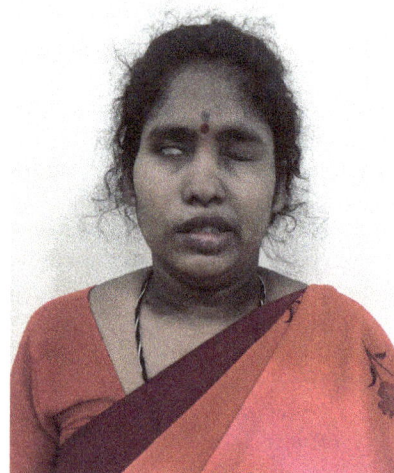

FIGURE 4: Contrast axial MRI shows the extension of the tumor into the internal auditory canal represents "shark fin" appearance (white arrow).

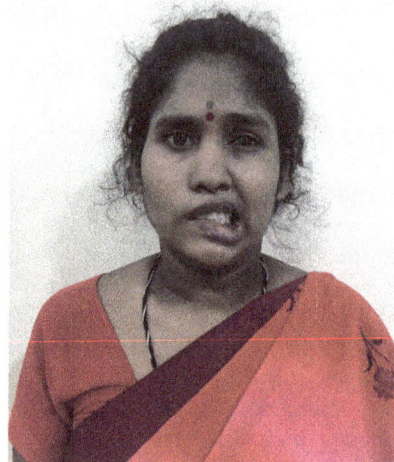

FIGURE 6: Postoperative image shows inability to close the right eyelid and upward rolling of right eyeball.

the patient reported advanced clinical features and AN, and diagnosis was made based on MRI imaging.

The AN originates from the Schwann cell, in the peripheral portion of superior and inferior vestibular nerves, and also from cochlear nerve [16]. The AN occurs in an incidence of about $1:100000$ inhabitants per year [17]. In most recent statistics, an increase of such incidence has been reported due to frequent use of more sensitive magnetic resonance (MR) techniques, diagnosing very small tumors [18]. It happens independently of ethnicity and is more frequently diagnosed in men within 50–60 years of age (61%) [5]. Orofacial pain as the sole symptom of an intracranial tumor is rare. When orofacial pain is caused by such a lesion, neurological abnormalities are usually present [19].

In the present case, initial clinical features suggested orofacial pain but late stages exhibit neurological abnormalities like trigeminal neuralgia. Although the patient exhibited the classic symptoms of acoustic neuroma, namely, tinnitus and loss of hearing, the patient's primary concern was neuralgic pain that became unbearable. These symptoms had only been diagnosed as part of the patient's dental follow-up. Upon limited success of treatment of orofacial pain and considering her young age, the patient was referred for MRI suspecting an intracranial tumor, which led to the diagnosis of trigeminal neuralgia secondary to acoustic neuroma.

Few case reports [5, 9, 20] were published with a confirmed diagnosis of AN mimicking orofacial pain, whereas most of the cases [21–23] in the literature are of trigeminal neuralgia secondary to acoustic neuroma. In our case, the

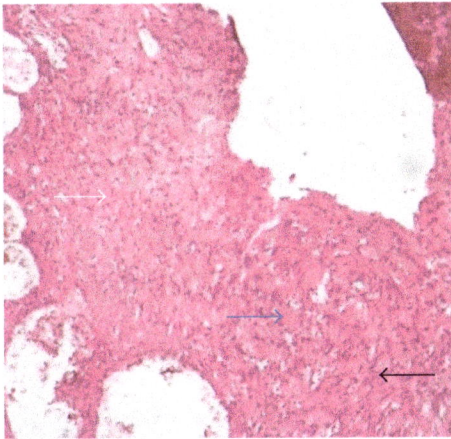

FIGURE 7: Histological features (H&D ×40) show Antoni-A areas (black arrow), Antoni-B areas (white arrow), and Verocay bodies (blue arrow).

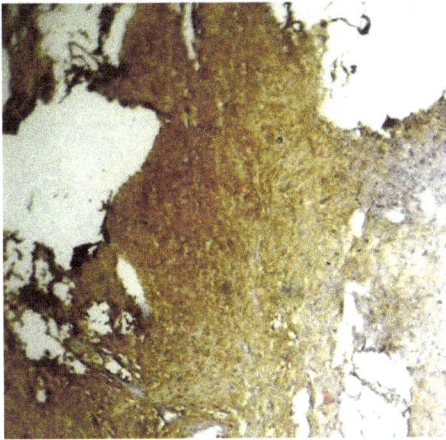

FIGURE 8: Immunohistochemistry (×40) positive for S-100.

patient manifested features of orofacial pain in early visits but in late stage clinical features suggested trigeminal neuralgia. This may be because some authors believe that as tumor size increases it pushes the trigeminal nerve root against the superior cerebellar artery, producing a neurovascular conflict similar to the vascular compression theory proposed for classic trigeminal neuralgia. Another school of thought suggests that the increasing pressure on the trigeminal root or ganglion may induce loss of myelination in the trigeminal sensory root resulting in ephaptic short-circuiting within the nerve root, which results in facial pain and sensory deficits [2].

MRI images of AN in the literature [24] show "trumpeted internal acoustic meatus sign" or "ice cream cone sign," which is a distinguishing feature between AN and other cerebellopontine angle entities. In our case, extension of the AN has a typical "shark fin" like appearance.

Early diagnosis of a vestibular schwannoma is key to preventing its serious consequences. There are three options for managing a vestibular schwannoma: observation, radiation, and surgical removal [25]. In the present case, right

retromastoid suboccipital craniotomy and total excision of lesion were done. Surgical access to this confined zone is difficult; there is a high likelihood of introducing new symptoms or exacerbating preexisting conditions. In our case, the patient developed facial paralysis, loss of taste sensation, and hearing loss on the right side. Facial paralysis and loss of taste sensation are due to damage to the facial nerve which resulted in reduced tonicity in the muscles of facial expression, as well as affecting taste in the anterior two-thirds of the tongue via the chorda tympani nerve. Due to encirclement of the vestibule-cochlear nerve around the tumor,, the patient suffered hearing loss on the right side. Literature [26] shows that about 68% of AN patients are diagnosed by otolaryngologists, 28% are diagnosed by neurosurgeons, 19% are diagnosed by neurologists, 5% are diagnosed by physicians, and less than 5% are diagnosed by dentists, a very low percentage.

4. Conclusion

Hence, the dentist should give more emphasis through history and clinical and radiological examination and also include AN in the differential diagnosis when considering orofacial pain, TMD, and trigeminal neuralgia in young age.

Competing Interests

The authors declare that they have no competing interests.

References

[1] B. Blasberg, E. Eliav, M. S. Greenberg, M. Glick, and J. A. Ship, "Orofacial pain," in *Burket's Oral Medicine*, M. S. Greenberg, M. Glick, and J. A. Ship, Eds., p. 257, BC Decker, Toronto, Canada, 11th edition, 2008.

[2] M. Horowitz, M. Horowitz, M. Ochs, R. Carrau, and A. Kassam, "Trigeminal neuralgia and glossopharyngeal neuralgia: two orofacial pain syndromes encountered by dentists," *Journal of the American Dental Association*, vol. 135, no. 10, pp. 1427–1433, 2004.

[3] S. Prasad and S. Galetta, "Trigeminal neuralgia: historical notes and current concepts," *Neurologist*, vol. 15, no. 2, pp. 87–94, 2009.

[4] G. V. Sowmya, B. S. Manjunatha, S. Goel, M. P. Singh, and M. Astekar, "Facial pain followed by unilateral facial nerve palsy: a case report with literature review," *Journal of Clinical and Diagnostic Research*, vol. 8, no. 8, pp. ZD34–ZD35, 2014.

[5] M. A. Bisi, C. M. P. Selaimen, K. D. Chaves, M. C. Bisi, and M. L. Grossi, "Vestibular schwannoma (acoustic neuroma) mimicking temporomandibular disorders: a case report," *Journal of Applied Oral Science*, vol. 14, no. 6, pp. 476–481, 2006.

[6] D. P. Malkin, "The role of TMJ dysfunction in the etiology of middle ear disease," *International Journal Of Orthodontics*, vol. 25, no. 1-2, pp. 20–21, 1987.

[7] J. R. Fricton, R. Kroening, D. Haley, and R. Siegert, "Myofascial pain syndrome of the head and neck: a review of clinical characteristics of 164 patients," *Oral Surgery, Oral Medicine, Oral Pathology*, vol. 60, no. 6, pp. 615–623, 1985.

[8] A. A. Moazzam and M. Habibian, "Patients appearing to dental professionals with orofacial pain arising from intracranial

tumors: a literature review," *Oral Surgery, Oral Medicine, Oral Pathology and Oral Radiology*, vol. 114, no. 6, pp. 749–755, 2012.

[9] E. Bullitt, J. M. Tew, and J. Boyd, "Intracranial tumors in patients with facial pain," *Journal of Neurosurgery*, vol. 64, no. 6, pp. 865–871, 1986.

[10] L. M. Jr. Tierney, *Current Medical Diagnosis and Treatment*, Mc Graw Hill, New York, NY, USA, 43th edition, 2004.

[11] M. Tos and J. Thomsen, "Epidemiology of acoustic neuromas," *Journal of Laryngology and Otology*, vol. 98, no. 7, pp. 685–692, 1984.

[12] J. D. Swartz, "Lesions of the cerebellopontine angle and internal auditory canal: diagnosis and differential diagnosis," *Seminars in ultrasound, CT, and MR*, vol. 25, no. 4, pp. 332–352, 2004.

[13] J. W. Ferguson and J. F. Burton, "Clinical presentation of acoustic nerve neuroma in the oral and maxillofacial region," *Oral Surgery, Oral Medicine, Oral Pathology*, vol. 69, no. 6, pp. 672–675, 1990.

[14] T. Hansen, *Netter's Clinical Anatomy*, Saunders, Philadelphia, Pa, USA, 3rd edition, 2014.

[15] S. H. Selesnick, R. K. Jacklor, and W. P. Lawrence, "The changing clinical presentation of acoustic tumors in the MRI era," *Laryngoscope*, vol. 103, no. 4, pp. 431–436, 1993.

[16] E. M. Tallan, S. G. Harner, and C. W. Beatty, "Does the distribution of Schwann cells correlate with the observed occurrence of acoustic neuromas?" *American Journal of Otology*, vol. 14, no. 2, pp. 131–134, 1993.

[17] Acoustic Neuroma, "National institutes of health consensus develoment conference," *Consens Statement*, vol. 9, pp. 1–24, 1991.

[18] S. J. Haines and S. C. Levine, "Intracanalicular acoustic neuroma: early surgery for preservation of hearing," *Journal of Neurosurgery*, vol. 79, no. 4, pp. 515–520, 1993.

[19] D. M. Feinerman and M. H. Goldberg, "Acoustic neuroma appearing as trigeminal neuralgia.," *The Journal of the American Dental Association*, vol. 125, no. 8, pp. 1122–1125, 1994.

[20] D. S. German, "A case report: acoustic neuroma confused with TMD," *The Journal of the American Dental Association*, vol. 122, no. 13, pp. 59–60, 1991.

[21] Y. Matsuka, E. T. Fort, and R. L. Merrill, "Trigeminal neuralgia due to an acoustic neuroma in the cerebellopontine angle," *Journal of Orofacial Pain*, vol. 14, no. 2, pp. 147–151, 2000.

[22] R. Gupta, S. S. Walia, and D. Thaman, "Acoustic neuroma presenting as refractory trigeminal neuralgia," *Indian Journal of Anaesthesia*, vol. 50, no. 3, pp. 218–219, 2006.

[23] N. Mehrkhodavandi, D. Green, and R. Amato, "Toothache caused by trigeminal neuralgia secondary to vestibular schwannoma: a case report," *Journal of Endodontics*, vol. 40, no. 10, pp. 1691–1694, 2014.

[24] J. Howard and A. Singh, "Neoplastic diseases," in *Neurology Image-Based Clinical Review*, p. 179, Demos Medical, New York, NY, USA, 2016.

[25] H. Gouveris, M. Zisiopoulou, and W. J. Mann, "Management of vestibular schwannoma: dependence on stakeholder's view for small and medium-sized tumors," *Otorhinolaryngology Clinics*, vol. 3, no. 1, pp. 7–13, 2011.

[26] D. E. Brackmann and D. M. Barrs, "Assessing recovery of facial function following acoustic neuroma surgery," *Otolaryngology—Head and Neck Surgery*, vol. 92, no. 1, pp. 88–93, 1984.

14

A Rare Tumor in the Cervical Sympathetic Trunk: Ganglioneuroblastoma

Ozan Erol, Alper Koycu, and Erdinc Aydin

Department of Otorhinolaryngology, Baskent University Faculty of Medicine, 06500 Ankara, Turkey

Correspondence should be addressed to Ozan Erol; ozzy.erol@gmail.com

Academic Editor: Abrão Rapoport

Ganglioneuroblastoma is a rare tumor with moderate malignancy, which is composed of mature ganglion cells and seen in sympathetic ganglia and adrenal medulla. The diagnosis is possible after cytological and immunohistochemical studies following a needle biopsy or surgical excision. There is no consensus regarding the need for chemo- or radiotherapy after surgery. In this case report, clinical behavior and diagnosis and treatment of the rare tumor cervical ganglioneuroblastoma were discussed.

1. Introduction

Neuroblastomas are malignant solid tumors. They emerge from out-of-control, immature cells of the sympathetic nervous system. Neuroblastomas can emerge in any place where sympathetic nervous tissues are present. They are most commonly seen in suprarenal gland and areas called truncus sympathicus on neural networks in each side of the spine. In cases where truncus sympathicus is involved, neuroblastomas can emerge in either side of the spine and in any area of it [1]. Different levels of microscopic differentiations are observed in the majority of neuroblastomas. The tumor may transform into ganglioneuroma on the basis of fibrous stroma. Various levels of differentiation may be observed between pure neuroblastoma and pure ganglioneuroma and these are called ganglioneuroblastoma [1, 2].

In this study, a 5-year-old patient with no complaints other than neck swelling and a positive pathology of ganglioneuroblastoma is presented.

2. Case Report

Five-year-old male patient was admitted to our clinic with complaint of swelling in the left side of the neck, which was not accompanied by any pain for four months. He had no other complaints like loss of weight, fever, night sweating, respiratory distress, or difficulty swallowing. In the physical examination, a hard, mobile mass with an approximate size of 2 * 3 cm was detected on the front of musculus sternocleidomastoideus in patient's neck. A neck ultrasonography, which had been conducted in the external center, had the result of a lymphadenopathy with the size of 28 * 21 mm and with no fat hilus on musculus sternocleidomastoideus anterior.

Magnetic resonance imaging of the neck showed a properly limited lesion with 2,8 * 2,3 cm size on the front of musculus sternocleidomastoideus and internal carotid artery. The lesion which pushes parotid gland towards the front was starting from the inferior part of the posterior digastric muscle and progressing up to the C4 level (Figure 1).

A fine-needle aspiration biopsy was offered but refused by the family. In his examination 1 month later, the mass in the neck was found to be approximately 4 * 4 cm. Patient's family was informed that the mass to be extracted by surgery is deep under large arteries in the neck, that it may cover nerves outside the lymph node, and that there are risks of possible lowering of the left eyelid and in operation of the left vocal cord. The family gave written consent for the surgery. The patient underwent the operation with provisional diagnosis of lymphadenopathy and a tumor of nerve origin.

The properly limited and encapsulated mass on musculus sternocleidomastoideus, which was pushing the carotid artery and internal jugular vein into lateral position, was separated from surrounding tissue by blunt dissection. It was observed that the mass had nerve continuity in its upper and

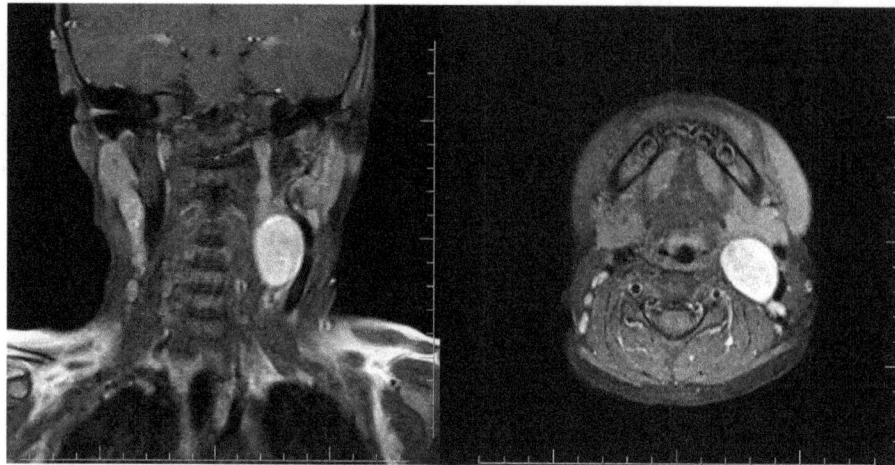

Figure 1: MRI of the head and neck: axial and coronal views of mass. The lesion with 2,8 * 2,3 cm size on the front of musculus sternocleidomastoideus and internal carotid artery.

lower regions and it was in fact of nerve origin. Nerves in the upper part were connected by clamping and the nerves which were severed during blunt dissection were made into another specimen. The total mass was extracted (Figure 2).

Pathological diagnosis was reported as intermixed type ganglioneuroblastoma. While there was no calcification on the encapsulated tumor which was rich in terms of stroma Schwann cells, it was found that ganglioneuromatosis component is over 50%. In addition, differentiation neuroblasts and immature and dysplastic ganglion cells were observed under microscopic examination (Figure 3).

Patient had developed ipsilateral Horner syndrome (miosis, ptosis, and anhidrosis) in the postoperative period. However, no sign of this was found in the 3rd-month control examination. Tests like abdominal and thorax imaging, complete blood count, bone marrow aspiration test, 24-hour urinary VMA, and N-myc protooncogene protein scan were conducted. No pathological findings were observed. After the I-131 Metaiodobenzylguanidine (I-131 MIBG) scan in the 6th-month control examination, an involvement was observed in the right cervical region, the opposite area of the operated region, and patient was directed to adjuvant chemotherapy. No evidence of any recurrence was found in the 12th-month control examination.

3. Discussion

Cervical masses are common pathologies in the pediatric population. While most of them are benign such as inflammatory or congenital ones, over 10% of biopsies extracted from suspicious masses are being reported as malign [2]. Ganglioneuroblastomas represent a histological subgroup of rare neuroblastic tumors with moderate malignancy potential, which originate from neural crest progenitor cells of sympathetic nerve cells. They are very difficult to diagnose using only physical examination and imaging methods. Generally, final diagnosis is possible after cytological and immunohistochemical studies following a surgical excision.

Neuroblastic tumors are divided into four types in International Neuroblastoma Pathology Classification: neuroblastoma, intermixed ganglioneuroblastoma, modular ganglioneuroblastoma, and ganglioneuroma [3]. The type our case study reports, intermixed ganglioneuroblastoma, was reported in several studies in the literature. While in those publications this type of mass was reported to cause respiratory distress and difficulties in swallowing, our case study reported none of these symptoms.

The International Neuroblastoma Risk Group (INRG) classification system was developed to establish a consensus approach for pretreatment risk stratification. The International Neuroblastoma Staging System (INSS) is a postsurgical staging system. In the INRG classification system, a combination of clinical, pathologic, and genetic markers is used to predict whether the tumor will grow and how it will respond to treatment. These markers are used to define risk. Using the following factors, neuroblastoma is classified into 1 of 4 categories: very low-risk, low-risk, intermediate-risk, or high-risk. INRG includes the following: the stage of the disease according to the INRG Staging System, age at the time of diagnosis, histologic category, such as maturing ganglioneuroma versus ganglioneuroblastoma, intermixed versus ganglioneuroblastoma, or nodular versus neuroblastoma, grade or how cells of the tumor are differentiated, MYCN gene status, chromosome 11q status, and tumor cell ploidy, which is the DNA content of tumor cells.

The INRG Staging System (INRGSS) was designed specifically for the INRG pretreatment classification system. It does not include surgical results or spread to lymph nodes to determine the stage. Knowledge regarding the presence or absence of image defined risk factors (IDRFs) is required for this staging system. Stage L1: the tumor is located only in the area where it started; no IDRFs are found on imaging scans, such as CT or MRI. Stage L2: the tumor has not spread beyond the area where it started and the nearby tissue; IDRFs are found on imaging scans, such as CT or MRI. Stage M: the tumor has spread to other parts of the body. Stage MS: the

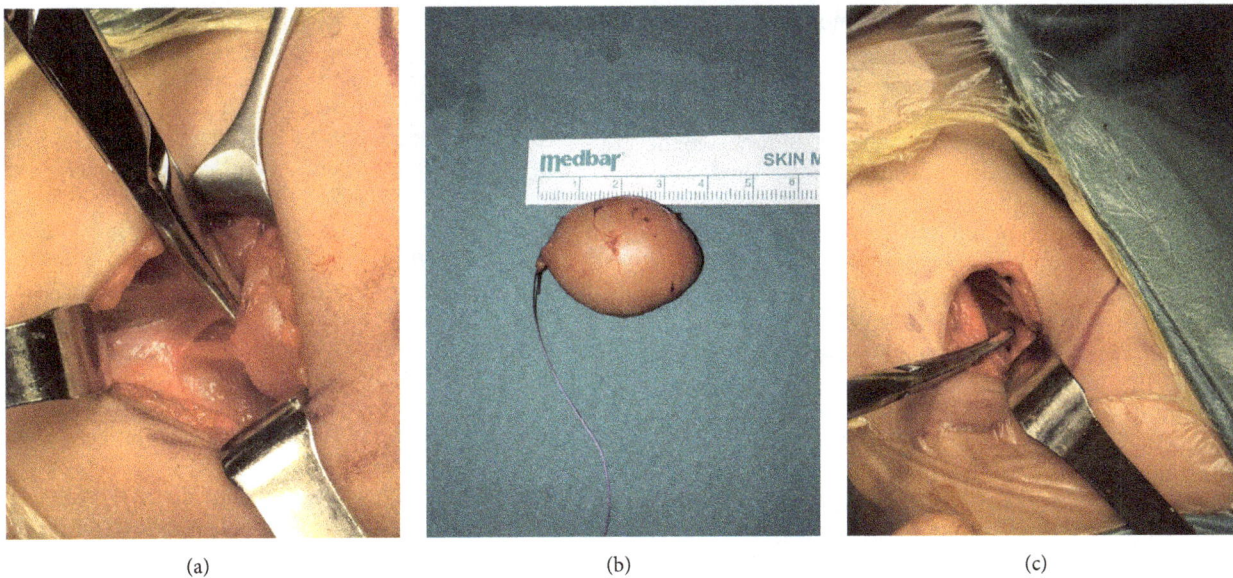

FIGURE 2: (a) Intraoperative view of the neurogenic mass. (b) The lesion with 4 cm size after the total excision. (c) Upper part of the nerve was held by the clamp.

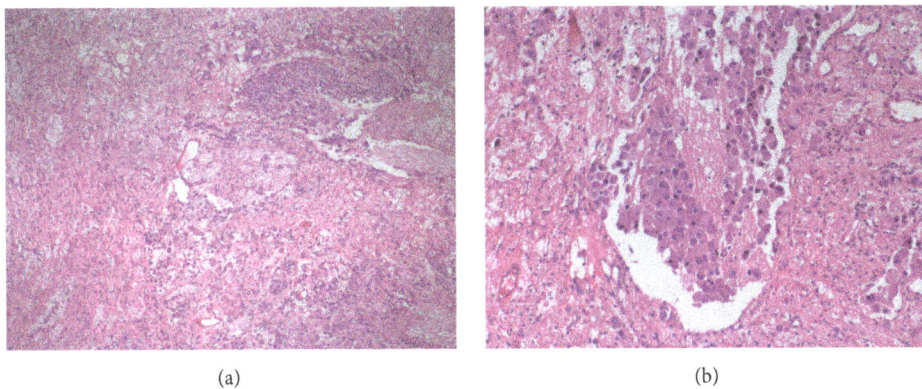

FIGURE 3: Photomicrographs showing more than 50% of tumor tissue in this case composed of Schwannian stroma and neuropil-like islands, differentiating neuroblasts, and immature and dysplastic ganglion cells. H&E (a and b), original magnification (a) 10x and (b) 40x.

tumor has spread to only the skin, liver, and/or bone marrow (less than 10% bone marrow involvement) in patients younger than 18 months [4].

Al-Jassim had stated that in his case study of 2-year-old patient with ganglioneuroblastoma the patient had developed postoperative Horner syndrome, but this had been resolved spontaneously over time [5]. Moukheiber et al. had reported in their study that 3 patients had primary cervical ganglioneuroblastoma and developed nerve paresis in the postoperative period [6]. Due to the risk of postoperative nerve palsy being high, parents and children should be informed in detail before the operation. As it happened in our case study, if the mass was found to be of nerve origin, the parents should absolutely be informed about possible complications (Horner syndrome due to sympathetic nerve chain incision, respiratory and nutrition problems due to vagal nerve incision, etc.) and their consent should be taken.

There is no doubt that imaging techniques are not enough for a definitive diagnosis. Magnetic resonance imaging is recommended. Ganglioneuroblastoma is typically heterogenous in imaging. Generally it shows high signal intensity in T1 images and low signal intensity in T2 images [5, 6]. However, as it happened in our case, it may show hypointense characteristics in T1 and hyperintense characteristics in T2, which may lead to misdiagnosis. First, a fine-needle biopsy should be offered for diagnosis. Following that, a staged treatment plan may be tailored according to histopathological diagnosis and body scan results [6, 7]. In our case, our patient's parents initially refused our suggestion of fine-needle aspiration and stated that they want to continue monitoring the situation. However, after the mass was found to have grown in size during control examination, patient was offered excisional biopsy with a prediagnosis of lymphadenopathy. After finding that the mass is of nerve origin, it was totally extracted and the examination of metastasis or primary tumor was conducted in postoperative period.

It is known that most neurogenic tumors secrete catecholamine. High levels of catecholamine may be an indication of recurrence or the presence of primary tumor. Genetic characteristics are also associated with tumor behavior. N-myc is a protooncogen, where its chromosome arm resides in far end of 2p. Detection of multiple N-myc copies indicates a fast tumor growth and negative prognosis in patients who show these histological characteristics and are over 1 year of age. Also a scintigraphic scan with MIBG should be conducted and invasion should be determined. In our patient, vanilmandelic acid (VMA) and N-myc protooncogene were found to be negative during the postoperative period [6–8].

The need for chemotherapy in postoperative period can be decided after a systematic scan was conducted. In one literature study, a myelogram of a patient, who was under 1 year of age, had showed metastatic cells and the patient had underwent postoperative chemotherapy. Some authors advocate giving chemotherapy even when there is no metastasis, due to ganglioneuroblastoma being a malignant tumor in nature [6–8]. In our patient, while there was no evidence of recurrence until the 6th month after the operation, PET-BT scan at the 6th month showed an involvement in the right side of the neck, and patient was given chemotherapy. After 2 sessions of chemotherapy, no recurrence was found in the 12th-month control examination of the patient.

4. Conclusion

In this case study, our aim was to discuss clinical behavior and diagnosis and treatment of primary cervical ganglioneuroblastoma together with the literature review. Ganglioneuroblastomas in cervical ganglions are rather rare tumors. They are usually asymptomatic, thus making preoperative diagnosis difficult. Clinicians should bear this in mind as this is found in the differential diagnosis of masses in parapharyngeal space.

Consent

Informed consent was obtained from individual participant included in the study.

Competing Interests

Authors have no financial relationships or conflict of interests to disclose.

References

[1] J. G. Manjaly, V. R. C. Alexander, C. M. Pepper, S. N. Ifeacho, R. J. Hewitt, and B. E. J. Hartley, "Primary cervical ganglioneuroblastoma," *International Journal of Pediatric Otorhinolaryngology*, vol. 79, no. 7, pp. 1007–1012, 2015.

[2] İ. Keskinöz, Ş. Erdem, E. Sert, and Ö. T. Selçuk, "Cervical ganglioneuroblastoma mimicking thyroid tissue in a young adult: differential diagnosis," *Turkiye Klinikleri Journal of Medical Sciences*, vol. 31, no. 4, pp. 1041–1045, 2011.

[3] H. Shimada, I. M. Ambros, L. P. Dehner, J.-I. Hata, V. V. Joshi, and B. Roald, "Terminology and morphologic criteria of neuroblastic tumors," *Cancer*, vol. 86, no. 2, pp. 349–363, 1999.

[4] S. L. Cohn, A. D. J. Pearson, W. B. London et al., "The International Neuroblastoma Risk Group (INRG) classification system: an INRG task force report," *Journal of Clinical Oncology*, vol. 27, no. 2, pp. 289–297, 2009.

[5] A. H. H. Al-Jassim, "Cervical ganglioneuroblastoma," *Journal of Laryngology and Otology*, vol. 101, no. 3, pp. 296–301, 1987.

[6] A. K. Moukheiber, R. Nicollas, S. Roman, C. Coze, and J.-M. Triglia, "Primary pediatric neuroblastic tumors of the neck," *International Journal of Pediatric Otorhinolaryngology*, vol. 60, no. 2, pp. 155–161, 2001.

[7] R. J. Brown, N. J. Szymula, and J. M. Lore Jr., "Neuroblastoma of the head and neck," *Archives of Otolaryngology*, vol. 104, no. 7, pp. 395–398, 1978.

[8] C. Kimber, A. Michalski, L. Spitz, and A. Pierro, "Primitive neuroectodermal tumours: anatomic location, extent of surgery, and outcome," *Journal of Pediatric Surgery*, vol. 33, no. 1, pp. 39–41, 1998.

15

Contralateral Cochlear Labyrinthine Concussion without Temporal Bone Fracture: Unusual Posttraumatic Consequence

I. M. Villarreal, D. Méndez, J. M. Duque Silva, and P. Ortega del Álamo

Otorhinolaryngology Department, "Móstoles" University Hospital, Madrid, Spain

Correspondence should be addressed to I. M. Villarreal; imvillarrealp@gmail.com

Academic Editor: Ingo Todt

Introduction. Labyrinthine concussion is a term used to describe a rare cause of sensorineural hearing loss with or without vestibular symptoms occurring after head trauma. Isolated damage to the inner ear without involving the vestibular organ would be designated as a cochlear labyrinthine concussion. Hearing loss is not a rare finding in head trauma that involves petrous bone fractures. Nevertheless it generally occurs ipsilateral to the side of the head injury and extraordinarily in the contralateral side and moreover without the presence of a fracture. *Case Report.* The present case describes a 37-year-old patient with sensorineural hearing loss and tinnitus in his right ear after a blunt head trauma of the left-sided temporal bone (contralateral). Otoscopy and radiological images showed no fractures or any abnormalities. A severe sensorineural hearing loss was found in his right ear with a normal hearing of the left side. *Conclusion.* The temporal bone trauma requires a complete diagnostic battery which includes a neurotologic examination and a high resolution computed tomography scan in the first place. Hearing loss after a head injury extraordinarily occurs in the contralateral side of the trauma as what happened in our case. In addition, the absence of fractures makes this phenomenon even more unusual.

1. Introduction

Labyrinthine concussion is a term used to depict a sensorineural hearing loss (SNHL) with or without vestibular symptoms occurring after head trauma. The temporal bone is at risk for injury in the setting of high-impact craniofacial trauma. Skull fractures due to blunt force trauma occur in 3% to 22% of patients with head trauma. 80% to 90% of cases with temporal bone trauma sustain unilateral injury [1–3]. Hearing loss secondary to head trauma, especially if a temporal bone fracture is associated, is not an unusual clinical consequence. There are several theories postulated to explain the phenomenon of deafness after head injury. Nevertheless, hearing loss in the contralateral side of the injury without evidence of a skull base fracture is a very exceptional finding [4, 5].

2. Clinical Case

We report a case of a 37-year-old male patient who presented to the emergency room with a left side head trauma after being hit with a hammer during an altercation. He complained of contralateral hearing loss and tinnitus denying any right side injury. No vertigo accompanied his deafness. The onset of the symptoms was immediately after the head trauma.

The patient had no personal or family history of previous hearing disorders, including hearing loss or anatomical alterations; hence we believe he had a normal hearing prior to trauma since we have no previous audiological records.

Otoscopic examination revealed normal bilateral intact tympanic membranes. A positive Rinne test in both ears and a Weber test lateralized to the left side in 256, 512, and 1024 Hz. Severe sensorineural hearing loss in the right ear and normal hearing in his left ear were demonstrated with a pure tone audiometry test (Figure 1(a)). Additionally, a tympanogram of his right ear was consistent with a type A pattern and a proper acoustic reflex was present (Figure 2). Regarding imaging studies, a high definition computed tomography (CT) scan showed no radiological evidence of temporal bone fractures, intact ossicular chains, no hemorrhages, and no

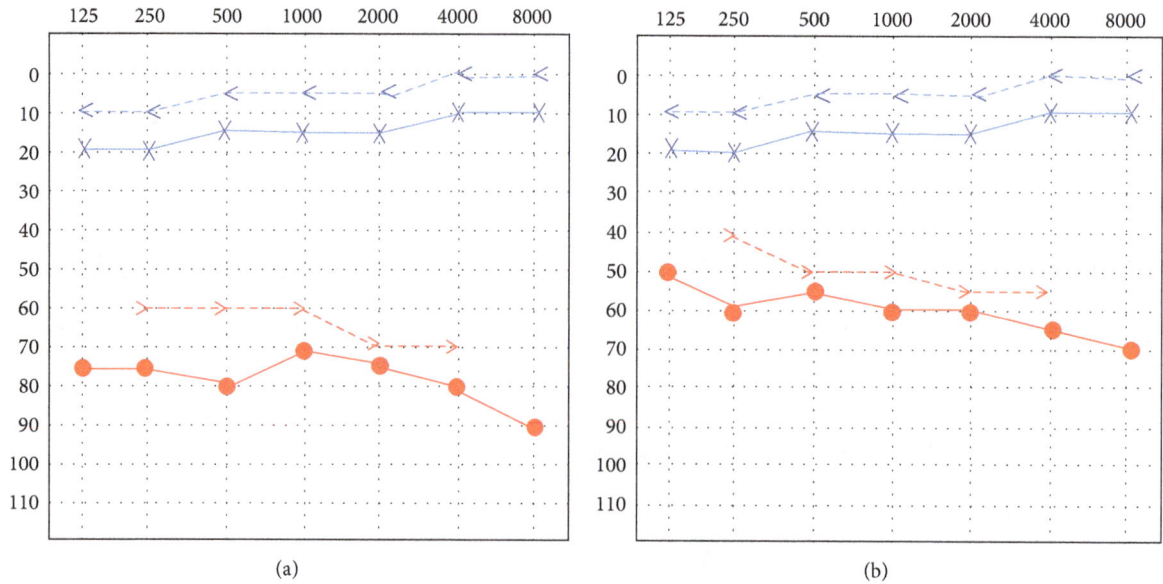

FIGURE 1: Pure tone audiometry: (a) Severe sensorineural hearing loss in the right ear and normal hearing in his left ear. (b) Treatment with oral corticosteroids was administered gaining approximately 15 dB in all frequencies after one week.

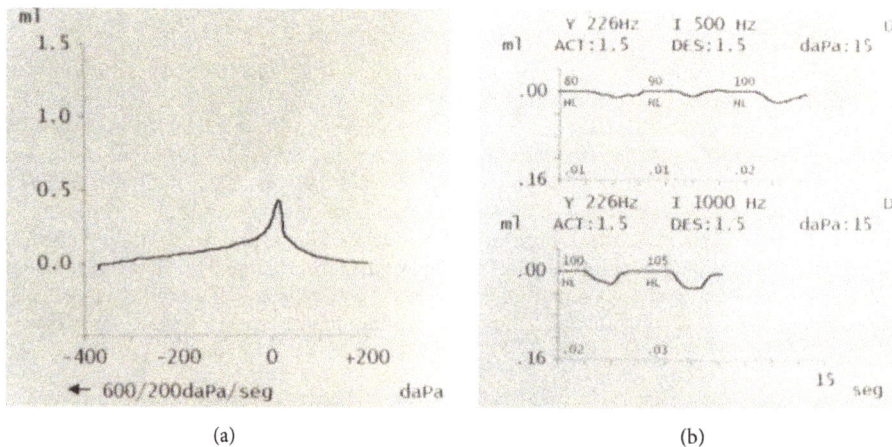

FIGURE 2: (a) Right ear tympanogram was consistent with a type A curve; (b) acoustic reflex was present.

obvious fistulas (Figure 3). No vestibular otoneurological tests were performed due to the lack of vestibular symptoms.

Treatment with oral corticosteroids (Deflazacort at a 1 mg/kg per day dose beginning with 70 mg and slowly tapering the dose) was administered gaining 15 dB in all frequencies within a week when follow-up was assessed. (Figure 1(b)). The patient refused to receive intravenous treatment and only accepted oral medication. The patient made only one follow-up visit in our department and moved out of town afterwards.

3. Discussion

Temporal bone fractures due to blunt head trauma are not an unusual finding. They are classified according to their anatomical orientation and moreover correlated with their clinical presentation. The three possibilities involve a longitudinal, a transversal, or a mixed type of fracture. These fractures may involve some complications or sequelae such as facial paralysis, conductive hearing loss, cerebrospinal fluid leakage (CSF), SNHL, vertigo, and vascular injury [2, 3]. Temporal fractures should be well recognized. A setback in the diagnosis of a temporal bone fracture may lead to a delay in the correct surgical treatment when needed (such as cases of a complete facial paralysis) or a conservative treatment with a strict vigilance in cases of CSF leak.

Longitudinal fractures account for the majority of the cases involving usually a conductive hearing loss and in very few cases facial paralysis or vertigo. Some studies have reported the mixed type of hearing loss as the most common. These fractures are usually associated with temporal or

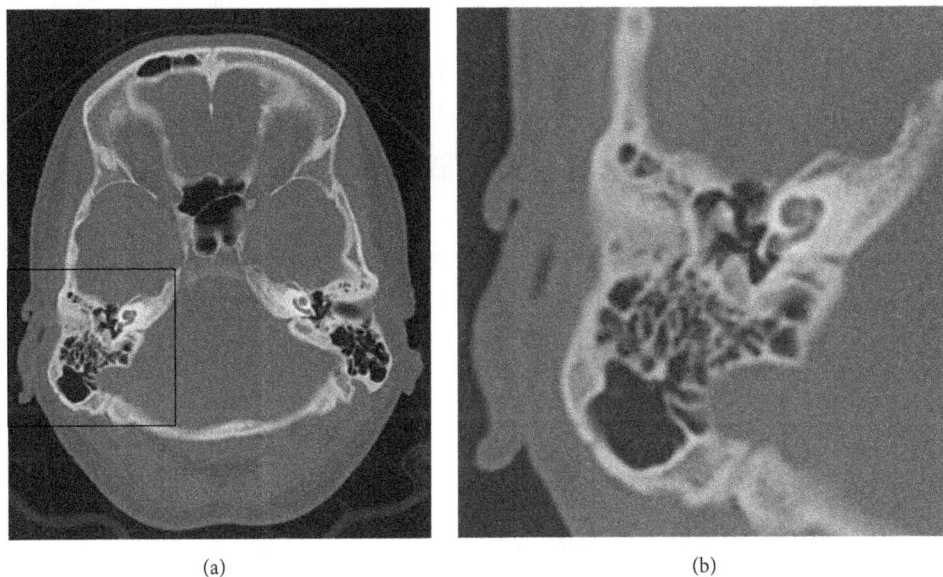

(a)   (b)

FIGURE 3: Computed tomography (CT) scan (axial section): No radiological evidence of temporal bone fracture, intact ossicular chains, no hemorrhages, and no obvious fistulas.

parietal bone trauma. Transversal fractures have a major incidence of facial paralysis and if accompanied by hearing loss it usually involves a sensorineural type due to its labyrinth involvement [1–3]. Nevertheless, since the arrival of high definition CT scan alternative classifications for temporal bone fractures have been proposed. Kelly and Tami suggested that the involvement of the otic capsule should be taken into account [4]. Otic capsule violating injuries have a higher incidence of CSF leak [2]. Some authors have classified them as petrous fractures or those involving the otic capsule or petrous apex and nonpetrous fractures which are subcategorized into middle ear involvement or mastoid involvement [1–3]. This classification according to the authors allows a better correlation regarding the related clinical findings.

Hearing loss is not a rare finding in head trauma that involves petrous bone fractures. It generally occurs ipsilateral to the side of the head injury. Hearing loss extraordinarily occurs in the contralateral side and moreover without the presence of a fracture as what happens in our case [5].

Several theories have been proposed to explain this circumstance such as labyrinthine concussion resulting from a fracture to the bony labyrinthine capsule. However the mechanism involving this phenomenon remains unclear. Labyrinthine concussion is a term used to depict a SNHL with or without vestibular symptoms occurring after head trauma [5–7]. A subclassification can be made regarding labyrinthine concussion. If there is an isolated damage to the inner ear it would be a cochlear labyrinthine concussion and if the damage involves the otolith organ a vestibular labyrinthine concussion would be the preferable designation [8, 9]. Labyrinthine concussion in most cases involves a SNHL with a notch in the 4–6 kHz resembling acoustic trauma, positional vertigo, or tinnitus [7, 8, 10]. Most cases show an accompanying tinnitus regardless of the presence of vertigo as what happened to our patient.

Disruption to the organ of Corti has been suggested involving a pattern seen when high-pressure waves of the intracranial CSF caused by intense airborne sounds transmitted to the cochlea. In the animal experiments from which this theory was built, hemorrhage sites and microcirculation disturbances in the cochlea destroying the sensory epithelium due to rupture of vessels in the membranous labyrinth were also seen [6, 7, 10]. Histopathological changes reported in cochlear labyrinthine concussion (cochlear concussion) vary from mild alterations in the internal or external hair cells to a complete degeneration of the organ of Corti. In cochlear labyrinthine concussion basilar membrane shearing and eventual auditory nerve fiber avulsion might also be described. Another hypothesis involves direct disruption of the membranous labyrinth with inflammatory changes resulting in fibrotic tissue and scarring accumulation and new bone formation. These changes are possible causes of a vestibular labyrinthine concussion [6, 7, 10].

One differential diagnosis may include a perilymph fistula but in this case we would expect the hearing loss to be accompanied not only by tinnitus but also by vestibular symptoms. This did not occur in our case [1, 6, 7]. A benign paroxysmal positional vertigo may also result from head trauma but vertigo must be present as the name indicates and no hearing loss is seen [7]. Another possibility is an isolated eighth nerve stretch injury which may be assessed by tests such as vestibular evoked myogenic potentials (VEMPs) or a severe crush injury or nerve transaction which is extremely rare and might be evaluated with a "promontory examination" test or a brainstem evoked response audiometry (BERA) [9, 10].

We have found only one case described similar to our case except for vestibular symptoms accompanying the SNHL [6]. Three cases of labyrinthine concussion characterized by SNHL in the contralateral side of the head injury without vestibular symptoms have been described [7]. Nevertheless, they were accompanied by fracture of the ipsilateral side making these cases different from ours. On the other hand, Chiaramonte et al. [9] presented a case of a patient with bilateral SNHL without temporal bone fractures but with the presence of severe vertigo making it different from our case based on these two details. Two other cases of head trauma without cranial base fractures with SNHL were reported but no details regarding other symptoms such as vertigo are described in these 2 specific cases nor if the SNHL was contralateral [11].

4. Conclusion

Temporal bone trauma requires a complete diagnostic battery which includes a neurotologic examination, a high resolution CT scan (in cases with clinical suspicion of temporal fracture), an electroneuronography if facial paralysis is present, audiometric tests, and vestibular tests if required [7].

There is no definitive treatment for labyrinthine concussion. Corticosteroids are controversial and most of them are managed expectantly. We administered steroids as described before to our patient and there was 15 dB improvement in all frequencies. Nevertheless, we have no evidence that the hearing improvement was a response to corticotherapy or it just occurred incidentally. Further studies have to be performed to prove the effectiveness of this treatment [12]. The prognosis of hearing recovery is disappointing in most cases.

Hearing loss after a head injury extraordinarily occurs in the contralateral side of the trauma as what happened in our case and moreover in the absence of fractures which makes this phenomenon even more unusual.

Competing Interests

The authors declare that there are no competing interests.

References

[1] T. A. Kennedy, G. D. Avey, and L. R. Gentry, "Imaging of temporal bone trauma," *Neuroimaging Clinics of North America*, vol. 24, no. 3, pp. 467–486, 2014.

[2] S. L. Ishman and D. R. Friedland, "Temporal bone fractures: traditional classification and clinical relevance," *Laryngoscope*, vol. 114, no. 10, pp. 1734–1741, 2004.

[3] A. F. Juliano, D. T. Ginat, and G. Moonis, "Imaging review of the temporal bone: part II. Traumatic, postoperative, and noninflammatory nonneoplastic conditions," *Radiology*, vol. 276, no. 3, pp. 655–672, 2015.

[4] K. Kelly and T. Tami, "Temporal bone and skull base trauma," in *Neurotology*, R. Jackler and D. Brackmann, Eds., p. 1127, Mosby, St. Louis, Mo, USA, 1994.

[5] M. K. M. Daud, M. Irfan, and S. Rosdan, "Traumatic head injury with contralateral sensorineural hearing loss," *Annals of the Academy of Medicine Singapore*, vol. 38, no. 11, pp. 1017–1018, 2009.

[6] A. Toh, E. C. Ho, and N. Turner, "Contralateral deafness post head injury without temporal bone fractures," *American Journal of Otolaryngology—Head and Neck Medicine and Surgery*, vol. 31, no. 1, pp. 54–56, 2010.

[7] T. Ulug and S. A. Ulubil, "Contralateral labyrinthine concussion in temporal bone fractures," *Journal of Otolaryngology*, vol. 35, no. 6, pp. 380–383, 2006.

[8] T. Brusis, "Sensorineural hearing loss after dull head injury or concussion trauma," *Laryngo-Rhino-Otologie*, vol. 90, no. 2, pp. 73–80, 2011.

[9] R. Chiaramonte, M. Bonfiglio, A. D'Amore, A. Viglianesi, T. Cavallaro, and I. Chiaramonte, "Traumatic labyrinthine concussion in a patient with sensorineural hearing loss," *Neuroradiology Journal*, vol. 26, no. 1, pp. 52–55, 2013.

[10] D. C. Fitzgerald, "Head trauma: hearing loss and dizziness," *Journal of Trauma—Injury, Infection and Critical Care*, vol. 40, no. 3, pp. 488–496, 1996.

[11] G. Singh, B. Singh, and D. Singh, "Prospective study of 'otological injury secondary to head trauma,'" *Indian Journal of Otolaryngology and Head and Neck Surgery*, vol. 65, no. 3, pp. S498–S504, 2013.

[12] R. Lawrence and R. Thevasagayam, "Controversies in the management of sudden sensorineural hearing loss: an evidence-based review," *Clinical Otolaryngology*, vol. 40, no. 3, pp. 176–182, 2015.

16

Primary Lymphangioma of the Palatine Tonsil in a 9-Year-Old Boy: A Case Presentation and Literature Review

Eleftheria Iliadou,[1] **Nektarios Papapetropoulos,**[1] **Eleftherios Karamatzanis,**[1]
Panagiotis Saravakos,[2] **and Konstantinos Saravakos**[1]

[1]*Department of Otorhinolaryngology, Head and Neck Surgery, Penteli Children Hospital, Athens, Greece*
[2]*Department of Otorhinolaryngology, Head and Neck Surgery, Siloah St. Trudpert Hospital, Pforzheim, Germany*

Correspondence should be addressed to Panagiotis Saravakos; psaravakos@yahoo.com

Academic Editor: Abrão Rapoport

Primary lymphangiomas or lymphangiomatous polyps of the palatine tonsil are rare benign lesions that are described infrequently in the literature. The majority of the published cases concern adults. We report a case of a lymphangiomatous lesion of the right palatine tonsil of a 9-year-old boy. Our clinical suspicion was confirmed by the histological examination after tonsillectomy and the diagnosis of primary lymphangioma of the tonsil was made. In this case we discuss the clinical and histopathological features of this lesion and present a short review of the current literature.

1. Introduction

Lymphangiomas or lymphagiomatous polyps of the palatine tonsil are rare benign tumors. They present as unilateral or bilateral tonsillar outgrowths and cause a large spectrum of symptoms related to local irritation and airway obstruction [1]. Their pathogenesis has not been clarified and multiple theories have been proposed. Here we report the case of a lymphangioma of the palatine tonsil in a 9-year-old boy and briefly review the existing literature.

2. Case Presentation

A 9-year-old boy presented to our hospital complaining of a foreign body feeling in the throat of a few months' duration, causing him a nonproductive cough, mild dysphagia, and sleep disturbance. His medical and surgical history were unremarkable. The examination of the oral cavity revealed a large, oval, pale mass protruding from the lower pole of the right tonsil, which was partially obstructing the airway (Figure 1). It was nontender, nonfriable and did not bleed on touch. It was attached to the lower pole of the right tonsil by a narrow elongated stalk. The patient underwent a bilateral tonsillectomy under general anesthesia. The right tonsil and the pedunculated mass were removed by dissection, and hemostasis was performed by ligation. The recovery was uneventful and the patient was discharged the following day. A postoperative follow-up after one month revealed no evidence of any residual or recurrent polypoid disease.ﻉﻉ£

The histopathological examination showed macroscopically a tonsil of 3.2 × 2 × 0.8 cm in size with an exophytic polypoid nodule measuring 1.8 × 1.2 × 1.2 cm (Figure 2). Under the microscope, the examination of the mass showed strong cellular proliferation without suspicion of malignancy, consistent with lymphangioma of the tonsil. Abnormal lymphatics did not involve the deep tissues of the tonsil and the tumor was removed in its entirety. The adjacent tonsil showed no significant abnormalities (Figures 3(a) and 3(b)).

3. Discussion

More than 90% of all lymphagiomatous lesions occur in the head and neck area, including the cheek, tongue, and floor of mouth [1]. However, lymphagiomatous lesions of the palatine tonsil are rarely reported in the literature [2–18]. The references are even less frequent in the pediatric population

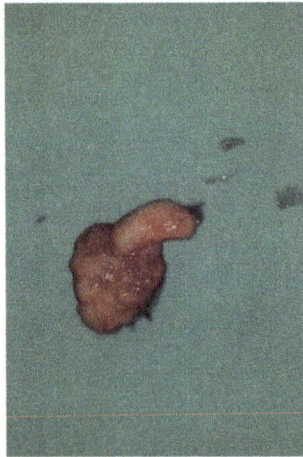

FIGURE 1: Large oval, pale, pedunculated mass protruding from the lower pole of the right tonsil, compatible to a lymphangioma of the tonsil.

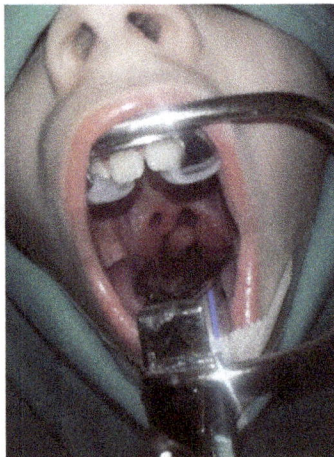

FIGURE 2: Exophytic polypoid nodule attached to the right tonsil by a stalk (pedunculated polypoid lesion) measuring 1.8 × 1.2 × 1.2 cm.

[1–3, 5, 9]. Many authors believe that the true incidence may be higher than reported [1, 2, 9].

Histologically, lymphangiomas are formed by abundant dilated lymphatic and blood channels mixed with a fibrous stroma of lymphoid and adipose elements [14]. There are several theories regarding the pathogenesis of this type of tonsillar disorder. The first one suggests that lymphangiomas arise due to sequestration of lymphatic tissue derived from primitive sacs, which retain their rapid and proliferative growth potential but fail to join the major lymph sac of the body. The second theory proposes that it arises from endothelial fibrillar membranes, which sprout from the walls of the cyst, penetrate the surrounding tissue, canalize, and then produce more cysts along lines of least resistance. These cysts maintain their ability to branch out and grow, and they do so in an uncontrolled, disorderly manner with a tendency to penetrate and destroy normal anatomic structures. This uncontrolled proliferation is thought to be caused by a dysregulation of growth factors involved in lymphangiogenesis

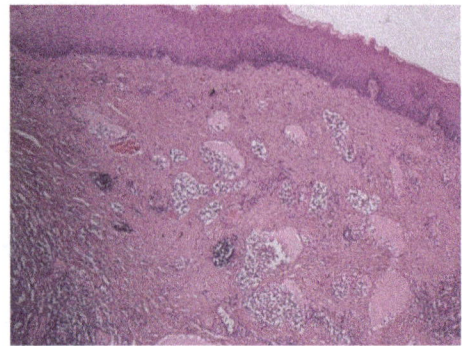

(a)

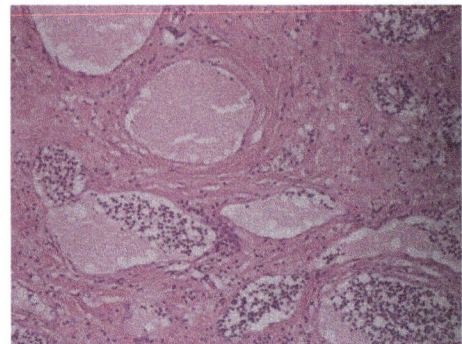

(b)

FIGURE 3: Overlying epithelium without signs of dysplasia. Presence of numerous lymphocytes, with round nuclei and condensed nuclear chromatin, and pedunculated proliferation of vascular channels within abundant fibrous stroma.

known as Prox-1 and vascular endothelial factor (VEGF-C) [1]. The third theory advances the hypothesis that the primitive lymphatic sac does not reach the venous system [1]. Finally, there is another pathogenetic theory, which suggests that chronic inflammation of the tonsil and the associated obstruction of the lymphatic channels cause mucosal congestion and subsequently polypoidal swelling [5]. However, this last theory is considerably unlikely because chronic tonsillitis is much more common than the lymphangiomatous tonsillar polyps, and because there are many patients, like our case, who do not have a history of recurrent tonsillitis [12, 16].

The clinical behavior of the tumor is largely unknown, because most of these lesions are diagnosed histologically after surgical excision of the tonsils. Common presenting symptoms include dysphagia, dyspnea, foreign body sensations, sore throat, and chronic tonsillitis. When the mass is very large, it can affect surrounding vital structures to produce rhinolalia clausa, respiratory difficulty, stridor, excessive saliva, or nausea [1]. In all reported cases, the disorder behaved in a benign fashion and no complications or recurrences have been reported. In our case, the main symptoms were foreign body sensation, interrupted sleep, and mild dysphagia, which were resolved after surgery.

The history and the clinical examination are important for the diagnosis, but a histological examination is required to establish the diagnosis. The differential diagnosis includes lymphangiectasia, hemangioma, arteriovenous malformation, fibroepithelial polyps, and papilloma. In our young patient's case, the preoperative suspicion was strong because of the typical appearance and the large size of the lesion. However, as a lymphangioma clinically may resemble a true neoplasm of the palatine tonsil, the lesion needed to be removed in order to complete an accurate histological diagnosis and to rule out malignancy.

Tonsillectomy is the curative procedure of choice for the management of these tonsillar polypoid lesions. An excision of the polypoid mass may be the only necessary procedure, while sclerosing therapy with OK-432 or radiotherapy is not suggested. Furthermore, a carbon dioxide laser has been frequently used to treat a group of pediatric patients with benign lesions of the upper aerodigestive tract exclusive of the larynx, but there have been no benefits compared to the cold steel tonsillectomy [1]. As our patient presented a bilateral tonsillar hypertrophy, we decided to proceed with a traditional bilateral tonsillectomy, with good results.

4. Conclusion

In summary, this case demonstrates a case of tonsillar lymphangiomatous polyp occurring in a 9-year-old boy. It is believed that the incidence of the tonsillar lymphangiomatous polyps is greater than what is reported in the literature, especially in the pediatric population. The aim of this case report is to consider this type of benign tumor in the differential diagnosis of tonsillar masses in childhood.

Ethical Approval

All procedures performed in studies involving human participants were in accordance with the ethical standards of the institutional and/or national research committee and with the 1964 Helsinki declaration and its later amendments or comparable ethical standards.

Competing Interests

The authors have no conflict of interests to disclose.

References

[1] H. H. Chen, M. A. Lovell, and K. H. Chan, "Bilateral lymphangiomatous polyps of the palatine tonsils," *International Journal of Pediatric Otorhinolaryngology*, vol. 74, no. 1, pp. 87–88, 2010.

[2] S. M. Al Samarrae, S. S. Amr, and V. J. Hyams, "Polypoid lymphangioma of the tonsil: report of two cases and review of the literature," *The Journal of Laryngology & Otology*, vol. 99, no. 8, pp. 819–823, 1985.

[3] F. Araujo, "Lymphangioma of the palatine tonsil (author's transl)," *Annales d'Oto-Laryngologie et de Chirurgie Cervico Faciale*, vol. 94, no. 3, pp. 111–116, 1977.

[4] D. G. Balatsouras, A. Fassolis, G. Koukoutsis, P. Ganelis, and A. Kaberos, "Primary lymphangioma of the tonsil: a case report," *Case Reports in Medicine*, vol. 2011, Article ID 183182, 3 pages, 2011.

[5] B. P. Cengiz, M. Acar, and E. Giritli, "A pedunculated lymphangiomatous polyp of the palatine tonsil. A case report," *Brazilian Journal of Otorhinolaryngology*, vol. 79, no. 3, article 402, 2013.

[6] D. M. Crockett, G. B. Healy, T. J. I. McGill, and E. M. Friedman, "Benign lesions of the nose, oral cavity, and oropharynx in children: excision by carbon dioxide laser," *Annals of Otology, Rhinology and Laryngology*, vol. 94, no. 5, part 1, pp. 489–493, 1985.

[7] G. I. Harrison and L. A. Johnson, "LXIX lymphangioma of the tonsil report of a case with a critical review of the literature," *Annals of Otology, Rhinology & Laryngology*, vol. 69, no. 4, pp. 961–968, 1960.

[8] D. E. Kardon, B. M. Wenig, D. K. Heffner, and L. D. R. Thompson, "Tonsillar lymphangiomatous polyps: a clinicopathologic series of 26 cases," *Modern Pathology*, vol. 13, no. 10, pp. 1128–1133, 2000.

[9] J. Kasznica and A. Kasznica, "Tonsillar polypoid lymphangioma in a small child," *New Jersey Medicine*, vol. 88, no. 10, pp. 729–731, 1991.

[10] T. L. Kennedy, "Cystic hygroma-lymphangioma: a rare and still unclear entity," *The Laryngoscope*, vol. 99, supplement 1, pp. 1–10, 1989.

[11] Y. Khatib, V. Gite, R. Patel, M. Shoeb, and A. Oraon, "Lymphangiomatous polyp of palatine tonsil in a child presenting with dysphagia and dysarthria," *Journal of Clinical and Diagnostic Research*, vol. 9, no. 5, pp. ED01–ED02, 2015.

[12] S. Mardekian and J. K. Karp, "Lymphangioma of the palatine tonsil," *Archives of Pathology and Laboratory Medicine*, vol. 137, no. 12, pp. 1837–1842, 2013.

[13] E. A. Pallestrini and M. Ameli, "Polypoid lymphangioma of the palatine tonsil," *Archivio Italiano di Otologia, Rinologia e Laringologia*, vol. 77, no. 3, pp. 343–348, 1966.

[14] E. Park, S. M. Pransky, D. M. Malicki, and P. Hong, "Unilateral lymphangiomatous polyp of the palatine tonsil in a very young child: a clinicopathologic case report," *Case Reports in Pediatrics*, vol. 2011, Article ID 451542, 3 pages, 2011.

[15] O. Raha, V. Singh, and P. Purkayastha, "Lymphangioma tonsil—rare case study," *Indian Journal of Otolaryngology and Head and Neck Surgery*, vol. 57, no. 4, pp. 332–334, 2005.

[16] M. Roth, "Lymphangiomatous polyp of the palatine tonsil," *Otolaryngology—Head and Neck Surgery*, vol. 115, no. 1, pp. 172–173, 1996.

[17] T. N. Ninh and T. X. Ninh, "Cystic hygroma in children: a report of 126 cases," *Journal of Pediatric Surgery*, vol. 9, no. 2, pp. 191–195, 1974.

[18] P. G. Visvanathan, "A pedunculated tonsillar lymphangioma," *Journal of Laryngology and Otology*, vol. 85, no. 1, pp. 93–96, 1971.

17

Lipoma of Piriform Sinus: A Case Report and Review of the Literature

Gilberto Acquaviva,[1] **Theodoros Varakliotis,**[1,2] **Stefano Badia,**[1] **Francesco Casorati,**[1] **Alberto Eibenstein,**[2] **and Gianluca Bellocchi**[1]

[1]*Department of Otolaryngology and Head & Neck Surgery, "San Camillo-Forlanini" Hospital, Rome, Italy*
[2]*Department of Applied Clinical Sciences and Biotechnology (DISCAB), L'Aquila University, L'Aquila, Italy*

Correspondence should be addressed to Theodoros Varakliotis; theo_va@hotmail.com

Academic Editor: Marco Berlucchi

The lipomas of oropharynx, hypopharynx, and larynx are so rare that up to now approximately there have been 100 cases reported. The lipomas are slow-growing lesions that are capable of reaching considerable dimensions and are often detected at a late stage. The symptoms can vary both in dimension and in location, semiobstructing the aerodigestive tract or exerting compression on adjacent structure. In this case, the lesion, which originated from the piriform sinus, was removed endoscopically urgently due to obvious signs of tissue suffering caused by stretching of the pedicle as a result of displacement of the mass. The two aims of this case report are to expose an interesting and rare case study mainly for an Emergency Room Specialist and an ENT (Ear, Nose, and Throat) Specialist involved in solving the problem and to demonstrate that the choice of an endoscopic approach is useful in order to have an optimal visualization of the lesion and to perform a total eradication. The use of endoscopic devices also allows a rapid postoperative recovery, compared to external access and optimum locoregional control in the follow-up procedures to prevent possible relapses.

1. Introduction

Lipomas are tumors that represent 4-5% of all benign tumors and they are predominantly found in the hypodermic layer [1].

These tumors are rare in the head and neck region and specifically for the upper aerodigestive tract represent 0.6% of all neoplasias [2, 3].

We present a rare case of a 63-year-old woman who arrived at the emergency room of our hospital with a pedunculated mass protruding from the buccal rhyme, emitted by coughing.

2. Case Report

In August of 2011 a 63-year-old woman suffering from multiple sclerosis and diabetes mellitus type I, in treatment with insulin since the age of 18, arrived at the emergency room with severe dyspneic syndrome. She presented a voluminous mass, partially protruding from the mouth and completely occupying the oral cavity, looking diverticular with a solid consistency and brownish-yellow color, cylindrical, and smooth, with a diameter of about 25 mm. The protruding portion from the mouth measured in length about 65 mm (Figure 1).

The relatives, who accompanied the patient, reported a sudden onset of dyspnea and the appearance from the mouth of the abovementioned lesion protruding after regurgitation and coughing. After the first examination it was clear that the tumor extended in the hypopharynx with slightly smaller dimensions. The patient was immediately submitted to an endotracheal intubation, and an urgent CT scan of the neck was carried out to identify the relationship and the cause of the neoformation.

The CT scan showed the presence of solid polypoid-like tissue that occupied the space from the hypopharynx to the oral cavity with a large extraoral hypodense component having thin branches of vascularity to the left of the center

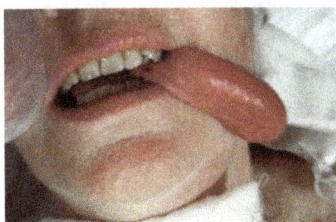

FIGURE 1

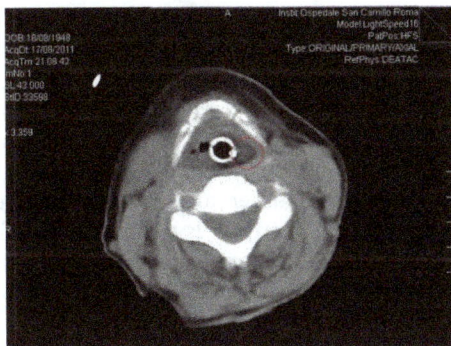

FIGURE 2

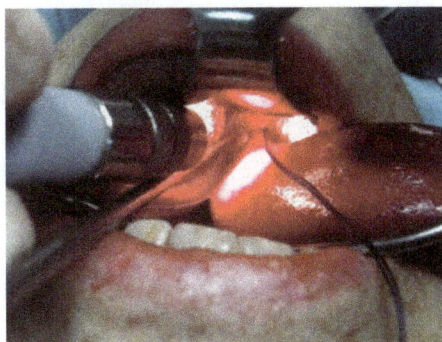

FIGURE 3

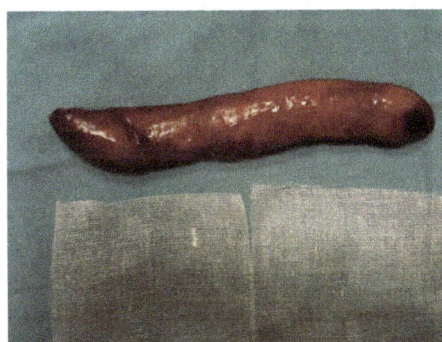

FIGURE 4

section; the first hypothesis could be defined as a fibrovascular polyp with the implantation on the left side of the hypopharynx (Figure 2).

The microlaryngoscopy exploration, performed immediately due to obvious signs of the insufficient blood supply of the neoformation with the risk of ulceration and consequent bleeding, showed instead that the base of implant, also cylindrical, but with a diameter of about 10 mm, was located in area of the medial wall of the piriform sinus on the right (Figure 3).

During the procedure, we used a Polysorb n.1 lace as a landmark and as point of traction at the base of implantation of the neoformation which was subsequently sutured with 2 stitches of Monocryl 2-0 and 2 stitches of Polysorb 2-0. With the aid of mechanical stapler Endo Gia Universal 12 mm used to dissect the neoformation at the base, it was consequently removed and the material was sent for a definitive histological examination (Figure 4); then a nasogastric tube was inserted ensuring its position towards the left piriform sinus.

The final histological examination described an oval shape lesion with a size of 15 × 2,5 × 2 cm, smooth in texture, soft in consistency, and yellowish in color. Fifteen blocks in paraffin, one centimeter in diameter, were obtained and were available for microscopic examination. Microscopic examination demonstrated a subepithelial neoplasm not encapsulated, composed of mature adipocytes with no cellular atypia. The diagnosis of lipoma was thus proposed (Figure 5).

The postoperative recovery period was quick and without complications, with resumption of oral feeding after 72 hours. Upon the patient's discharge from the hospital the examination with fibrolaryngoscope showed the absence of

residual disease and the advanced state of reepithelialization of the implant site.

3. Discussion

Lipomas are benign tumors of mesenchymal originating from mature fat cells (adipocytes) in adipose component tissue. The adipose tissue in the larynx is represented in epiglottis, in the ventricular and aryepiglottic fold.

In this case the origin of the adipose tissue was located in the lateral submucosa to the arytenoid cartilage.

Lipomas generally are slow-growing sessile or pedunculated lesions having a rough surface, yellowish color, and soft consistency.

Histologically these lesions can be classified into several subtype groups based on their stroma: angiomyolipoma, spindle cell lipomas, myolipoma, chondrolipoma, and myxolipoma [4].

However among the possible malignant histotypes we find liposarcoma having well-differentiated cells [5].

The microscopic histological characteristics that allow differentiating benign from malignant neoformation are the following: presence of pleomorphism, atypical cells, and infiltration of surrounding tissues and lipoblasts.

The suspicion of malignancy growth can be defined in the case of the presence of one or more relapses after surgical removal [6]; however the malignant transformation is rare in cases of single lipoma, considering that an association to

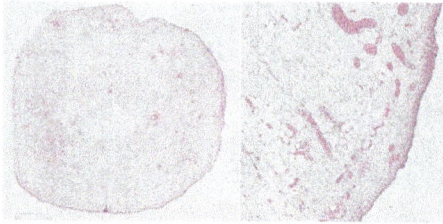

FIGURE 5

multiple pharyngolaryngeal lipomas or relapsing lipomas has been described.

The etiology of lipomas is unknown; however some authors have suggested that they derive from lipoblasts or by a metaplasia of muscle cells, while others have suggested a possible etiopathological role of familiar and endocrine factors or conditions such as trauma, infection, or chronic diseases. Nowadays some risk factors such as abuse of alcohol, tobacco, and environmental and work conditions, which involve toxic chemicals, have not been recognized as a possible cause [1, 6].

Clinically the lipomas remain asymptomatic for a long time, but once they reach large dimensions, symptoms may arise in relation to the size and lead to the compression of adjacent structures [7].

Lipomas of the upper aerodigestive tract occur with continuous or intermittent symptoms over the course of a few months or years, which include dysphagia, hoarseness, feeling of discomfort in the throat like the feeling of a mass in the pharynx, and, in case of airway obstruction, stridor and dyspnea [8]. In severe but rare cases it is necessary to perform an emergency tracheostomy to prevent asphyxia and possible episodes of respiratory arrest [9].

The diagnosis of these lesions starts with a local physical examination (lipomas may appear as sessile or pedunculated lesions or as a retention cyst with a rough surface, encapsulated and covered by a yellowish-pink mucosa) [6]; and consequently, using endoscopic techniques (fibrolaryngoscopy and esophagoscopy), a lipoma may appear as a submucosal mass or a polyp sometimes pedunculated.

Imaging techniques such as CT and MRI are helpful for the diagnosis and allow an acceptable preoperative evaluation of the lesion. On CT images lipoma appears as a homogeneous lesion with low attenuation values of ionizing radiation with a density lower than water [10, 11]. The accuracy rate of CT ranges from 75% to 90%.

MRI is preferable to CT because it allows a better study of the soft tissues, the patient is not exposed to ionizing radiation, and it does not require iodinated radiocontrast agents. Furthermore MRI also allows a more accurate and specific diagnosis of the lesion with a better indication of position of the peduncle or of the extension of the lesion and its relationship with the surrounding structures [12].

In this case CT scan, performed in urgency, helped to identify the caudal limit of the lesion and therefore identifying its place of origin, but not showing its position. The choice of using an endoscopic access [13], despite the difficulties

arising due to small dimensions of the surgical field, caused by the tumor mass, rather than a lateral pharyngotomy [14], has been proved correct for best framing and also effective for the purposes of treatment [15].

4. Conclusions

The lipomas are benign tumors, but because of their rare location found in the upper aerodigestive tract, they must be taken seriously by the Emergency Room Specialist, the ENT Specialists, and Maxillofacial Surgeons. In fact often these lesions are very voluminous and their rapid displacement from the area, in which they have been growing for a long time, may endanger the life of the patient due to obstruction of upper airways. After the stabilization of the patient, ensuring good and safe ventilation, it is necessary to proceed with a quick imaging study and then to perform an endoscopy exam in order to plan a correct treatment. When the endoscopic approach is technically possible, with ablation of the neoformation at the base of the root, it is possible to apply an effective treatment and to obtain a rapid postoperative recovery period.

Competing Interests

The authors declare that there is no conflict of interests regarding the publication of this paper.

References

[1] R. B. Lucas, "Tumors of adipose tissue," in *Pathology of Tumors of Oral Tissue*, R. B. Lucas, Ed., pp. 176–179, Churchill-Livingstone, London, UK, 4th edition, 1984.

[2] F. M. Enzinger and S. W. Weiss, "Benign lipomatous tumours," in *Soft Tissue Tumours*, F. M. Enzinger and S. W. Weiss, Eds., pp. 381–430, Mosby, St. Louis, Mo, USA, 3rd edition, 1995.

[3] P. M. Som, M. P. Scherl, V. M. Rao, and H. F. Biller, "Rare presentations of ordinary lipomas of the head and neck: a review," *American Journal of Neuroradiology*, vol. 7, no. 4, pp. 657–664, 1986.

[4] H. E. Eckel and M. Jungehulsing, "Lipoma of the hypopharynx: preoperative diagnosis and transoral resection," *Journal of Laryngology and Otology*, vol. 108, no. 2, pp. 174–177, 1994.

[5] B. M. Wenig, "Lipomas of the larynx and hypopharynx: a review of the literature with the addition of three new cases," *The Journal of Laryngology & Otology*, vol. 109, no. 4, pp. 353–357, 1995.

[6] J. E. Mitchell, S. J. Thorne, and J. D. Hern, "Acute stridor caused by a previously asymptomatic large oropharyngeal spindle cell lipoma," *Auris Nasus Larynx*, vol. 34, no. 4, pp. 549–552, 2007.

[7] M. L. Som and L. Wolff, "Lipoma of the hypopharynx producing menacing symptoms," *Archives of Otolaryngology*, vol. 56, no. 5, pp. 524–531, 1952.

[8] R. A. P. Persaud, R. Kotnis, C. C. Ong, and D. A. Bowdler, "A rare case of a pedunculated lipoma in the pharynx," *Emergency Medicine Journal*, vol. 19, no. 3, pp. 275–276, 2002.

[9] J. R. Di Bartolomeo and A. R. Olsen, "Pedunculated lipoma of the epiglottis. Second known case reported," *Archives of Otolaryngology*, vol. 98, no. 1, pp. 55–57, 1973.

[10] M. H. A. El-Monem, A. H. Gaafar, and E. A. Magdy, "Lipomas of the head and neck: presentation variability and diagnostic work-up," *The Journal of Laryngology & Otology*, vol. 120, no. 1, pp. 47–55, 2006.

[11] T. D'Auria, S. Santoro, A. Gambardella, A. D'Amico, and F. Di Salle, "Lipoma of the hypopharynx: role of computerized tomography in the diagnosis protocol," *Acta Otorhinolaryngologica Italica*, vol. 10, no. 1, pp. 87–92, 1990.

[12] R. D. Tien, J. R. Hesselink, P. K. Chu, and J. Szumowski, "Improved detection and delineation of head and neck lesions with fat suppression spin-echo MR imaging," *American Journal of Neuroradiology*, vol. 12, no. 1, pp. 19–24, 1991.

[13] P. Zbaren, H. Lang, and M. Becker, "Rare benign neoplasms of the larynx: rhabdomyoma and lipoma," *Journal for Oto-Rhino-Laryngology*, vol. 57, no. 6, pp. 351–355, 1995.

[14] K. Sakamoto, K. Mori, H. Umeno, and T. Nakashima, "Surgical approach to a giant fibrolipoma of the supraglottic larynx," *The Journal of Laryngology & Otology*, vol. 114, no. 1, pp. 58–60, 2000.

[15] N. Jesberg, "Fibrolipoma of the pyriform sinuses: thirty-seven year follow-up," *Laryngoscope*, vol. 92, no. 10, pp. 1157–1159, 1982.

18

Synovial Sarcoma of the Larynx: Report of a Case and Review of Literature

Geetha Narayanan,[1] **Anto Baby,**[2] **Thara Somanathan,**[3] **and Sreedevi Konoth**[4]

[1]*Department of Medical Oncology, Regional Cancer Centre, Trivandrum 695011, India*
[2]*St. Gregorios Medical Mission Hospital, Parumala, Pathanamthitta 689626, India*
[3]*Department of Pathology, Regional Cancer Centre, Trivandrum 695011, India*
[4]*Department of Radiology, Lourdes Hospital, Kochi 682012, India*

Correspondence should be addressed to Geetha Narayanan; geenarayanan@yahoo.com

Academic Editor: Marco Berlucchi

Sarcomas account for less than 1% of malignant neoplasms arising in the head and neck in adults. Laryngeal synovial sarcoma is an extremely rare form of laryngeal malignancy with less than 20 cases reported in the literature. We report the case of a 48-year-old man with synovial sarcoma of the larynx. He underwent excision of the tumor followed by radiation. He is alive in remission at 36 months. The literature on synovial sarcoma of the larynx is reviewed.

1. Introduction

Sarcomas account for less than 1% of malignant neoplasms arising in the head and neck in adults and less than 5% of soft tissue sarcomas in adults occur in the head and neck region [1–3]. Larynx is a rare primary site in which sarcomas comprise less than 1% of all laryngeal tumors [1]. Synovial sarcoma likewise represents a rare sarcoma histology of which only 3% arise in the head and neck [4]. We report the case of a young man with synovial sarcoma of the larynx.

2. Case Report

A 48-year-old man presented with a history of hoarseness of voice since 5 months, dyspnea since 3 months, and dysphagia since 2 months. He consulted an ENT surgeon where a fibre optic laryngoscopy showed a pedunculated mass occupying the laryngeal inlet and extending up to base of tongue (Figure 1). A computed tomogram (CT) showed a well-defined heterogeneously enhancing lesion, $2.7 \times 2.0 \times 2.6$ cm in the laryngeal inlet in the supraglottic compartment, almost filling it (Figures 2(a), 2(b), and 3). Small cervical lymph nodes were present bilaterally. Patient underwent excision of the mass and tracheostomy. Intraoperatively, a globular pedunculated mass attached to posterior pharyngeal wall and arytenoids was seen. Histopathology examination of the biopsy specimen showed spindle cell sarcoma with hemangiopericytic pattern of intermediate grade, which on immunohistochemistry (IHC) was focally positive for cytokeratin and Bcl 2 (Figures 4, 5(a), and 5(b)). A diagnosis of synovial sarcoma was made. His haemogram, serum chemistries, and CT scan of chest were normal. He was given postoperative external beam irradiation 60 Gy/30#. No chemotherapy was given since it was an intermediate grade tumor. The patient is alive in remission at 36 months.

3. Discussion

Laryngeal synovial sarcoma is an extremely rare form of laryngeal malignancy with less than 20 cases reported in the literature (Table 1 [5–23]). Synovial sarcoma is an aggressive malignant soft tissue tumor that is thought to arise from pluripotent mesenchymal cells and usually involve the lower extremities [24]. Sarcomas occur uncommonly in the head and neck region in adults and synovial sarcoma is extremely rare in this site. Squamous cell carcinoma accounts for over

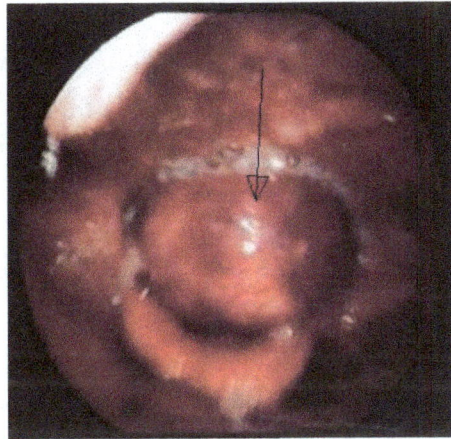

FIGURE 1: Laryngoscopy showing a pedunculated mass coming from laryngeal inlet.

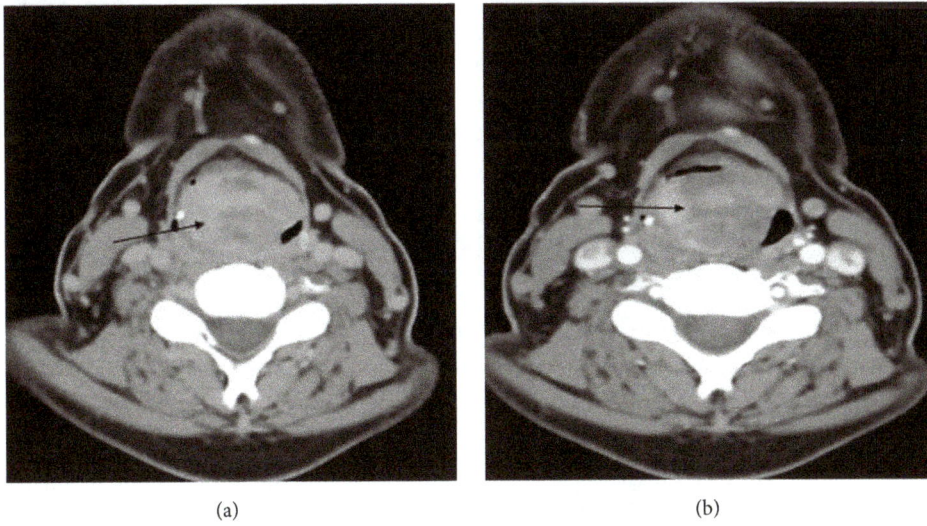

(a)   (b)

FIGURE 2: (a) Plain CT scan of the neck showing soft tissue mass at the region of epiglottis with tiny specks of calcifications in the periphery. (b) Postcontrast image showing heterogenous enhancement.

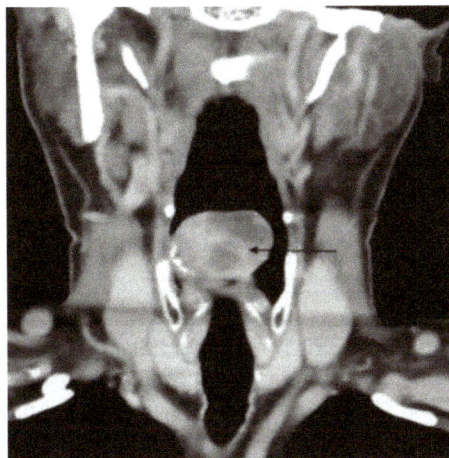

FIGURE 3: Coronal postcontrast image showing the mass lesion with nonenhancing areas.

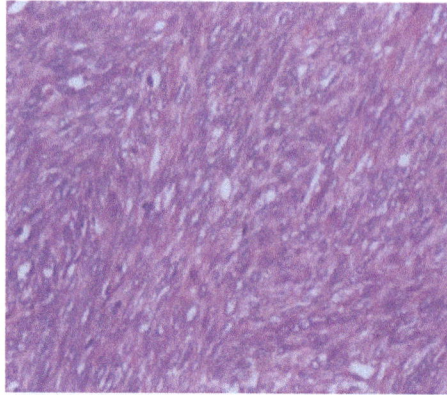

FIGURE 4: H&E ×40 showing spindle cell sarcoma with hemangiopericytic pattern.

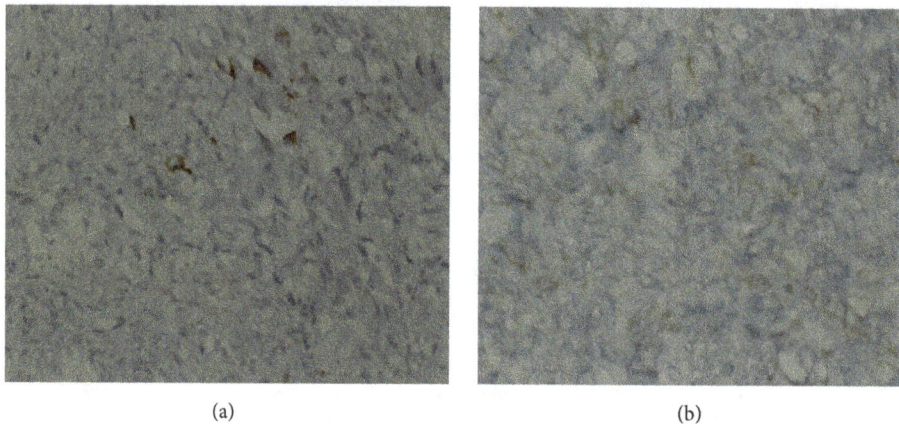

(a)

(b)

FIGURE 5: (a) Section showing focal positivity for cytokeratin. (b) Section showing focal positivity for Bcl 2.

90% of all laryngeal cancers [24]. The median age of patients at diagnosis of the disease is the third decade of life and there is male predominance [25].

Sarcoma of the head and neck commonly presents as painless submucosal or subcutaneous mass and symptoms vary according to the location. Similar to primary squamous cell carcinomas of the larynx, sarcomas in this location produce symptoms secondary to mechanical interference with function dependent on the size. Hoarseness is usually the first symptom; stridor and dyspnea occur subsequently. Dysphagia usually occurs only when the tumor becomes large enough and protrudes into the hypopharynx [26]. In majority of the reported cases the gross appearance has been polypoidal and sometimes infiltrative. Ulceration is rare, in contrast with the early ulceration commonly present in carcinoma of the larynx. Sarcomas may originate in any part of the larynx but most often involve the vocal cords [3, 26]. Our patient also had a similar presentation.

Synovial sarcoma acquired its name due to its microscopic resemblance to developing synovium but is immunophenotypically and ultrastructurally distinct from normal synovium, only rarely arising in joint cavities, and usually occurs in association with para-articular regions of the extremities, with no relation to synovial structures [27].

Histologically, the 2 predominant forms are biphasic and monophasic forms. A branching hemangiopericytoma-like vascular pattern is characteristic and a common finding in both types is the presence of stromal calcification, which ranges from focal to extensive and is an important diagnostic clue [28]. Immunohistochemically, synovial sarcoma is characterised by coexpression of mesenchymal and epithelial markers (cytokeratins and epithelial membrane antigen) [11]. 90% of synovial sarcomas harbour a specific translocation between the SYT gene on chromosome 18 and either the SSX1 or SSX2 gene on the X chromosome [24]. The type of fusion product correlates with the histological pattern; those with SYT-SSX1 are usually biphasic and those with SYT-SSX2 are monophasic. Genetic testing is particularly useful in the poorly differentiated tumors. Our case was positive for cytokeratin and Bcl 2.

The optimal treatment of synovial sarcoma is multimodal. The treatment for sarcoma of the larynx depends on its size, location, and grade. Radical surgical excision is generally accepted as the mainstay of therapy. Because most of the patients can be diagnosed early, conservative surgery with laryngeal preservation is usually possible. Radiotherapy (RT) is an important adjunct in the treatment of soft tissue sarcoma to diminish the incidence of local recurrence [29].

TABLE 1: Review of literature of synovial sarcoma of larynx.

Sl.lno	Reference	Age/sex	Site	Treatment	Survival status
1	[5]	28 F	Left hemilarynx hypopharynx	Pharyngolaryngectomy, 1 year lung metastasis, XRT + chemo	2.5 years DIED
2	[6]	23 F	Interarytenoid and left arytenoid area	Supraglottic laryngectomy and total laryngopharyngectomy	12 years NED
3	[7]	76 M	Rt supraglottic area	Laryngectomy	3 years NED
4	[8]	28 F	Rt aryepiglottic fold	Tumorectomy + XRT	3 years NED
5	[9]	28 M	Supraglottis	Supraglottic laryngectomy + RtND + XRT	16 years NED
6	[10]	14 M	Left arytenoid	Excision tumor, local recurrence at 3 years, total laryngectomy + CT + XRT	10 m NED
7	[11]	27 M	Supraglottis	Surgery, local recurrence 3 m, CT + XRT, 3 m hemilaryngectomy	9 m NED
8	[12]	68 F	Cricoids	Laryngopharyngectomy + neck dissection, cervical oesophagectomy	NA
9	[13]	24 M	Supraglottis	Hemilaryngectomy, recurrence at 12 m, total laryngectomy + XRT, lung mets, chemotherapy	42 m NED
10	[14]	16 M	Supraglottis	CO_2 laser surgery + XRT	24 m NED
11	[15]	54 M	Supraglottis	Laryngopharyngectomy + modified neck dissection	24 m NED
12	[16]	NA	Rt aryepiglottic fold	CO_2 laser surgery	36 m NED
13	[17]	26 M	Supraglottis	CO_2 laser surgery	NA
14	[18]	79 M	Supraglottis	Total laryngectomy	3 m NED
15	[19]	57 M	Supraglottis	CO_2 laser surgery	14 m NED
16	[20]	12 M	Supraglottis	Surgery + chemo	4 m NED
17	[21]	26 M	Larynx	Surgery + XRT	20 m NED
18	[22]	37 M	Supraglottis	Surgery + XRT + chemo	41 m DIED
19	[23]	20 M	Supraglottic larynx	Total laryngectomy, left hemithyroidectomy, left modified radical neck dissection + XRT + chemotherapy	18 m NED
20	Present case	48 M	Supraglottic larynx	Surgery + XRT	36 m NED

The major indications for postoperative RT are high grade lesions, positive surgical margins, larger tumor (>5 cm), and recurrent lesions [30]. Our patient received postoperative RT.

Adjuvant chemotherapy has been utilized for high grade synovial sarcoma. Doxorubicin and ifosfamide have been shown to demonstrate improvement in disease specific survival in the treatment of soft tissue sarcomas [31, 32]. Our patient was not given chemotherapy since it was an intermediate grade lesion. Disease recurrence is a significant problem, with up to 45% of patients with head and neck synovial sarcoma developing a local recurrence and 33%

developing distant metastatic disease [33]. Liu et al. in their review on treatment results of sarcoma of the larynx reported that the 5-year OS of patients with soft tissue sarcoma of the head and neck ranged from 32% to 75% [34]. Our literature review on 20 patients with synovial sarcoma of larynx shows that the survival of these patents ranged from 3 months to 16 years, with 50% alive at 2 years.

In summary, synovial sarcoma of larynx is a rare entity. Surgery is the mainstay of treatment with conservative surgery and organ preservation considered for early cases. Postoperative radiation is reserved for those with positive margins and high grade tumors and chemotherapy for high grade tumors.

Competing Interests

There is no conflict of interests or any financial disclosures.

Authors' Contributions

All authors have read and approved the manuscript.

References

[1] A. I. Farhood, S. I. Hajdu, M. H. Shiu, and E. W. Strong, "Soft tissue sarcomas of the head and neck in adults," *The American Journal of Surgery*, vol. 160, no. 4, pp. 365–369, 1990.

[2] R. A. Eeles, C. Fisher, R. P. A'pHern et al., "Head and neck sarcomas: prognostic factors and implications for treatment," *British Journal of Cancer*, vol. 68, pp. 201–207, 1993.

[3] S. G. Patel, A. R. Shaha, and J. P. Shah, "Soft tissue sarcomas of the head and neck: an update," *American Journal of Otolaryngology—Head and Neck Medicine and Surgery*, vol. 22, no. 1, pp. 2–18, 2001.

[4] S. Pai, R. F. Chinoy, S. A. Pradhan, A. K. D'cruz, S. V. Kane, and J. N. Yadav, "Head and neck synovial sarcomas," *Journal of Surgical Oncology*, vol. 54, no. 2, pp. 82–86, 1993.

[5] W. M. Gatti, C. C. G. Strom, and E. Orfei, "Synovial Sarcoma of the Laryngopharynx," *Archives of Otolaryngology*, vol. 101, no. 10, pp. 633–636, 1975.

[6] L. H. Miller, L. Santaella Latimer, and T. Miller, "Synovial sarcoma of the larynx," *Transactions of the American Academy of Ophthalmology and Otolaryngology*, vol. 80, no. 5, pp. 448–451, 1975.

[7] H. J. Quinn, "Synovial sarcoma of the larynx treated by partial laryngectomy," *Laryngoscope*, vol. 94, no. 9, pp. 1158–1161, 1984.

[8] M. Pruszczynski, J. J. Manni, and F. Smedts, "Endolaryngeal synovial sarcoma: case report with immunohistochemical studies," *Head and Neck*, vol. 11, no. 1, pp. 76–80, 1989.

[9] A. Ferlito and G. Caruso, "Endolaryngeal synovial sarcoma: an update on diagnosis and treatment," *ORL*, vol. 53, no. 2, pp. 116–119, 1991.

[10] B. Morland, G. Cox, C. Randall, A. Ramsay, and M. Radford, "Synovial sarcoma of the larynx in a child: case report and histological appearances," *Medical and Pediatric Oncology*, vol. 23, no. 1, pp. 64–68, 1994.

[11] A. P. Dei Tos, R. Sciot, C. Giannini et al., "Synovial sarcoma of the larynx and hypopharynx," *Annals of Otology, Rhinology and Laryngology*, vol. 107, no. 12, pp. 1080–1085, 1998.

[12] S. M. Taylor, D. Ha, R. Elluru, S. El-Mofty, B. Haughey, and M. Wallace, "Synovial sarcoma of the pericricoidal soft tissue," *Otolaryngology—Head and Neck Surgery*, vol. 126, no. 4, pp. 428–429, 2002.

[13] B. Bilgic, Ö. Mete, A. S. Öztürk, M. Demiryont, N. Keles, and M. Basaran, "Synovial sarcoma: a rare tumor of larynx," *Pathology and Oncology Research*, vol. 9, no. 4, pp. 242–245, 2003.

[14] S. Papaspyrou, G. Kyriakides, and M. Tapis, "Endoscopic CO2 laser surgery for large synovial sarcoma of the larynx," *Otolaryngology—Head and Neck Surgery*, vol. 129, no. 6, pp. 630–631, 2003.

[15] K. Szuhai, J. Knijnenburg, M. Ijszenga et al., "Multicolor fluorescence in situ hybridization analysis of a synovial sarcoma of the larynx with a t(X;18)(p11.2;q11.2) and trisomies 2 and 8," *Cancer Genetics and Cytogenetics*, vol. 153, pp. 48–52, 2004.

[16] V. Boniver, P. Moreau, and P. Lefebvre, "Synovial sarcoma of the larynx: case report and literature review," *B-ENT*, vol. 1, no. 1, pp. 47–51, 2005.

[17] H. A. Abou Zeid, S. A. Arab, A. M. Al-Ghamdi, A. A. Al-Qurain, and K. M. Mokhazy, "Airway management of a rare huge-size supraglottic mass," *Saudi Medical Journal*, vol. 27, no. 5, pp. 711–713, 2006.

[18] P. Mhawech-Fauceglia, P. Ramzy, W. Bshara, S. Sait, and N. Rigual, "Synovial sarcoma of the larynx in a 79-year-old woman, confirmed by karyotyping and fluorescence in situ hybridization analysis," *Annals of Diagnostic Pathology*, vol. 11, no. 3, pp. 223–227, 2007.

[19] M. Capelli, G. Bertino, P. Morbini, M. Proh, C. E. Falco, and M. Benazzo, "CO2 laser in the treatment of laryngeal synovial sarcoma: a clinical case," *Tumori*, vol. 93, no. 3, pp. 296–299, 2007.

[20] M. J. Fernández-Aceñero, F. Larach, and C. Ortega-Fernández, "Non-epithelial lesions of the larynx: review of the 10-year experience in a tertiary Spanish hospital," *Acta Oto-Laryngologica*, vol. 129, no. 1, pp. 108–112, 2009.

[21] A. Al-Nemer and M. A. El-Shawarby, "Laryngeal synovial sarcoma: case report and literature review," *Gulf Journal of Oncology*, vol. 1, no. 9, pp. 52–56, 2011.

[22] Y.-Y. Bao, Q.-Y. Wang, S.-H. Zhou, K. Zhao, L.-X. Ruan, and H.-T. Yao, "Poor outcome of comprehensive therapy in a case of laryngeal synovial sarcoma," *Radiology and Oncology*, vol. 47, no. 2, pp. 111–118, 2013.

[23] C. Saxby, R. Bova, and M. Edwards, "Laryngeal synovial sarcoma: a rare clinical entity," *Case Reports in Otolaryngology*, vol. 2013, Article ID 578606, 4 pages, 2013.

[24] E. M. Sturgis and B. O. Potter, "Sarcomas of the head and neck region," *Current Opinion in Oncology*, vol. 15, no. 3, pp. 239–252, 2003.

[25] M. F. Okcu, M. Munsell, J. Treuner et al., "Synovial sarcoma of childhood and adolescence: a multicenter, multivariate analysis of outcome," *Journal of Clinical Oncology*, vol. 21, no. 8, pp. 1602–1611, 2003.

[26] H. L. Levine and R. Tubbs, "Nonsquamous neoplasms of the larynx," *Otolaryngologic Clinics of North America*, vol. 19, pp. 475–488, 1986.

[27] Enzinger and Weiss's, *Soft Tissue Tumors*, Mosby Elsevier, 5th edition, 2008.

[28] C. D. M. Fletcher, *Diagnostic Histopathology of Tumors*, Churchill Livingstone Elsevier, 3rd edition, 2007.

[29] Q.-T. X. Le, K. K. Fu, S. Kroll et al., "Prognostic factors in adult soft-tissue sarcomas of the head and neck," *International Journal of Radiation Oncology Biology Physics*, vol. 37, no. 5, pp. 975–984, 1997.

[30] P. K. Pellitteri, A. Ferlito, P. J. Bradley, A. R. Shaha, and A. Rinaldo, "Management of sarcomas of the head and neck in adults," *Oral Oncology*, vol. 39, no. 1, pp. 2–12, 2003.

[31] R. Lor Randall, K. L. S. Schabel, Y. Hitchcock, D. E. Joyner, and K. H. Albritton, "Diagnosis and management of synovial sarcoma," *Current Treatment Options in Oncology*, vol. 6, no. 6, pp. 449–459, 2005.

[32] J. F. Tierney, "Adjuvant chemotherapy for localised resectable soft-tissue sarcoma of adults: meta-analysis of individual data," *The Lancet*, vol. 350, no. 9092, pp. 1647–1654, 1997.

[33] W. J. Harb, M. A. Luna, S. R. Patel, M. T. Ballo, D. B. Roberts, and E. M. Sturgis, "Survival in patients with synovial sarcoma of the head and neck: association with tumor location, size, and extension," *Head and Neck*, vol. 29, no. 8, pp. 731–740, 2007.

[34] C. Liu, M. Wang, W. Li, S. Chang, and P. Chu, "Sarcoma of the larynx: treatment results and literature review," *Journal of the Chinese Medical Association*, vol. 69, no. 3, pp. 120–124, 2006.

19

Rhinosporidiosis: A Rare Cause of Proptosis and an Imaging Dilemma for Sinonasal Masses

Amit Kumar Dey, Rajaram Sharma, Kartik Mittal, Puneeth Kumar, Vivek Murumkar, Sumit Mitkar, and Priya Hira

Department of Radiology, King Edward Memorial Hospital and Seth G.S. Medical College, Room No. 107, KEM Main Boy's Hostel, Parel, Mumbai 400012, India

Correspondence should be addressed to Amit Kumar Dey; amit5kem@gmail.com

Academic Editor: Guangwei Zhou

Background. Rhinosporidiosis is a common disease entity in tropical countries; however, it can be encountered in other parts of the world as well due to increasing medical tourism. It may mimic other more malignant and vigorous pathologies of the involved part. *Case Report.* We present a case of a 36-year-old male presenting with proptosis due to involvement of nasolacrimal duct which is rare. We will discuss typical CT and MRI features of the disease which were present in the case. *Conclusion.* For a surgeon and a radiologist, this is a necessary differential to be kept in mind for sinonasal masses. CT and MRI are invaluable investigations. However, FNAC is confirmatory. Both clinical and radiological aspects are required to reach correct diagnosis.

1. Introduction

Rhinosporidiosis is mainly prevalent in south Asian countries. Frequent bathing in stagnant water ponds is a risk factor for this infection [1]. It is a chronic granulomatous disease caused by the fungus *Rhinosporidium seeberi*. Pathologically, there is nasal polyposis and other manifestations like hyperplasia of nasal mucosa [2]. Recurrence is quite common after surgical excision [3]. This is primarily a disease of orofacial region. In decreasing frequency, it involves nasal cavity, nasopharynx, oropharynx, and nasolacrimal duct. However, other viscera, trachea, bones, brains, and orbits have also been involved [4].

Here, we are presenting a case of a 36-year-old male patient presenting with proptosis due to involvement of nasolacrimal duct which is rare. We will discuss typical CT and MRI features of the disease which were present in the case.

2. Case Report

A 36-year-old male presented with long standing history of proptosis of right eye since 1 year and foul smelling nasal discharge since 2 months. The patient also gave history of spells of nasal itching. There is no history of constitutional symptoms. There is no history of similar complaints in the family. He works as a farmer in rice fields. Local examination of the eye showed proptosis of lower eyelid and there was a firm and round swelling near medial canthus of right eye. Local examination of the nasal cavity showed friable polypoidal reddish mass in inferior turbinate which was extending into opening of nasolacrimal duct.

In nasopharynx multiple polypoidal reddish friable mass which would bleed on touching was seen originating from the base of the skull. Biochemical and haematological tests done on the patient were normal.

A CT scan of paranasal sinuses and orbits was ordered which showed intensely enhancing extraconal mass lesion in inferior portion of right eye. There was rarefaction of inferior orbital wall and bony portion of nasolacrimal duct. Nasolacrimal duct was enlarged with rarefaction of bony walls.

Similarly, enhancing mass was seen in inferior turbinate and nasopharynx. There were few areas of air specs and calcification within the lesion. There was a leash of blood

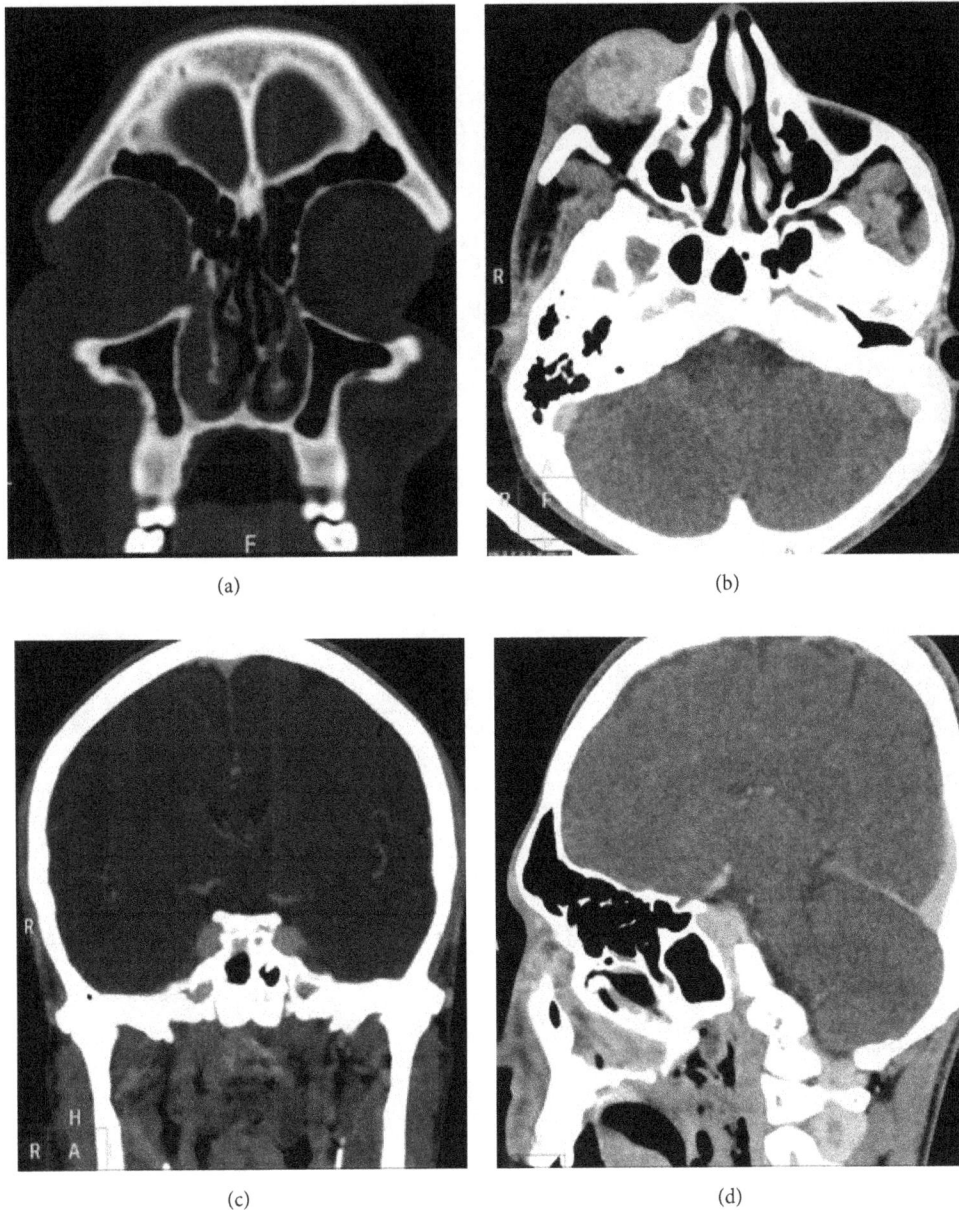

(a)

(b)

(c)

(d)

FIGURE 1: (a) Coronal image of CT paranasal sinuses in bone window showing soft tissue density mass lesion in inferior portion of right eye with extension into nasolacrimal duct. Nasolacrimal duct is expanded with rarefaction of its walls. Mass is reaching up to inferior turbinate. (b) CT postcontrast axial view in soft tissue window at the level of maxillary antrum showing well-defined, intensely enhancing mass lesion anteroinferior to right globe. (c) CT coronal image in maximum intensity projection showing abnormally hypertrophied vessels originating from nasopharyngeal mucosa and supplying the lesion. (d) CT postcontrast sagittal view in soft tissue window showing extension of the lesion through the expanded nasolacrimal duct into inferior turbinate.

vessels seen originating from the nasopharyngeal wall and supplying the mass (Figure 1). Following this, MRI was done which showed the following (Figure 2):

(a) T2-weighted sagittal section showing heterogeneously hyperintense multilobulated mass originating from nasal cavity and nasopharynx and extending into oropharynx. Lesion shows few flow voids within

(b) Postcontrast T1-weighted coronal section showing enhancing mass lesion in inferior portion of right orbit. There are few nonenhancing areas within. Lesion is extending into the inferior turbinate via nasolacrimal duct

(c) Postcontrast T1-weighted sagittal section showing intensely enhancing multilobulated mass originating

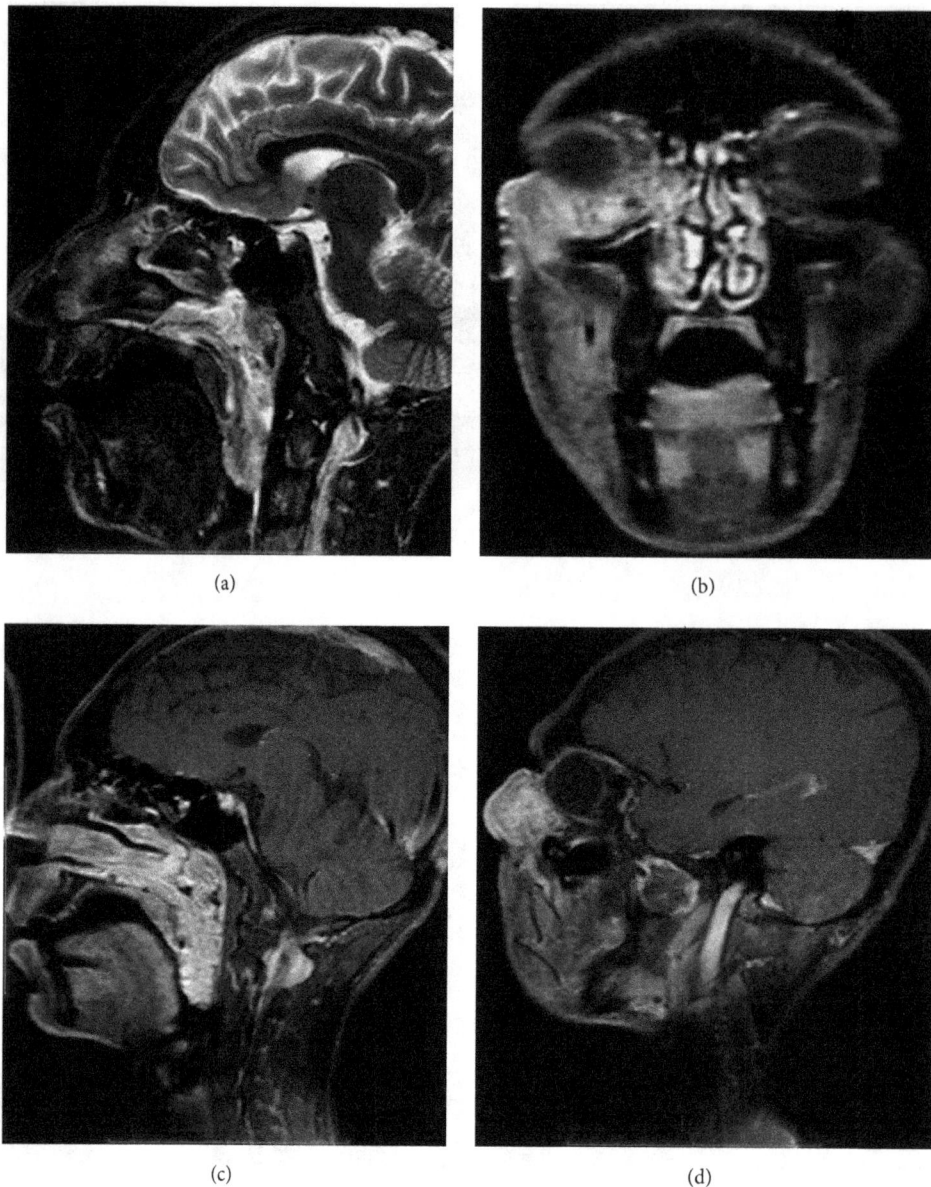

FIGURE 2: (a) T2-weighted MRI sagittal section showing heterogeneously hyperintense multilobulated mass originating from nasal cavity and nasopharynx and extending into oropharynx. Lesion shows few flow voids within. (b) Postcontrast T1-weighted MRI coronal section showing enhancing mass lesion in inferior portion of right orbit. There are few nonenhancing areas within. Lesion is extending into the inferior turbinate via nasolacrimal duct. (c) Postcontrast T1-weighted MRI sagittal section showing intensely enhancing multilobulated mass originating from nasal cavity and nasopharynx and extending into oropharynx. Lesion shows few nonenhancing areas within. Lesion shows multilobulated external surface mimicking cerebriform appearance of inverted papilloma. (d) Postcontrast T1-weighted MRI sagittal section showing extraconal, intraorbital, intensely enhancing mass extending into the nasal cavity via nasolacrimal duct. The mass is protruding outside of the orbital margins causing proptosis.

from nasal cavity and nasopharynx and extending into oropharynx. Lesion shows few nonenhancing areas within. Lesion shows multilobulated external surface mimicking cerebriform appearance of inverted papilloma

(d) Postcontrast T1-weighted sagittal section showing extraconal, intraorbital, intensely enhancing mass extending into the nasal cavity via nasolacrimal duct.

The mass is protruding outside of the orbital margins causing proptosis

Finally, FNAC (H&E staining) of the orbital lesion was done, which showed groups of spore of rhinosporidium of varying sizes (Figure 3). Following this, wide excision of the nasolacrimal duct/orbital lesion and electric cauterization of the base of the orbital lesion were done. Endoscopic sinus surgery of the nasopharyngeal lesion was done and to prevent

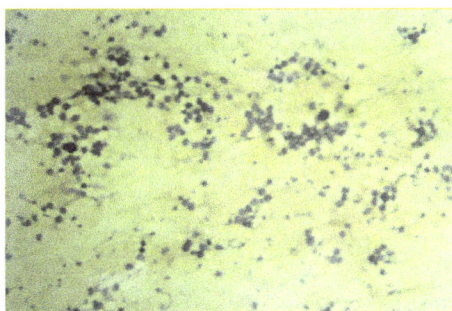

FIGURE 3: H&E slide prepared by fine-needle aspiration cytology from the lesion showing groups of spore of rhinosporidium of varying sizes.

recurrence patient was put on dapsone therapy. The patient did remarkably well and showed no signs of recurrence on follow-up.

3. Discussion

Rhinosporidiosis is a chronic granulomatous disease caused by *Rhinosporidium seeberi* presently classified in class Mesomycetozoea [5]. The pathogen enters the host primarily by abraded skin or mucosa via transepithelial spread [6]. This explains nose as being the most common site in involvement of the disease. However, other methods like autoinoculation, haematogenous spread, and direct inoculation have been described for other visceral involvements [7, 8]. Nasal involvement can be a single pedunculated polyp or multiple sessile polyps arising from mucosa [9]. Other manifestations like multiple cutaneous reddish polyps, bone lesions, and corneal mass are described by few case reports. Diagnosis in the cases affecting nose and throat can be done by clinical examination. However, atypical presentation like ours and lower respiratory tract involvement require radiological examination. CT and MRI are also needed for depiction of extent of the lesion and complications and in cases of recurrence to plan surgery.

On CT, it looks like irregular or lobulated lesions of soft tissue density showing moderate-to-intense postcontrast enhancement. Small foci of calcification and air can be seen within the lesions. Multiple dilated vessels can be also seen arising from nasopharyngeal mucosa which can be seen supplying the lesion. Lesions arising from oropharynx or trachea can be relatively hypoenhancing compared to the lesions at other sites. Bony involvement may appear as thinning of wall, rarefaction, or complete erosion [10].

MRI shows heterogeneous mixed density mass lesion with prominent flow voids on T2-weighted imaging. Postcontrast imaging shows intense enhancement of the mass. Multilobulated appearance may give rise to cerebriform appearance as described for inverted papilloma in the literature. The main imaging differentials are inverted papilloma, juvenile angiofibroma, lobular capillary hemangioma, angiomatous polyp, and sinonasal malignancy [10].

Diagnosis can be done by FNAC and examination under 10% KOH or Papanicolaou smear. However, usually

histopathological examination is required. Both of the above methods show pathogen in its various stages of development [11, 12].

Surgical removal with wide margins remains the main cornerstone of the treatment with electrocautery of the base. Dapsone can be added as adjuvant medical therapy; however, no definite benefits of dapsone therapy have been proven. Even after the treatment with wide excision, there are high chances of recurrence probably due to hematogenous spread of the disease during surgery [13–15].

4. Conclusion

Rhinosporidiosis is a common disease entity in tropical countries; however, it can be encountered in other parts of the world as trend of medical tourism is increasing. It may mimic other more malignant and vigorous pathologies of the involved part. For a surgeon and for a radiologist, this is a necessary differential to be kept in mind for sinonasal masses. Both clinical and radiological aspects are required to reach correct diagnosis.

Inferior meatus is a common site of involvement in the nasal cavity because of its close proximity with the nasolacrimal duct. It is more likely that lesion began in the nasal cavity and then extended into the orbit via the nasolacrimal duct. The presence of other lesions in the nasopharynx may further support this.

Consent

Informed consent was obtained for experimentation with human subjects.

Disclosure

No animals have been experimented upon. Amit Kumar Dey and Rajaram Sharma are joint first authors of the paper.

Competing Interests

The authors declare that they have no competing interests.

Authors' Contributions

Amit Kumar Dey and Rajaram Sharma are first authors as they have contributed equally. All the authors were associated in conceiving the idea of the case as well as in the preparation of the manuscript.

References

[1] A. A. Mallick, T. K. Majhi, and D. K. Pal, "Rhinosporidiosis affecting multiple parts of the body," *Tropical Doctor*, vol. 42, no. 3, pp. 174–175, 2012.

[2] R. Kumari, C. Laxmisha, and D. M. Thappa, "Disseminated cutaneous rhinosporidiosis," *Dermatology Online Journal*, vol. 11, p. 19, 2005.

[3] H. Banjara, R. K. Panda, A. V. Daharwal, V. Sudarshan, D. Singh, and A. Gupta, "Bronchial rhinosporidiosis: an unusual presentation," *Lung India*, vol. 29, no. 2, pp. 173–175, 2012.

[4] G. O. Echejoh, A. N. Manasseh, M. N. Tanko et al., "Nasal rhinosporidiosis," *Journal of the National Medical Association*, vol. 100, no. 6, pp. 713–715, 2008.

[5] S. K. D. Thakur, S. P. Sah, and B. P. Badhu, "Oculosporidiosis in Eastern Nepal: a report of five cases," *Southeast Asian Journal of Tropical Medicine and Public Health*, vol. 33, no. 2, pp. 362–364, 2002.

[6] W. A. Karunaratne, "The pathology of rhinosporidiosis," *Journal of Pathology and Bacteriology*, vol. 42, pp. 193–202, 1934.

[7] W. A. Karunaratne, *Rhinosporidiosis in Man*, The Athlone Press, London, UK, 1964.

[8] R. V. Rajam and G. C. Viswanathan, "Rhinosporidiosis: a study with a report of a fatal case with systemic dissemination," *Indian Journal of Surgery*, vol. 17, pp. 269–298, 1955.

[9] A. M. Dick, "Nasal rhinosporidiosis; report of a case in natal," *South African Medical Journal*, vol. 25, no. 16, pp. 270–271, 1951.

[10] S. M. Prabhu, A. Irodi, H. L. Khiangte, V. Rupa, and P. Naina, "Imaging features of rhinosporidiosis on contrast CT," *The Indian Journal of Radiology & Imaging*, vol. 23, no. 3, pp. 212–218, 2013.

[11] S. Agrawal, K. D. Sharma, and J. B. Shrivastava, "Generalized rhinosporidiosis with visceral involvement; report of a case," *Archives of Dermatology*, vol. 80, no. 1, pp. 22–26, 1959.

[12] D. M. Thappa, S. Venkatesan, C. S. Sirka, T. J. Jaisankar, Gopalkrishnan, and C. Ratnakar, "Disseminated cutaneous rhinosporidiosis," *Journal of Dermatology*, vol. 25, no. 8, pp. 527–532, 1998.

[13] M. Vijaikumar, D. M. Thappa, K. Karthikeyan, and S. Jayanthi, "Verrucous lesion of the palm," *Postgraduate Medical Journal*, vol. 78, no. 919, pp. 302–306, 2002.

[14] K. K. Nair, "Clinical trial of diaminodiphenylsulfone (DDS) in nasal and nasopharyngeal rhinosporidiosis," *Laryngoscope*, vol. 89, no. 2, pp. 291–295, 1979.

[15] A. Job, S. Venkateswaran, M. Mathan, H. Krishnaswami, and R. Raman, "Medical therapy of rhinosporidiosis with dapsone," *Journal of Laryngology and Otology*, vol. 107, no. 9, pp. 809–812, 1993.

20

Acute Vision Loss Following Endoscopic Sinus Surgery

Serena Byrd, Adnan S. Hussaini, and Jastin Antisdel

Department of Otolaryngology-Head and Neck Surgery, Saint Louis University School of Medicine, Saint Louis, MO, USA

Correspondence should be addressed to Serena Byrd; sbyrd7@slu.edu

Academic Editor: Rong-San Jiang

A 41-year-old female with a history of uterine cancer and Celiac and Raynaud's Disease presented to our institution with frequent migraines and nasal congestion. She underwent functional endoscopic sinus surgery (FESS) and experienced acute unilateral vision loss postoperatively. Rapid recognition of the etiology and effective treatment are paramount given the permanent and irreversible vision loss that can result. Arterial vasospasm following FESS is rare. Patients with autoimmune diseases have perhaps an increased risk for vasospasm secondary to an increased vasoreactive profile. We present the first documented case of nitroglycerin sublingual therapy to successfully treat ophthalmic artery vasospasm following FESS. Nitroglycerin sublingual therapy is a promising treatment for ophthalmic vasospasm secondary to its ability to cross the blood-ocular barrier, its rapid onset of action, and its ability to promote relaxation of vascular smooth muscle.

1. Introduction

Acute postoperative vision loss is a rare but devastating complication of functional endoscopic sinus surgery (FESS). The most feared orbital complication following routine sinus surgery is orbital hematoma. Orbital hematoma is oftentimes obvious to recognize on physical examination by rapid unilateral orbital swelling and thus is easily treated with decompression (i.e., lateral canthotomy and cantholysis). Injury to orbital structures, thromboembolic event, retinal migraine, and ophthalmic artery vasospasm are other etiologies of unilateral vision loss that are oftentimes more difficult to recognize clinically [1]. Rapid identification of the underlying etiology of vision loss is paramount because permanent and irreversible vision loss often occurs within 60–90 minutes following vascular compromise and treatment differs based on etiology.

Our patient underwent topical decongestion with oxymetazoline (Afrin). Oxymetazoline is a long-acting imidazoline derivative with an onset of action under 10 minutes and duration of action of 6 hours or longer. It acts locally as a sympathomimetic vasoconstrictor, causing shrinkage of the nasal mucosa [2, 3]. There are few documented cases of suspected retinal artery branch occlusion and segmental cerebral vasoconstriction following excessive home use of oxymetazoline [4] and no reports to suggest vasoconstriction to the ocular vasculature following endoscopic sinus surgery. However, there have been several documented cases of ophthalmic artery vasospasm following FESS thought to be secondary to direct injection of epinephrine into the ethmoidal artery [5].

This case report is unique in that it is the first documented case of acute vision loss without local injection or associated orbital hematoma and the first reported case of nitroglycerin sublingual therapy to successfully treat suspected ophthalmic artery vasospasm.

2. Case Presentation

A 41-year-old female with a history of Raynaud's disease and self-reported Celiac disease presented to our institution with frequent migraines and nasal congestion. She was found to have a recurrent inverting papilloma of the left frontal and ethmoid sinuses (Figure 1). She had previously undergone resection of this inverting papilloma at an outside hospital, which was complicated by a delayed CSF leak requiring placement of a lumbar drain. On initial presentation to our institution, her physical exam was unremarkable except for nasal endoscopy revealing a polypoid mass emanating from the left frontal sinus outflow tract.

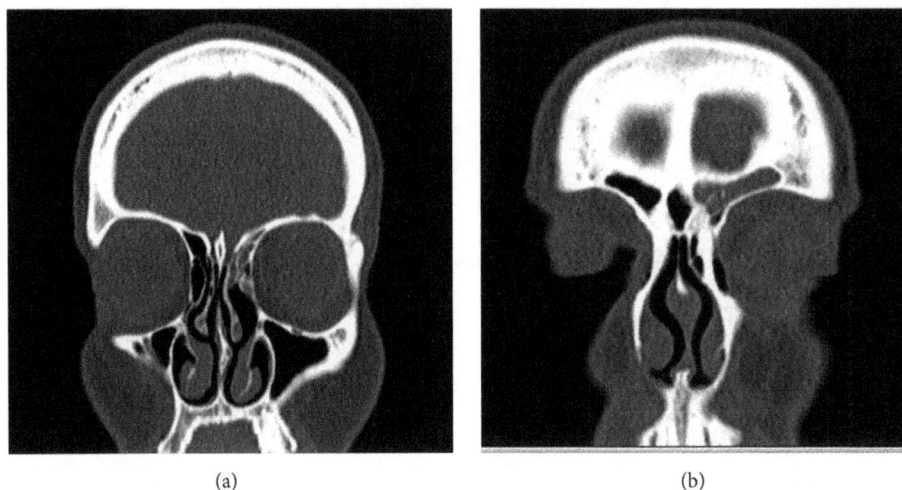

(a)   (b)

FIGURE 1: Preoperative coronal CT scan demonstrating evidence of soft tissue density consistent with known inverting papilloma in ethmoid (a) and frontal (b) sinuses.

She underwent an uncomplicated endoscopic modified Lothrop for approach and resection of the tumor. Perioperatively, topical oxymetazoline was used with no injection of local anesthetic. The patient was noted to have tumor superior to the anterior ethmoid artery and pedicled off the lamina papyracea. In order to completely remove the tumor, the anterior ethmoidal artery required ligation using bipolar followed by monopolar cautery. The superior aspect of the lamina papyracea was drilled away with only a small amount of orbital fat protruding from the foramen of the anterior ethmoidal artery. The lesion was completely removed with no significant blood loss and no CSF leak.

The patient remained hemodynamically stable throughout her postoperative course. However, approximately 12 hours after her surgery, she began to experience left sided eye pain and slight eye pressure but denied visual changes or other symptoms. This progressed over the next several hours to left sided blurry vision and prompted immediate ENT evaluation. Physical exam showed soft, moderate fullness of the left periorbital region, intact extraocular movement, and no proptosis. Ophthalmology was immediately consulted and fundoscopic exam showed pallor of the left retina and optic disk with an inferior visual loss and an afferent pupillary defect.

This was treated immediately with one nitroglycerin sublingual tablet with prompt return of her vision within several minutes of administration. Repeat fundoscopic examination after nitroglycerin treatment revealed a normal appearing retina and optic disk.

3. Discussion

Our case report is unique in that it is the first documented case of nitroglycerin sublingual therapy to successfully treat suspected ophthalmic artery vasospasm. Informed consent was obtained from the patient prior to writing of this manuscript.

In our patient, the etiology of her unilateral vision loss was felt to be most consistent with retinal artery vasospasm. It was felt that an orbital hematoma was unlikely given that the patients symptoms developed long after the completion of her surgery (>12–18 hours). Although the patient does have a prior history of uterine cancer, a thromboembolic event was also felt to be an unlikely etiology given that she has remained cancer free, is otherwise young and healthy, and experienced a prompt response to nitroglycerin treatment. Carotid artery disease (CAD) was also not felt to contribute as our patient had no preceding history or risk factors for such disease. Given that her symptoms did not start until more than 12 hours after surgery (at which time oxymetazoline should no longer be present) and the fact that our patient had such a rapid improvement in her symptoms and ophthalmologic exam after sublingual nitroglycerin treatment, we find it most likely that retinal vasospasm was the cause of her vision loss.

The anterior and posterior ethmoidal arteries provide a direct connection of the nasal cavity and orbit via their continuity with the ophthalmic artery. This vascular connection demonstrates how local anesthetic with epinephrine injected within the nasal cavity could cause retrograde flow, vasoconstriction to the blood supply of the optic nerve, and subsequent vision loss [5]. Although no injection of local anesthetic was performed in our patient, perhaps drilling of the lamina at the region of the ethmoid artery foramen to control bleeding could have contributed to vasospasm and compromised optic nerve perfusion. Retinal vasospasm may also occur in patients with migraines or migraine risk factors [6].

Studies have also suggested that patients with a history of migraine headaches and Raynaud's Disease, both comorbidities that our patient experienced, are more likely to suffer from vasospastic syndrome. Vasospastic syndrome is characterized by a more vasoreactive response to stimuli such as cold, emotional stress, or possibly vasoconstrictive medications. It has also been reported to occur more frequently in women of childbearing age. Some patients suffer from migraines, but the relationship between vasospastic syndrome and migraines is rather weak [7]. Choroidal and optic nerve circulation involvement in vasospastic syndrome has been previously described. While the exact pathophysiology of focal retinal vasospasm remains unknown, it has been speculated that endothelin-1 (ET-1), which increases in all diseases related to vasospasm, contributes to retinal vasoconstriction by inducing vascular hyperresponsiveness to various stimuli rather than being the direct cause of vasospasm [7].

The regulation of metabolic substrates and oxygen to the retina is a complex process due to the presence of two vascular systems, which differ anatomically and physiologically: the retinal and the choroidal systems. These systems form what is known as the blood-ocular barrier. The blood-ocular barrier is a highly selective barrier formed by tight junctions along the endothelial cells and is similar in composition to the blood-brain barrier. Physical or oxidative stress, as well as inflammatory events, may affect the permeability of the intercellular junctions. The extraocular and choroidal vessels are autonomically innervated. The retinal vessels lack autonomic supply, such that blood flow is controlled solely by local vascular control mechanisms determined by a balance of ET-1 and endothelium-derived nitric oxide (NO) [8].

Vasospasm has been described extensively in the neurosurgery and vascular literature. It is often diagnosed by a high level of clinical suspicion and can be confirmed by angiography. "Triple-H" (hypertension, hypervolemia, and hemodilution) therapy and calcium channel blockers have been shown to improve treatment outcomes. Catheter angiography with infusion of vasodilators and balloon angioplasty to mechanically open the stenosed vessel and break the vasospasm cycle have also been described. Treatment of acute monocular vision loss related to vasospasm includes prompt treatment with calcium channel blockers, which improves blood flow by reducing the vasoconstrictive effects of ET-1 [9]. If standard therapy for vasospasm fails to correct the underlying problem/symptom, typically other etiologies such as thromboembolic event, migraine, or surgical injury should be considered and further investigated [10].

In our particular case report, nitroglycerin was used for the treatment of retinal vasospasm. This drug is well known for its treatment of coronary artery spasm, angina, and myocardial infarction [11]. It often produces a severe headache shortly after administration because nitroglycerin readily crosses the blood-brain barrier and causes vasodilation. In addition, nitroglycerin offers a rapid onset of action, which is extremely important as permanent irreversible vision loss is typically seen at 60–90 minutes after vascular compromise. Given the similarities of the blood-ocular barrier to the blood-brain barrier, it seems that a rationale and effective treatment of retinal vasospasm is nitroglycerin sublingual therapy.

In summary, arterial vasospasm following FESS is rare. However, prompt recognition and effective treatment are vital in preserving vision. Patients with Raynaud's Disease and/or a history of migraines are perhaps more at risk for vasospasm secondary to a more vasoreactive profile [7]. Nitroglycerin sublingual therapy is a promising treatment for ophthalmic

vasospasm secondary to its ability to cross the blood-ocular barrier, its rapid onset of action, its relative good safety profile, and its ability to promote relaxation of vascular smooth muscle. This medication, although not previously documented for the treatment of ophthalmic artery vasospasm, should be considered as an alternative treatment or in addition to standard calcium channel blockers therapy.

Competing Interests

The authors declare that there is no conflict of interests regarding the publication of this paper.

Acknowledgments

This paper was presented at the 2015 American Academy of Otolaryngology Rhinologic Society Meeting in Dallas, Texas.

References

[1] J. H. Pula, K. Kwan, C. A. Yuen, and J. C. Kattah, "Update on the evaluation of transient vision loss," *Clinical Ophthalmology*, vol. 10, pp. 297–303, 2016.

[2] T. S. Higgins, P. H. Hwang, T. T. Kingdom, R. R. Orlandi, H. Stammberger, and J. K. Han, "Systematic review of topical vasoconstrictors in endoscopic sinus surgery," *Laryngoscope*, vol. 121, no. 2, pp. 422–432, 2011.

[3] M. İ. Şahin, K. Kökoğlu, Ş. Güleç, İ. Ketenci, and Y. Ünlü, "Premedication methods in nasal endoscopy: A Prospective, Randomized, Double-Blind Study," *Clinical and Experimental Otorhinolaryngology*, 2016.

[4] G. D. Fivgas and N. J. Newman, "Anterior ischemic optic neuropathy following the use of a nasal decongestant," *American Journal of Ophthalmology*, vol. 127, no. 1, pp. 104–106, 1999.

[5] P. J. Savino, R. M. Burde, and R. P. Mills, "Visual loss following intranasal anesthetic injection," *Journal of Clinical Neuro-Ophthalmology*, vol. 10, no. 2, pp. 140–144, 1990.

[6] R. W. Evans and B. M. Grosberg, "Retinal migraine: migraine associated with monocular visual symptoms," *Headache*, vol. 48, no. 1, pp. 142–145, 2008.

[7] J. Flammer, M. Pache, and T. Resink, "Vasospasm, its role in the pathogenesis of diseases with particular reference to the eye," *Progress in Retinal and Eye Research*, vol. 20, no. 3, pp. 319–349, 2001.

[8] C. E. Riva et al., "Ocular circulation," in *Adler's Physiology of the Eye*, pp. 243–73, Elsevier, Amsterdam, Netherlands, 11th edition, 2011.

[9] P. Meyer, M. G. Lang, J. Flammer, and T. F. Lüscher, "Effects of calcium channel blockers on the response to endothelin-1, bradykinin and sodium nitroprusside in porcine ciliary arteries," *Experimental Eye Research*, vol. 60, no. 5, pp. 505–510, 1995.

[10] A. R. Naylor, T. G. Robinson, D. Eveson, and J. Burns, "An audit of management practices in patients with suspected temporary monocular blindness," *British Journal of Ophthalmology*, vol. 98, no. 6, pp. 730–733, 2014.

[11] M.-J. Hung, P. Hu, and M.-Y. Hung, "Coronary artery spasm: review and update," *International Journal of Medical Sciences*, vol. 11, no. 11, pp. 1161–1171, 2014.

21

Blue Ear Cyst: A Rare Eccrine Hidrocystoma of the Ear Canal and Successful Endoscopic Excision

Taha A. Mur,[1] Ronald Miick,[2] and Natasha Pollak[3]

[1]*Lewis Katz School of Medicine, Temple University, Philadelphia, PA, USA*
[2]*Department of Pathology and Laboratory Medicine, Einstein Medical Center, Philadelphia, PA, USA*
[3]*Department of Otolaryngology-Head & Neck Surgery, Lewis Katz School of Medicine, Temple University, Philadelphia, PA, USA*

Correspondence should be addressed to Natasha Pollak; pollakn1@hotmail.com

Academic Editor: M. Tayyar Kalcioglu

Aims. Hidrocystomas are benign cystic growths of the apocrine and eccrine sweat glands. These cystic lesions have been well documented on the face, head, and neck, but rarely in the external auditory canal. *Presentation of Case*. A 67-year-old woman presented with a bluish cystic mass partially occluding the external auditory canal and interfering with hearing aid use. Lesion was excised completely via a transcanal endoscopic approach with excellent cosmetic results, no canal stenosis, and no recurrence at 1-year follow-up. *Discussion*. We present a rare eccrine hidrocystoma of the external auditory canal and successful excision of this benign lesion. We describe the surgical management using a transcanal endoscopic approach and follow-up results. An eccrine gland cyst that presents as a mass occluding the external auditory canal is quite rare. There are only a few such cases reported in the literature. These masses can be mistaken for basal cell carcinomas or cholesterol granulomas but can be easily differentiated using histopathology. *Conclusion*. Eccrine hidrocystoma is a cystic lesion of sweat glands, rarely found in the external auditory canal. A characteristic bluish hue aids in diagnosis and surgical excision using ear endoscopy provides excellent control.

1. Introduction

The skin of the external auditory canal, just like skin elsewhere in the body, contains several types of adnexal secretory glands, including eccrine (common sweat glands), apocrine (modified sweat glands), and holocrine (sebaceous) glands. The external canal skin also contains ceruminous glands, essentially apocrine glands, which, in combination with the sebaceous glands, create cerumen [1]. The balance of secretory functions creates a slightly acidic (pH 6) microenvironment in the ear canal that supports a balanced and healthy skin flora.

Several types of solid tumors have been reported to originate from these glands, both benign, such as ceruminous adenomas, and malignant, such as ceruminous adenocarcinomas [2]. Cystic masses originating from these secretory glands are rarely seen in the external auditory canal (EAC). Cystic lesions associated with the apocrine glands have been documented in the literature to occur within the eyelid, axillae, and groin [2]. These cysts, also known as apocrine

hidrocystomas, occasionally present as bluish masses [3, 4]. Similarly, cystic tumors associated with the eccrine glands or eccrine hidrocystomas are extremely rare in the ear canal, with only a few cases reported in the literature [1, 2, 4].

Here, we present a rare case of an eccrine hidrocystoma, confined to the external auditory canal in an adult patient. The lesion was surgically excised using endoscopic ear surgery techniques. There was no recurrence, EAC stenosis, or other complications.

2. Presentation of Case

A 67-year-old woman presented to our otolaryngology clinic complaining of a lesion in her left ear canal that had been growing slowly for approximately 10 years. She had prior bilateral mastoidectomies (intact canal wall) for chronic otitis media as a child. Over the past 20+ years, her ear symptoms have been quiescent and there is no ongoing inflammatory process in her ears. She has some mixed hearing loss and

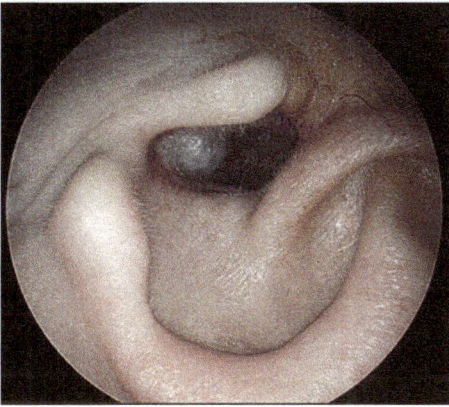

FIGURE 1: A bluish lesion is seen in the external auditory canal inferiorly, partially blocking the canal lumen.

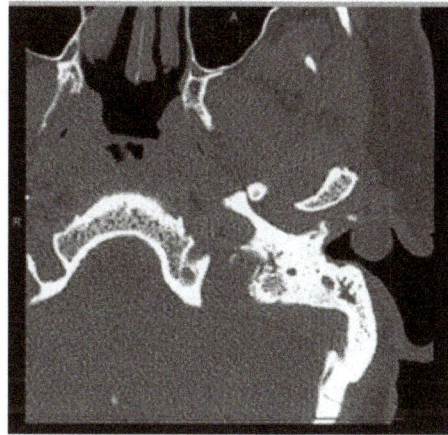

FIGURE 2: CT of the temporal bones shows a well-defined cystic lesion originating from the anterolateral portion of the left external auditory canal. The lesion has no deep extension, does not show any bone erosion, and does not involve the middle ear cleft.

wears bilateral hearing aids. Recently, the lesion in her left ear canal has interfered with hearing aid placement. On otoscopic examination, a soft, nontender, ovoid, smooth, bluish mass about 1 cm in diameter was noted partially blocking the left EAC meatus (Figure 1).

Her tympanic membrane, which could still be partially visualized past the lesion, appeared grossly intact with normal landmarks. Audiometry was consistent with a severe to profound mixed hearing loss bilaterally. Tympanometry was normal (type A) on the right, but on the left ear, a seal could not be achieved.

To evaluate the deep extent of the lesion, the patient underwent a CT scan of the temporal bones without contrast, which revealed a well-circumscribed 1.0 × 0.8 cm sessile cystic lesion arising from the floor of the lateral portion of the left external auditory canal. A thin rim of calcification could be seen along the inferior margin of the lesion. There was no evidence of invasion of surrounding soft tissues or bone. The tympanic membrane, middle ear cleft, and ossicular chain were intact and normal. Prior mastoidectomies were evident on CT images (Figure 2).

Because of the benign features of the lesion on history, examination, and imaging, decision was made to proceed with local excision of the lesion with minimal margins. The patient was taken to the operating room for excision of this lesion under general anesthesia, using the otologic endoscope and binocular otomicroscopy. The mass was completely enucleated via a transcanal approach. The lesion was broadly attached to the anteroinferior surface of the external auditory canal but did not involve the bony canal or the tragal cartilage. Minimal bleeding was encountered which was controlled with simple pressure. No skin closure was needed for the resultant defect of less than 10 mm diameter. Bacitracin ointment was applied to the wound. After excision, the bluish smooth cystic lesion was opened and dark brown liquid was seen emanating from the lumen (Figure 3).

Histopathological examination showed skin with multiple small dermal cysts ranging from 2 to 5 millimeters, with scattered normal sweat glands present between the cysts (Figure 4). On higher magnification, the cysts are

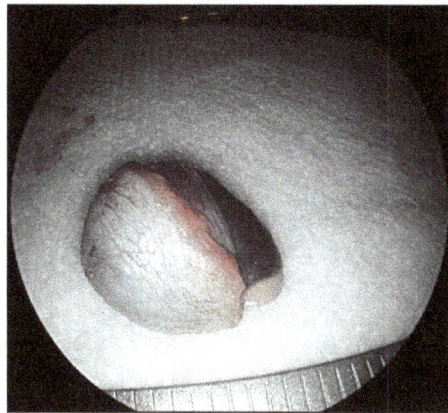

FIGURE 3: A bluish smooth cystic lesion is excised with some overlying skin. The lesion contains brown liquid.

lined by a flattened cuboidal double-layered epithelium. Apocrine features, such as columnar cell epithelium with dense eosinophilic cytoplasm and decapitation secretion, are not identified (Figure 5). The histologic features are consistent with an eccrine hidrocystoma.

The patient did well postoperatively with no complications. A postoperative audiogram revealed stable hearing and normal tympanometry (type A) bilaterally. The wound site epithelialized well and the surgical site healed without scarring or stenosis. The lesion did not recur during the 12-month follow-up period. The patient was now able to use her hearing aids without difficulty.

3. Discussion

Hidrocystomas of the external ear canal are rare, benign cystic lesions and are generally categorized as apocrine or eccrine [3, 5]. They usually present as papular or nodular firm cystic lesions with a smooth surface and bluish appearance. The clinical presentation can be variable and is dependent

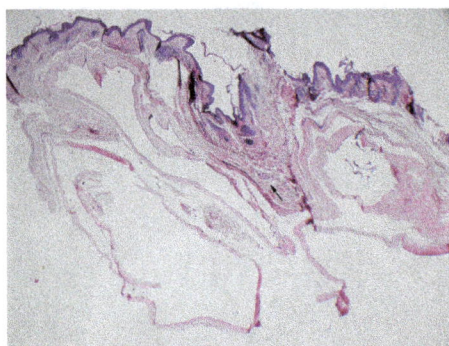

FIGURE 4: Histopathologic examination shows external auditory canal skin with multiple dermal cysts. A focus of normal sweat glands is present between the cysts in the middle of the photomicrograph (arrow). *Hematoxylin and eosin stain, 20x.*

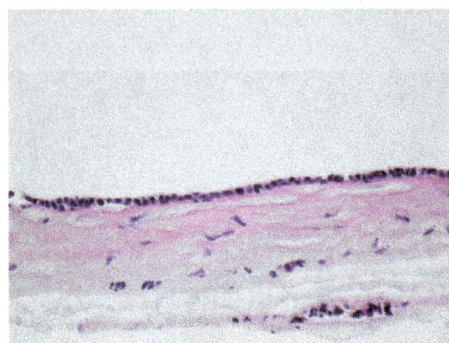

FIGURE 5: Close-up of a cyst wall demonstrates a cuboidal double-layered epithelium, consistent with an eccrine hidrocystoma. *Hematoxylin and eosin stain, 400x.*

on the lesion's anatomic location and impact on surrounding structures. These masses can obstruct the lumen of the ear canal, interfere with hearing aid use, and may be mistaken for basal cell carcinomas or cholesterol granulomas but can be easily differentiated from the others by examining their histopathologic features. As in a cholesterol granuloma, the bluish hue is an optical illusion. The cystic space of an eccrine hidrocystoma contains either clear or brown fluid. The presence of multiple hidrocystomas may be associated with focal dermal hypoplasia, a genetic disorder, formerly referred to as Jessner-Cole syndrome or Goltz-Gorlin syndrome. Our patient had a solitary hidrocystoma.

Eccrine hidrocystomas are characterized by the presence of cysts lined with attenuated double-layered epithelium which lack features of apocrine cell differentiation, such as decapitation secretion and tall columnar cells with eosinophilic cytoplasm. Scattered benign sweat glands are often found admixed with the cystic glands. Some authors suggest that eccrine hidrocystomas may actually be of apocrine type, with the typical apocrine features attenuated due to the intraluminal pressure of the cyst fluid [6].

Surgical excision is the treatment of choice. In patients with multiple hidrocystomas, or lesions that are not easily

accessible to surgery, alternative treatments exist, such as topical atropine, scopolamine cream, botulinum toxin injection, or CO_2 laser ablation [7]. The choice of surgical approach is largely dictated by the tumor location and relationship to surrounding structures. For lesions limited to the external auditory canal, without involvement of the tympanic membrane or mastoid, endoscopic transcanal approaches are becoming increasingly popular. The advantage of an endoscopic approach is superior visualization of the tumor due to the wide-angle view provided by the Hopkins rod endoscope. In our patient, the mass was completely surgically excised with endoscopic assistance, and the patency of the EAC was maintained without any surgical complications or recurrences.

4. Conclusion

While hidrocystomas are generally uncommon cystic lesions of the sweat glands, it is quite rare to find an eccrine hidrocystoma originating from the skin of the external auditory canal. The slow growing nature and smooth, solitary, cystic appearance, in addition to the bluish tint, can provide valuable diagnostic clues [3]. Complete excision with no margins is curative and can be done via a transcanal endoscopic approach.

Consent

Written informed consent was obtained from the patient for publication of this report and images. A copy of the written consent is available for review upon request.

Competing Interests

There are no competing interests to report for any of the three authors.

Authors' Contributions

Taha Mur participated in choosing the study design, reviewed the literature, wrote the manuscript, and edited the manuscript. Ronald Miick is the pathologist who reviewed the pathology slides, reviewed the literature, wrote the histopathology related parts of the manuscript, and edited the manuscript. Natasha Pollak is the senior author who cared for the patient. She chose the study design, reviewed the literature, wrote parts of the manuscript, and edited the entire manuscript.

References

[1] M. Stoeckelhuber, C. Matthias, M. Andratschke et al., "Human ceruminous gland: ultrastructure and histochemical analysis of antimicrobial and cytoskeletal components," *Anatomical Record—Part A Discoveries in Molecular, Cellular, and Evolutionary Biology*, vol. 288, no. 8, pp. 877–884, 2006.

[2] N. A. Obaidat and D. M. Ghazarian, "Bilateral multiple axillary apocrine hidrocystomas associated with benign apocrine

hyperplasia," *Journal of Clinical Pathology*, vol. 59, no. 7, p. 779, 2006.

[3] K. Sarabi and A. Khachemoune, "Hidrocystomas—a brief review," *MedGenMed Medscape General Medicine*, vol. 8, no. 3, article 57, 2006.

[4] M. Haro-García, T. Corzón-Pereira, J. M. Morales-Puebla, and T. Figueroa-García, "Eccrine hidrocystoma of the external auditory canal," *Acta Otorrinolaringologica Espanola*, vol. 66, no. 4, pp. 241–242, 2015.

[5] D. G. Ioannidis, E. I. Drivas, C. E. Papadakis, A. Feritsian, J. G. Bizakis, and C. E. Skoulakis, "Hidrocystoma of the external auditory canal: a case report," *Cases Journal*, vol. 2, no. 1, article 79, 2009.

[6] D. Weedon, *Weedon's Skin Pathology*, Elsevier, Philadelphia, Pa, USA, 3rd edition, 2010.

[7] M. R. Lee and W. Ryman, "Multiple eccrine hidrocystomas," *Australasian Journal of Dermatology*, vol. 45, no. 3, pp. 178–180, 2004.

22

Bilateral Non-Hodgkin's Lymphoma of the Temporal Bone: A Rare and Unusual Presentation

Sanjay Vaid,[1] Jyoti Jadhav,[1] Aparna Chandorkar,[1] and Neelam Vaid[2]

[1]Head and Neck Imaging Division, Star Imaging and Research Center, Pune 411001, India
[2]Department of Otorhinolaryngology, KEM Hospital, Pune 411011, India

Correspondence should be addressed to Sanjay Vaid; svaidhn@gmail.com

Academic Editor: Abrão Rapoport

Primary lymphoma of the temporal bone is an unusual finding in clinical practice and bilateral affection is even more rare. To the best of our knowledge, there are no reports of bilateral primary temporal bone lymphoma without middle ear involvement in the English medical literature so far. We report, for the first time, a case of primary lymphoma involving both temporal bones which presented with left-sided infranuclear facial palsy. A combination of contrast enhanced magnetic resonance imaging (MRI) and high resolution computed tomography (HRCT) was used to characterize and to map the extent of the lesion, as well as to identify the exact site of facial nerve affection. An excision biopsy and immunohistochemistry revealed diffuse large B-cell non-Hodgkin's lymphoma (DLBCL). Whole body fluorodeoxyglucose (FDG) positron emission tomography-computed tomography study (PET-CT) was performed to stage the disease. The patient was treated with chemotherapy and radiation therapy and is now on regular follow-up. The patient is alive and asymptomatic without disease progression for the last twenty months after initial diagnosis.

1. Introduction

Malignancies of the temporal bone are rare with an incidence of less than 0.2% [1, 2] amongst all head and neck cancers. Non-Hodgkin's lymphoma (NHL) is the second most common malignancy found in the head and neck region after squamous cell carcinoma [3, 4]. Involvement of the temporal bone as part of generalized lymphoma has been reported [5, 6]; however, primary involvement of temporal bone without systemic involvement is extremely rare [7]. High resolution multiplanar CT and MRI were useful in demonstrating the local infiltration into overlying soft tissues as well as extension to intracranial compartment. Facial nerve entrapment within the extracranial soft tissue was also well demonstrated using the imaging modalities. Early diagnosis made after an excision biopsy and immunohistochemistry work-up enabled prompt initiation of chemotherapy followed by radiation therapy. Follow-up imaging (MRI and PET-CT) revealed significant regression of the pathology.

2. Case Presentation

A 50-year-old male presented to the Department of Otorhinolaryngology with left facial asymmetry of two months duration. Clinical examination revealed an infranuclear facial palsy on left side with associated bilateral postauricular and occipital region scalp swellings. The scalp swellings were firm and nontender and margins could not be well identified. No neck nodes were palpable on clinical examination. Routine laboratory investigations were within normal limits. The patient was referred to the Department of Imaging to identify the cause of the facial palsy and determine extent of the scalp swellings. A noncontrast HRCT scan of the temporal bones and a contrast enhanced MRI scan of the temporal bones/brain was performed. HRCT of the temporal bones showed extensive irregular permeative osteolytic destruction of the right temporal bone and adjacent right occipital bone. Similar lesions were also noted involving the base of the left temporal bone (Figures 1(a) and 1(b)). HRCT also revealed

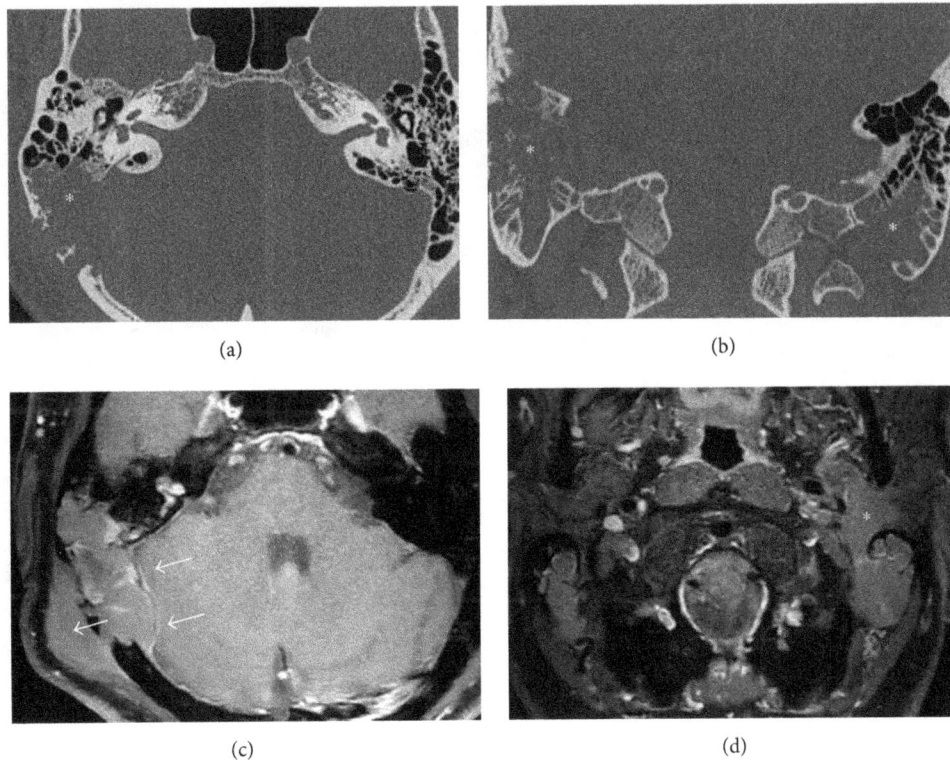

FIGURE 1: Axial (a) and coronal (b) HRCT images reveal extensive permeative destructive lesions involving both temporal bones (white asterisks). Axial postcontrast fat suppressed T1W axial (c) and coronal (d) images reveal postcontrast enhancement of large associated subgaleal and extracranial intradural soft tissue mass (arrows) on the right side and a moderately large lobulated soft tissue mass along undersurface of left temporal bone (asterisk) causing compression of the extracranial segment of left facial nerve.

soft tissue opacification of the mastoid air cells on both sides with erosion of the intercellular septae. Internal and external bony cortical erosions were seen on both sides with erosion of the descending mastoid segment of the left facial nerve canal. The middle and inner ear structures were normal on both sides. MRI scan showed diffuse signal alteration in both temporal bones with associated lobulated, extradural, and subgaleal enhancing soft tissue lesions (Figures 1(c) and 1(d)). The lesions were hypointense on both T1 weighted and T2 weighted images with heterogeneous postcontrast enhancement and showed restricted diffusion on diffusion weighted images (DWI). No calcification or hemorrhagic foci were noted. On the left side, the soft tissue was seen extending along the styloid process into the stylomandibular tunnel up to the deep lobe of parotid gland, involving the extracranial segment of the left facial nerve below the level of stylomastoid foramen. There was no enhancement of the facial nerve seen within the left temporal bone or left internal auditory canal. This finding ruled out retrograde perineural spread of the pathology. On the right side, the intracranial extradural enhancing soft tissue component was seen extending into the middle and posterior cranial fossa. Subgaleal extension of the soft tissue was seen through a defect in the right occipital bone. There was no significant cervical lymph node enlargement detected on the MRI scan. Based on the age of the patient, the clinical presentation, and examination as well as the imaging findings the differential diagnosis included

multiple myeloma, metastases, and lymphoma. The clinical presentation and imaging findings were not suggestive of an infective aetiology and hence this diagnosis was not considered.

An excision biopsy of the right subgaleal swelling was performed. Microscopy showed sheets of medium to large lymphoid cells with hyperchromatic nuclei and scanty cytoplasm (Figures 2(a)–2(d)). These cells stained positive for CD3 (Figure 2(e)), CD20 (Figure 2(f)), Ki67 (Figure 2(g)), LCA1, (Figure 2(h)), and LCA 2 (Figure 2(i)) and negative for CyclinD1 (clone Polyclonal), CD5 (Clone 4C7), and CD138 (clone MI-15). The tumor was also positive for Mum-1 and Bcl6 and negative for EBVLMP-1. The above results are suggestive of diffuse large B-cell non-Hodgkin's lymphoma (DLBCL), activated B-cell phenotype. Other blood and bone marrow investigations did not reveal any abnormality.

A whole body fluorodeoxyglucose (FDG) positron emission tomography-computed tomography study (PET-CT) was performed for staging purposes. The PET-CT scan revealed FDG-avid lesions (SUV max. 3.6) in both mastoids, in the extradural soft tissue mass on the right side and extracranial mass along left styloid process (Figures 3(a) and 3(b)). No other FDG-avid lesions were detected in the rest of the body (Figure 3(c)). This confirmed a primary extranodal involvement of the temporal bones by DLBCL.

The patient was treated with six cycles R+CHOP chemotherapy (one cycle of 21 days). This consisted of

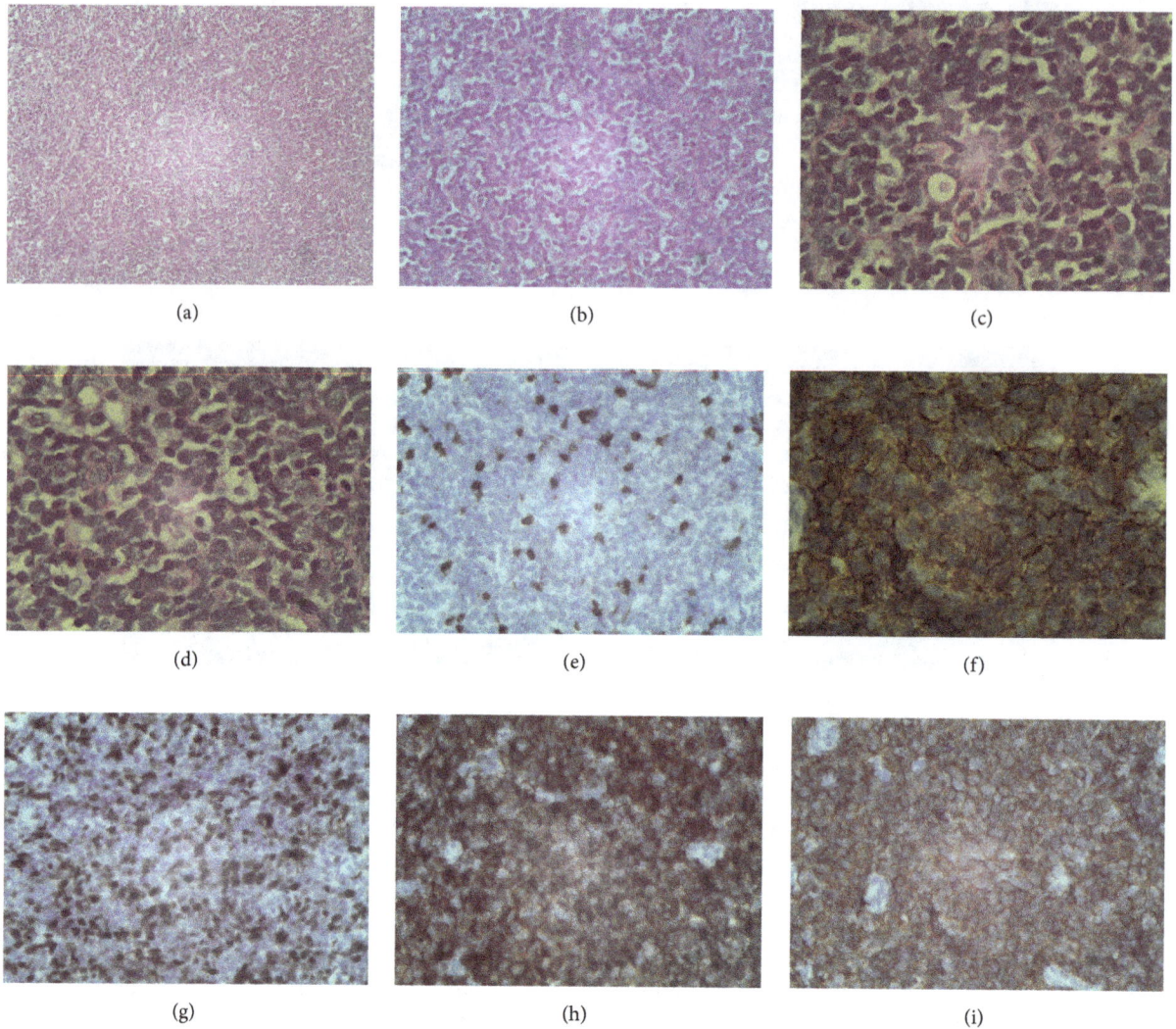

FIGURE 2: Microscopy showing sheets of medium to large lymphoid cells with hyperchromatic nuclei and scanty cytoplasm (a–d). The cells stained positive for CD3 (e), CD20 (f), Ki67 (g), LCA1 (h), and LCA2 (i).

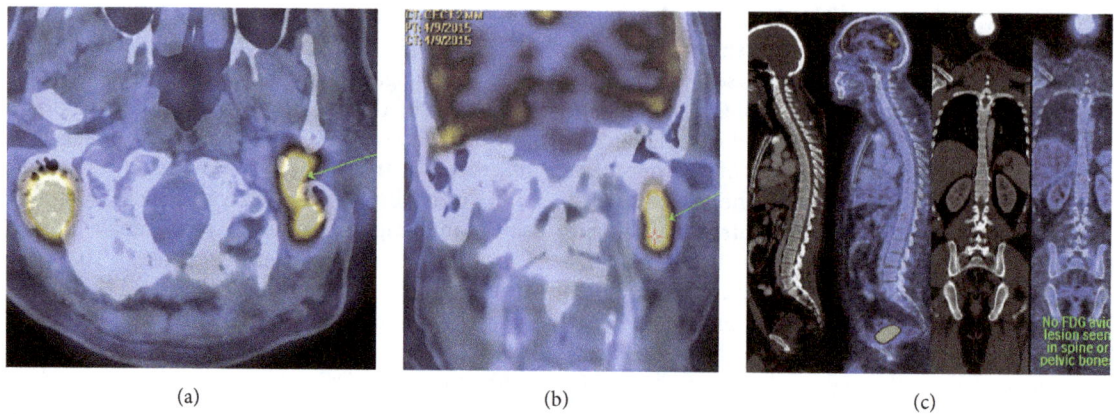

FIGURE 3: Whole body PET-CT scan revealed FDG-avid lesions (SUV max. 3.6) in both mastoids and along left styloid process (a, b). No other FDG-avid lesions were detected in the rest of the body (c).

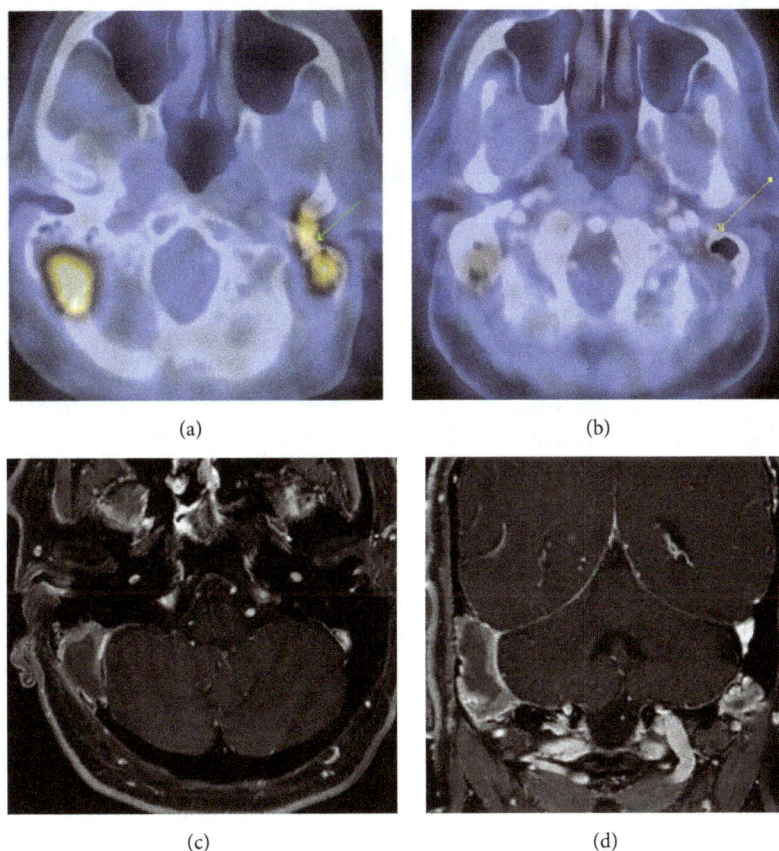

FIGURE 4: Posttherapy PET-CT scan (a, b) showing significant resolution in the metabolic activity of the mastoid lesions. Contrast enhanced MRI scan (c, d) also showed regression in the size of the enhancing soft tissue masses on both sides.

rituximab at $375 \, \text{mg/m}^2$, cyclophosphamide at $750 \, \text{mg/m}^2$, doxorubicin at $50 \, \text{mg/m}^2$, vincristine at $1.4 \, \text{mg/m}^2$, and prednisolone at $100 \, \text{mg/m}^2$. This was supplemented by prophylactic intrathecal methotrexate at 12.5 mg on day 2 of each cycle and G-CSF (granulocyte colony stimulating factor) at $300 \, \mu\text{gm}$ from day 3 to day 7 of each cycle. After six cycles of chemotherapy, patient was treated with six cycles of radiotherapy (45 Gy, 20 fractions). A PET-CT scan was performed three months after the end of radiation therapy which showed significant resolution in the metabolic activity of the mastoid lesions. (Figures 4(a) and 4(b)). The repeat MRI scan also showed regression in the size of the enhancing soft tissue masses on both sides (Figures 4(c) and 4(d)).

Patient also showed signs of clinical improvement and has been placed on routine surveillance protocol which includes a follow-up visit to the Oncology outpatient department once every 6 months for the first 2 years and then once every one year for next 3 years. At the time of the visit the patient will undergo a whole body FDG PET-CT scan, a 2D Echocardiogram (to look for cardiotoxic side effects of Adriamycin), and routine laboratory investigations. Till date the patient is in clinical remission as documented on the last outpatient department visit. The patient is alive and asymptomatic without disease progression for the last twenty months after initial diagnosis, without any evidence of local or systemic recurrence.

3. Discussion

Lymphoma, malignant monoclonal proliferation of lymphoid cells, is the second most frequent malignant tumor (incidence 2.5%) in the head and neck region [8, 9]. Most primary lymphomas of the head and neck are of the NHL variety and are generally extranodal in location at initial presentation occurring most commonly in the nasopharynx, lacrimal sac, and the temporal bone [10]. Primary lymphoma of the temporal bone involves the mastoid, middle ear most commonly, and the external/internal auditory canals to a lesser degree [6]. A layer of lymphoid tissue located deep to the epithelium of the mucosa lining the mastoid antrum, tympanic cavity, and tympanic orifice of the eustachian tube acts as the site of origin of the primary lymphoma. Bilateral affection by primary B-cell NHL involving mastoids without middle ear cavity affection is extremely uncommon and to the best of our knowledge the imaging features of this entity have not been reported in medical literature. Osteolytic permeative lesions involving temporal bones should be viewed with a high degree of suspicion for malignancy as similar appearances in adults can be seen with multiple myeloma, metastatic pathology, and aggressive infective pathologies like fulminant coalescent mastoiditis (especially in diabetic patients) and mycosis fungoides [11]. Differentiation based on clinical presentation may be difficult at times as patients present with similar complaints like ear pain, swelling in pre- and postauricular regions, and facial palsy [12–14]. Facial nerve palsy is rare in lymphoma because the nerve sheath is resistant to tumor invasion. Nerve palsy occurs when the bony facial canal is destroyed by the tumor and nerve fibers are infiltrated by the tumor cells [15]. Affection of the facial nerve by the tumor is usually seen in the region of the geniculate ganglion [14]. In this particular case, the left facial nerve infranuclear palsy was due to erosion of the bony descending mastoid segment of the left intratemporal facial nerve canal and direct nerve involvement by the tumor mass at and distal to the stylomastoid foramen. HRCT and contrast enhanced MRI scans are essential for a comprehensive evaluation of malignancies affecting the temporal bone. HRCT depicts bony details including type of bone destruction, status of middle ear cavity involvement, ossicular chain evaluation, integrity of the tegmen tympani, and exact site/extent of the intratemporal bony facial canal involvement. MRI is useful in identifying leptomeningeal and brain parenchymal invasion as well as mapping the entire extent of extracranial soft tissue involvement. Contrast enhanced MRI scans also provide information about perineural spread on the facial nerve [16]. PET-CT is essential to stage the disease, document pathology elsewhere in the body, and assess response to therapy. Biopsy and immunohistochemistry help in planning a cell targeted chemotherapeutic regime.

4. Conclusion

Our case report highlights the need to have a high degree of suspicion for malignancy even in bilateral temporal bone pathologies (which are more commonly seen in infective conditions). Primary lymphoma of the temporal bone, though rare, should be considered in the differential diagnosis of patients presenting with ear related symptoms and associated facial nerve palsy especially in the elder age group. HRCT and contrast enhanced MRI are essential to comprehensively evaluate such cases in order to effectively plan further management. As there may not be specific imaging criteria to make a definitive diagnosis, this can only be confirmed by histopathology and immunohistochemistry. PET-CT is useful in staging the disease and scrupulous surveillance is needed to monitor response to therapy and to identify early signs of tumor recurrence.

Competing Interests

The authors have no competing interests.

Acknowledgments

The authors wish to acknowledge Mr. Rishabh Vaid, SKN Medical College, Pune, India, for his help in literature search and manuscript editing.

References

[1] W. I. Kuhel, C. R. Hume, and S. H. Selesnick, "Cancer of the external auditory canal and temporal bone," *Otolaryngologic Clinics of North America*, vol. 29, no. 5, pp. 827–852, 1996.

[2] S. A. Moody, B. E. Hirsch, and E. N. Myers, "Squamous cell carcinoma of the external auditory canal: an evaluation of a staging system," *American Journal of Otology*, vol. 21, no. 4, pp. 582–588, 2000.

[3] J. Y. Suen and E. N. Myers, *Cancer of the Head and Neck*, Churchill Livingstone, New York, NY, USA, 1981.

[4] J. G. Batsakis, *Tumors of the Head and Neck: Clinical and Pathological Considerations*, Williams & Wilkins, Baltimore, Md, USA, 2nd edition, 1979.

[5] J. T. Fierstein and S. E. Thawley, "Lymphoma of the head and neck," *Laryngoscope*, vol. 88, no. 4, pp. 582–593, 1978.

[6] S. P. Hersh, W. G. Harrison, and D. J. Hersh, "Primary B cell lymphoma of the external auditory canal," *Ear, Nose and Throat Journal*, vol. 85, no. 9, pp. 597–599, 2006.

[7] S. Ogawa, I. Tawara, S. Ueno et al., "De novo CD5-positive diffuse large B-cell lymphoma of the temporal bone presenting with an external auditory canal tumor," *Internal Medicine*, vol. 45, no. 11, pp. 733–737, 2006.

[8] C. A. DePena, P. Van Tassel, and Y.-Y. Lee, "Lymphoma of the head and neck," *Radiologic Clinics of North America*, vol. 28, no. 4, pp. 723–743, 1990.

[9] P. Merkus, M. P. Copper, M. H. J. Van Oers, and P. F. Schouwenburg, "Lymphoma in the ear," *ORL*, vol. 62, no. 5, pp. 274–277, 2000.

[10] R. C. Jordan and P. M. Speight, "Extranodal non-Hodgkin's lymphomas of the oral cavity," *Current Topics in Pathology*, vol. 90, pp. 125–146, 1996.

[11] M. L. Paige and J. R. Bernstein, "Transcalvarial primary lymphoma of bone. A report of two cases," *Neuroradiology*, vol. 37, no. 6, pp. 456–458, 1995.

[12] J. Baar, R. L. Burkes, R. Bell, M. E. Blackstein, B. Fernandes, and F. Langer, "Primary non-Hodgkin's lymphoma of bone. A clinicopathologic study," *Cancer*, vol. 73, no. 4, pp. 1194–1199, 1994.

[13] U. Bockmuhl, K.-L. Bruchhage, and H. Enzmann, "Primary non-Hodgkin's lymphoma of the temporal bone," *European Archives of Oto-Rhino-Laryngology*, vol. 252, no. 6, pp. 376–378, 1995.

[14] D. L. Tucci, P. R. Lambert, and D. J. Innes Jr., "Primary lymphoma of the temporal bone," *Archives of Otolaryngology—Head and Neck Surgery*, vol. 118, no. 1, pp. 83–85, 1992.

[15] H. Saito, K. Chinzei, and M. Furuta, "Pathological features of peripheral facial paralysis caused by malignant tumour," *Acta Oto-Laryngologica. Supplementum*, vol. 446, pp. 165–171, 1988.

[16] W. R. Nemzek, S. Hecht, R. Gandour-Edwards, P. Donald, and K. McKennan, "Perineural spread of head and neck tumors: how accurate is MR imaging?" *American Journal of Neuroradiology*, vol. 19, no. 4, pp. 701–706, 1998.

23

Lymphoepithelial Cyst in the Palatine Tonsil

Fatih Bingöl,[1] **Hilal Balta,**[2] **Buket Özel Bingöl,**[1]
Recai Muhammet Mazlumoğlu,[3] **and Korhan Kılıç**[1]

[1]*Erzurum Research and Training Hospital, Department of Otorhinolaryngology, Erzurum, Turkey*
[2]*Erzurum Research and Training Hospital, Department of Pathology, Erzurum, Turkey*
[3]*Palandöken State Hospital, Department of Otorhinolaryngology, Erzurum, Turkey*

Correspondence should be addressed to Fatih Bingöl; drfbingol@gmail.com

Academic Editor: Abrão Rapoport

Lymphoepithelial cyst (LEC) is the most commonly encountered congenital neck pathology in the lateral part of the neck. A 66-year-old woman presented to the ENT clinic due to difficulty in swallowing persisting for approximately 1 year. Magnetic resonance imaging revealed a cystic mass at right tonsil. Surgery was performed due to this unilateral tonsillar mass, which was excised together with the right tonsil. LEC was diagnosed at histopathological examination. LEC in the palatine tonsil is rare, and only a few cases have been reported in the literature. We report a rare case of LEC in the palatine tonsil.

1. Introduction

Lymphoepithelial cyst (LEC), otherwise known as the branchial cleft cyst, is the most commonly encountered congenital neck pathology in the lateral part of the neck [1]. Branchial structures which develop at the 3rd to 7th weeks of life consist of the mesodermal arches and external clefts and the internal pounces separating these two structures [2]. If these clefts are not obliterated, they emerge as branchial cysts in the postnatal period. If the outer ends of the branchial clefts are not closed and open into this cyst, this is known as branchial sinus. If the ends of both the branchial pouches and the branchial clefts are not closed and are interconnected, the result is a branchial fistula connecting the skin and the fossa tonsillaris or pharynx [3].

Branchial cysts are divided into four types depending on their anatomical location. First branchial cleft cysts occur in the region of the ear. Second branchial cleft cysts are the most common type, at a level of 95%, and occur in the lateral part of the neck anteriorly to the sternocleidomastoideus muscle. Third branchial cleft cysts connected to the pharynx lie deep inside the carotid artery system. Fourth branchial cleft cysts appear in the thyroid region, generally on the left side [3].

In addition to the neck, LECs may rarely be observed in the oral cavity in the tongue, nasogenian sulcus, the floor of

the mouth, the soft palate, or the retromolar region [4, 5]. LEC in the palatine tonsil is rare, and only a few cases have been reported in the literature [6]. We report a case of LEC in the palatine tonsil.

2. Case Presentation

A 66-year-old woman presented to the ENT clinic due to difficulty in swallowing persisting for approximately 1 year. At ENT examination the right tonsil was hypertrophic and the inferior pole was bilobulated. A mass with the density of soft tissue obstructing the oropharyngeal air column at the level of the inferior lobe of the tonsillar palatine was observed at magnetic resonance imaging (MRI) (Figure 1). A cystic mass, hypointense on T1 images and hyperintense on T2, was observed inside the right tonsil at MRI. Surgery was performed due to this unilateral tonsillar mass, which was excised together with the right tonsil. A lesion in which diffuse nonkeratinized epithelial cells were observed in the lumen of the cystic space was observed on histopathological sections. The cyst wall was lined with a stratified squamous epithelium surrounding the stroma consisting of lymphoid follicle structures with germinal centers. Fibroconnective tissue, adipose tissue, vascular structures, seromucous glands, and muscle tissue at the most external part were also observed

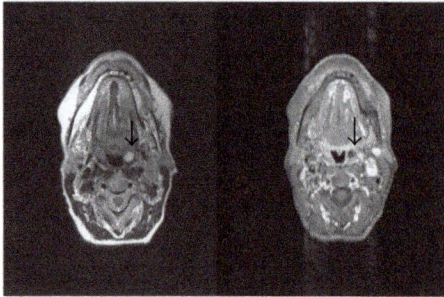

FIGURE 1: A cystic mass (black arrow) hypointense on T1 images and hyperintense on T2 was observed inside the right tonsil at magnetic resonance imaging (MRI).

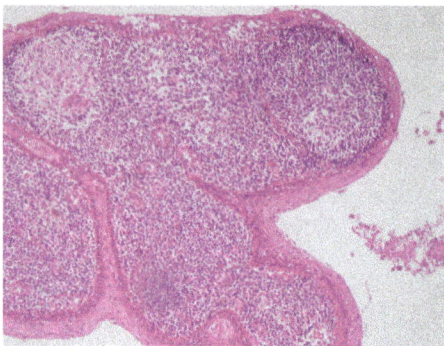

FIGURE 2: The cyst wall was lined with a stratified squamous epithelium surrounding the stroma consisting of lymphoid follicle structures with germinal centers. Fibroconnective tissue, adipose tissue, vascular structures, seromucous glands, and muscle tissue at the most external part were also observed in the stroma (H&E ×20).

in the stroma (Figure 2). LEC was diagnosed at histopathological examination.

3. Discussion

LEC is the most common congenital head and neck lesion after thyroglossal cyst. LECs occur due to the incomplete closure of embryological branchial clefts. Second LEC, the most common form (95%), is localized along the anterior margin of the sternocleidomastoid (SCM) muscle. First arch branchial cysts constitute 1–4% of cases, while third and fourth arch clefts are very rare [7]. Various theories have been proposed to account for the pathogenesis of LEC. Bhaskar and Bernier attributed LEC to proliferation of glandular epithelial cell. In contrast, Knapp suggested that these cysts in the oral cavity, more properly described as pseudocysts, derive from submucosal lymphoid aggregates in the sublingual region, the anterior lingual surface, and the soft palate, rather than from lymph nodes. Giunta and Cataldo suggested that LECs may be caused by obstruction of a tonsillar crypt, leading to an expanded space lined by epithelium communicating with the external environment and with keratin and desquamated cells observed in the lumen [6].

They are generally detected in late adulthood but are very rare at advanced age. LEC becomes conspicuous as a painless,

fluctuating neck mass. Rapid growth or pain may be present in the branchial cyst in association with upper respiratory tract infection. Differential diagnosis is diverse, and cystic hygroma, hemangioma, and metastasis should be considered [8].

Ultrasonography (USG) is the imaging technique of choice in lesions of a cystic nature. LEC appears with a hypo- or anechoic thin wall with well-determined margins at USG. At CT they are hypodense, thin-walled lesions. At MRI, they appear hypointense on T1 weighted sequences and hyperintense on T2 weighted sequences [9].

In addition to the neck, LECs may rarely be observed in the oral cavity in the tongue, in the floor of the mouth in the soft palate or in the retromolar region. A few case reports have been published of LEC in the tonsillar region. As with cervical branchial cysts, the therapeutic option in oral LECs is total excision. Injection of sclerosing material may be an alternative to surgical excision in the treatment of LECs [10].

4. Conclusions

Since LECs are more common at pediatric age group, they can be observed at any ages. Our patient was sixty-six years old. Although LECs usually occur in the neck, they can be seen in the oral cavity. While evaluating the tonsillar masses LECs should be kept in mind.

Competing Interests

The authors declare that they have no competing interests.

References

[1] S. Muller, A. Aiken, K. Magliocca, and A. Y. Chen, "Second branchial cleft cyst," Head and Neck Pathology, vol. 9, no. 3, pp. 379–383, 2014.

[2] J. H. T. Waldhausen, "Branchial cleft and arch anomalies in children," Seminars in Pediatric Surgery, vol. 15, no. 2, pp. 64–69, 2006.

[3] Y. Bajaj, S. Ifeacho, D. Tweedie et al., "Branchial anomalies in children," International Journal of Pediatric Otorhinolaryngology, vol. 75, no. 8, pp. 1020–1023, 2011.

[4] D. McDonnell, "Spontaneous regression of a yellow sublingual swelling: a case report," Pediatric dentistry, vol. 12, no. 6, pp. 388–389, 1990.

[5] C. Hupin, B. Weynand, and P. Rombaux, "Lymphoepithelial cyst of the nasogenian sulcus: a case report," B-ENT, vol. 6, no. 1, pp. 49–51, 2010.

[6] J. G. L. Castro, G. M. Ferreira, E. F. Mendonça, and L. A. de Castro, "A rare occurrence of lymphoepithelial cyst in the palatine tonsil: a case report and discussion of the etiopathogenesis," International Journal of Clinical and Experimental Pathology, vol. 8, no. 4, pp. 4264–4268, 2015.

[7] A. Adams, K. Mankad, C. Offiah, and L. Childs, "Branchial cleft anomalies: a pictorial review of embryological development and spectrum of imaging findings," Insights into Imaging, vol. 7, no. 1, pp. 69–76, 2016.

[8] C. Hart, D. A. Opperman, E. Gulbahce, and G. Adams, "Branchial cleft cyst: a rare diagnosis in a 91-year-old patient," Otolaryngology—Head and Neck Surgery, vol. 135, no. 6, pp. 955–957, 2006.

[9] M. Valentino, C. Quiligotti, and L. Carone, "Branchial cleft cyst,"
     Journal of Ultrasound, vol. 16, no. 1, pp. 17–20, 2013.

[10] M.-G. Kim, N.-H. Lee, J.-H. Ban, K.-C. Lee, S.-M. Jin, and S.-
     H. Lee, "Sclerotherapy of branchial cleft cysts using OK-432,"
     Otolaryngology—Head and Neck Surgery, vol. 141, no. 3, pp. 329–
     334, 2009.

24

Internal Jugular and Subclavian Vein Thrombosis in a Case of Ovarian Cancer

Hiroto Moriwaki,[1] Nana Hayama,[1] Shouko Morozumi,[1] Mika Nakano,[1] Akari Nakayama,[1] Yoshiomi Takahata,[1] Yuusuke Sakaguchi,[1] Natsuki Inoue,[1] Toshiki Kubota,[1] Akiko Takenoya,[1] Yoshiko Ishii,[1] Haruka Okubo,[1] Souta Yamaguchi,[1] Tsuyoshi Ono,[2] Toshiaki Oharaseki,[3] and Mamoru Yoshikawa[1]

[1]*Department of Otorhinolaryngology, Toho University Ohashi Medical Center, Tokyo, Japan*
[2]*Division of Cardiovascular Medicine, Toho University Ohashi Medical Center, Tokyo, Japan*
[3]*Department of Pathology, Toho University Ohashi Medical Center, Tokyo, Japan*

Correspondence should be addressed to Hiroto Moriwaki; hiroto.moriwaki@med.toho-u.ac.jp

Academic Editor: Nicolas Perez-Fernandez

Central venous catheter insertion and cancer represent some of the important predisposing factors for deep venous thrombosis (DVT). DVT usually develops in the lower extremities, and venous thrombosis of the upper extremities is uncommon. Early diagnosis and treatment of deep venous thrombosis are of importance, because it is a precursor of complications such as pulmonary embolism and postthrombotic syndrome. A 47-year-old woman visited our department with painful swelling on the left side of her neck. Initial examination revealed swelling of the region extending from the left neck to the shoulder without any redness of the overlying skin. Laboratory tests showed a white blood cell count of 5,800/mm^3 and an elevated serum C-reactive protein of 4.51 mg/dL. Computed tomography (CT) of the neck revealed a vascular filling defect in the left internal jugular vein to left subclavian vein region, with the venous lumina completely occluded with dense soft tissue. On the basis of the findings, we made the diagnosis of thrombosis of the left internal jugular and left subclavian veins. The patient was begun on treatment with oral rivaroxaban, but the left shoulder pain worsened. She was then admitted to the hospital and treated by balloon thrombectomy and thrombolytic therapy, which led to improvement of the left subclavian venous occlusion. Histopathologic examination of the removed thrombus revealed adenocarcinoma cells, indicating hematogenous dissemination of malignant cells.

1. Introduction

Cancer is the second cause of upper extremity deep venous thrombosis (UEDVT), only surpassed by central venous catheter (CVA) insertion [1]. Other predisposing factors include surgery, intravenous drug use, and infection; UEDVT has also been described as an acute complication of pharyngeal bacterial infection, known as Lemierre's syndrome. The percentage of patients with UEDVT among admitted patients with a CVC is relatively high [2], so that the disorder can be diagnosed without difficulty in patients having a CVC and presenting with neck swelling and/or pain. It is

of importance, however, to note that occasional cases are asymptomatic. Since it is difficult to immediately entertain the suspicion of UEDVT in patients without a CVC, interpretation of the symptoms and meticulous history taking are important to avoid overlooking the diagnosis. UEDVT, like lower-extremity venous thrombosis (LEDVT), can lead to complications such as pulmonary embolism (PE), sepsis with septic emboli, intracranial propagation of the thrombus with cerebral edema, and postthrombotic syndrome. PE reportedly occurs in 36% of patients with UEDVT [2]; therefore, the importance of prompt and appropriate treatment of UEDVT cannot be overemphasized.

Existence of a relationship between malignant disease and thromboembolic disorders has been known for a number of decades, having first been reported by Trousseau in 1865 [3]. Tumor cells express tissue factors that activate the clotting cascade, tumor procoagulants, fibrinolytic proteins and receptors for these factors, promoting interactions between the tumor cells, platelets and endothelial cells via cytokines, tumor antigens, and their immune complexes to facilitate thrombogenesis [4]. Phlebothrombosis is a known complication of cancer [5], and many published studies have reported cases in which the detection of venous thrombosis led to the diagnosis of cancer, even in patients without a history of malignancy [6]. Thus, in patients diagnosed as having DVT, systematic medical workup is necessary to identify any occult cancer. In cancer patients, death from DVT is second in frequency only to death from the tumor per se [7]. Therefore, it is of vital importance to effectively control DVT, as it influences the vital prognosis. We recently encountered a patient with left internal jugular and subclavian vein thrombosis that developed during anticancer chemotherapy following surgery for ovarian cancer and report the case herein.

2. Case Presentation

The patient, a 47-year-old woman, visited our hospital with a 2-day history of a painful swelling on the left side of her neck, which was of sudden onset.

On initial examination, a swelling, tender to palpation, involving the region extending from the left neck to the shoulder was noted, with no redness of the overlying skin. The patient was receiving postoperative periodic chemotherapy following total hysterectomy with bilateral adnexectomy and omentectomy performed elsewhere 2 years earlier for ovarian cancer. The patient was not obese (body mass index: 22.3 kg/m^2) and had no past history of central venous catheter insertion, ischemic disease, hypertension, diabetes, or hyperlipidemia. On initial examination, there were no abnormal findings in the oral cavity, and fiber-optic laryngoscopy did not reveal any evidence of inflammation, such as reddening or edema, nor was any tumor evident in the pharyngolaryngeal region. Hematologic examination showed the following: white blood cell count, 5,800/mm^3; hemoglobin, 11.8 g/dL; platelet count, 234,000/mm^3. The liver and kidney function test results were within normal limits, while the serum C-reactive protein was elevated to 4.51 mg/dL. Contrast-enhanced computed tomography (CT) of the neck, as part of the systematic medical workup, revealed a filling defect in the left internal jugular vein to left subclavian vein region, with the venous lumina filled with dense soft tissue. On the basis of the above findings, we diagnosed the patient as having thrombosis of the left internal jugular and left subclavian veins (Figures 1(a), 1(b), and 1(c)). With the diagnosis of UEDVT, blood coagulation tests were performed, which revealed that the prothrombin time, activated partial thromboplastin time, and antithrombin III levels were within normal limits, while the plasma d-dimer level was elevated to 1.5 g/mL (normal range: <1.0 g/mL). The patient was begun on treatment with oral rivaroxaban at the dose of 15 mg q.d. for the UEDVT on the 3rd hospital day. The left-sided neck

pain improved with the treatment; however, the left shoulder pain became worse on the 19th hospital day, at which time the plasma d-dimer level was found to have further increased to 3.9 g/mL. On the 27th hospital day, catheter thrombectomy was performed because of failure of the rivaroxaban therapy to provide sufficient benefit. Removal of the thrombus via an 8 Fr catheter inserted through the left brachial vein and left internal jugular vein dilation with a 6 mm balloon resulted in a 50% reduction of the complete left subclavian vein occlusion. As elevation of the left upper extremity led to reocclusion of the left subclavian vein (even though the blood flow in the left upper limb remained intact when the limb was not elevated), an infusion catheter was placed in the vein for 2-day thrombolytic therapy with urokinase at 480,000 units/day. Angiographic examination on the 29th hospital day showed a collapsed left internal jugular vein and appearance of a collateral circulatory pathway. The thrombus in the left subclavian vein was found to have diminished in size, and while the blood flow in the left subclavian vein was interrupted upon elevation of the left upper extremity, the flow in the vein had improved to such an extent that the vessel became reperfused and unoccluded when the left upper limb was hung down (Figures 2(a) and 2(b)). Histopathologic examination of the removed thrombus revealed the presence of adenocarcinoma cells that showed positive staining for cytokeratin (AE1/AE3), ER, and PgR expressions, indicating hematogenous dissemination of malignant cells (Figures 3(a), 3(b), and 3(c)). The patient was then discharged from the hospital on oral rivaroxaban at 15 mg q.d.

3. Discussion

DVT occurs more frequently in the lower extremities and is unusual in the upper extremities, the latter accounting for only about 4% to 10% of all cases of DVT [1]. As for the etiology of secondary UEDVT, CVC is the most common cause (70%), while more than about 40% of cases of secondary UEDVT are reported to be cancer-related. The disorder is of unknown cause in 20% of the cases [8]. According to a systematic review by Bleker et al., secondary UEDVT is CVC-related in 53% of cases and cancer-related in 44%; hence, CVC and cancer, accounting for most of the cases, represent the most important predisposing factors for secondary UEDVT [1]. One large cohort study conducted previously showed that tumors of the bone, ovary, brain, and pancreas were associated with the highest risk of DVT [9]. Girolami et al. reported that idiopathic UEDVT was more frequently associated with occult cancers as compared to LEDVT and that lung cancer and lymphomas represented the majority of cancers associated with UEDVT [10].

Other factors also reported as independent risk factors for the development of DVT are as follows (in decreasing order of the odds ratio): surgery, trauma, hospital or nursing home confinement, malignancy, venous catheter or pacemaker insertion, superficial venous thrombosis, and neurological disease with extremity paresis [11].

Venous thrombosis is a paraneoplastic syndrome, where stasis of the regional blood flow is prone to occur because of direct tumor invasion or compression of the blood vessels by

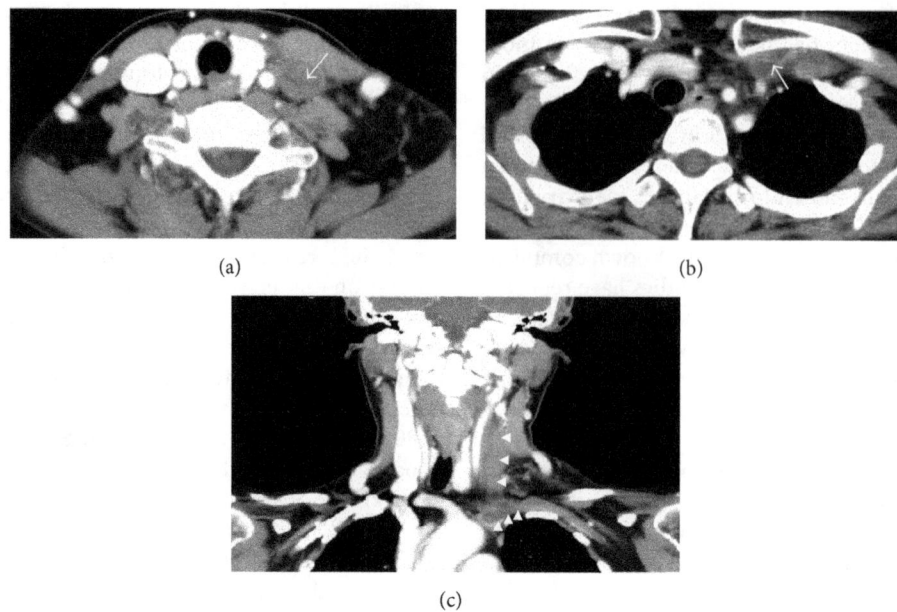

(a)

(b)

(c)

FIGURE 1: Axial enhanced CT image of soft tissue of the neck (a), the chest (b), and coronal enhanced CT image of soft tissue of the neck (c). There are filling defect in the left internal jugular vein (a) and subclavian vein (b), with the lumen filled with dense soft tissue (arrow). A vascular filling defect is noted in the region extending from the left internal jugular vein to the left subclavian vein, and the venous lumina are filled with dense soft tissue (arrowhead).

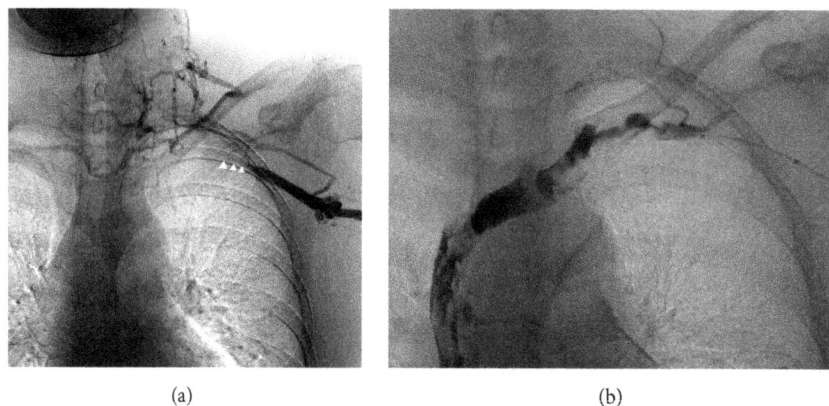

(a)

(b)

FIGURE 2: Left subclavian vein angiogram before (a) and after (b) dilation. Blood flow in the left subclavian vein to the left internal jugular vein is interrupted, while inflow of contrast medium is noted into the right subclavian vein via a collateral vessel (arrowhead in (a)). The left subclavian vein is visualized as a contrast-enhanced image after the balloon dilatation (b).

the tumor itself or by metastatic lymph nodes; in addition, hypercoagulability of the blood and vessel wall damage may also be involved. The hypercoagulable state may be attributed to the generation of clotting intermediates (e.g., tissue factor [TF], factor Xa, and thrombin), clotting or platelet function inhibitors (e.g., COX-2), or fibrinolysis inhibitors (e.g., plasminogen activator inhibitor, type 1 [PAI-1]) [12].

The risk of DVT is 4- to 7-fold greater in cases of malignancy and 6.5-fold higher in malignancy patients receiving chemotherapy as compared to that in those not receiving chemotherapy (4.1-fold higher) [9, 13]. The reported average incidence of recurrent DVT in cancer patients is 3.8% over a follow-up period of 3 to 13 months according to the results of a prospective study, with a 2- to 3-fold higher risk of recurrence

in cancer patients as compared to noncancer patients [1, 14, 15]. In cancer patients, the average mortality rate is 18% at 3 months after the onset of UEDVT and 47% at 1 year after the onset. The risk of mortality at 3 months after the onset of UEDVT in cancer patients is reportedly 8 times as high as that in noncancer patients; thus DVT associated with cancer poses a life-threatening problem [1, 14].

Several excellent guidelines for the treatment of DVT have been published in recent years [16, 17]. It is recommended in the American College of Chest Physicians (ACCP) guideline that treatment of UEDVT be conducted on the basis of the treatment rationale for LEDVT, observational studies, and the results of studies on understanding of the natural history of UEDVT, since there have been no randomized

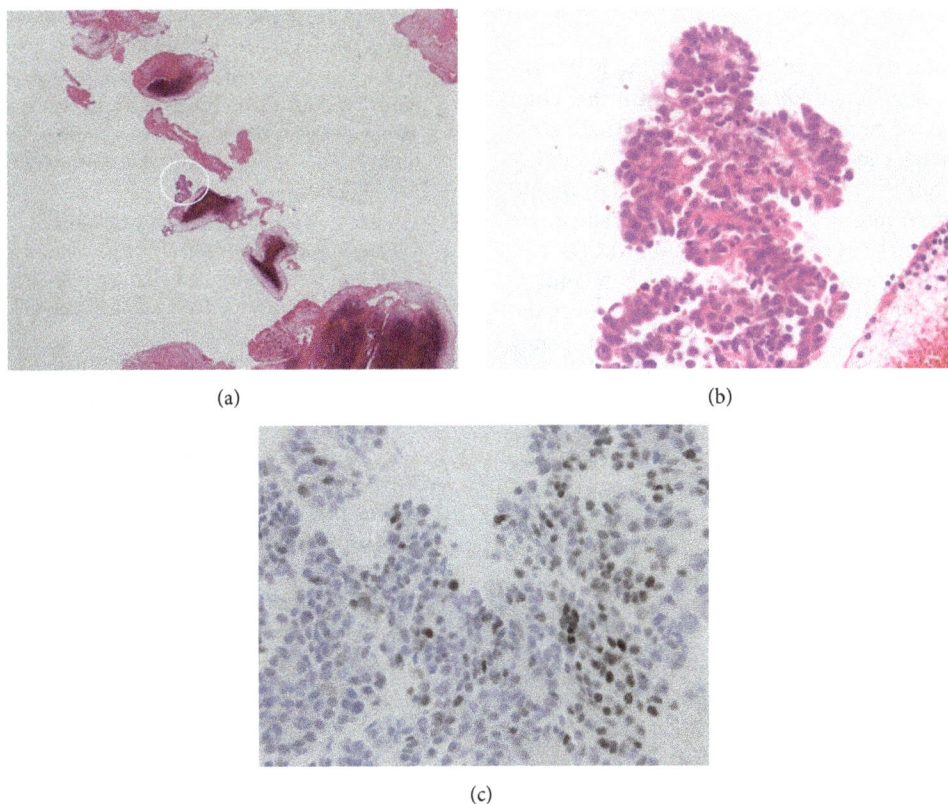

(a)

(b)

(c)

FIGURE 3: Histology of tumor cells in the blood clot (a)–(c). Tumor cells are seen in the blood clot (hematoxylin and eosin stain, ×100 (a)). Atypical cells with eosinophilic cytoplasm showing a high N/C ratio proliferating in a papillary pattern (hematoxylin and eosin stain, ×400 (b)). Note the positive (brownish) staining for estrogen receptors (Immunostaining for estrogen receptors (c)).

controlled trials for the treatment of UEDVT [16]. The ACCP guideline recommends initial parenteral anticoagulant therapy or initial anticoagulation with rivaroxaban in patients with acute DVT, and we prescribed oral rivaroxaban in our present case documented herein [16]. It has been shown that single-drug therapy with rivaroxaban yields similar efficacy to that of standard therapy for DVT consisting of low-molecular-weight heparin (LMWH) combined with a vitamin K antagonist (VKA) and that the risk of major bleeding in patients receiving rivaroxaban therapy is significantly lower as compared to that in patients receiving LMWH [18]. Ageno et al. also reported that rivaroxaban is a safe and effective alternative to standard anticoagulant therapy and is highly advantageous in that it can be managed even at the outpatient service, whereas the standard therapy requires hospitalization for laboratory monitoring and dose adjustment [19]. In the present case, the left shoulder pain became worse on day 17 of the oral medication (19th hospital day), associated with elevation of the plasma d-dimer level despite the ongoing rivaroxaban therapy, suggestive of aggravation of the DVT. Because of the apparent failure of the rivaroxaban therapy to provide sufficient efficacy, we performed catheter thrombectomy and balloon angioplasty. On account of the potential difficulty in balloon angioplasty of the left internal jugular vein in this case, we conducted the procedure on the left subclavian vein, whereby a 50%

reduction of the complete stenosis of the vein was achieved. However, mere elevation of the left upper extremity promptly resulted in reocclusion of the vessel, due in part to the rather extensive thrombosis. Since it is often the case that catheter thrombectomy and balloon angioplasty alone are insufficient to completely remove a venous thrombus, thrombolytic therapy was considered necessary as the next step of treatment in this case, and we decided to administer the thrombolytic therapy in consultation with the treating gynecologist. After placement of an infusion catheter, the patient was administered thrombolytic therapy for 2 days using urokinase, which resulted in reperfusion of the left subclavian vein, although angiography revealed interruption of the blood flow through the left internal jugular vein and inflow of contrast medium into the right subclavian vein via a collateral vessel. Pathologic examination of the removed thrombus revealed adenocarcinoma cells, suggestive of hematogenous dissemination from the ovarian cancer. Although needless to mention, it is ideal to accomplish radical cure of the primary disease in order to control the DVT; this was difficult to accomplish in the present case, because the patient already showed evidence of hematogenous tumor cell dissemination to the peritoneum. Therefore, as the risk of DVT recurrence is expected to persist, we propose to manage the patient with further continuation of the anticoagulant therapy as well as chemotherapy.

4. Conclusion

We recently encountered a case of UEDVT in a patient who presented to our outpatient service with the chief complaints of left-sided neck pain and swelling. There are a variety of disorders that can produce neck swelling, including inflammation and tumor. UEDVT is a rare disorder among outpatients without an inserted CVC, and its incidence rate is much lower (4% to 10%) as compared to that of LEDVT. It would presumably be difficult to promptly make a diagnostic differentiation of UEDVT from other disorders. However, the diagnosis of UEDVT should not be overlooked, as it may give rise to serious complications such as PE, and thus have a great impact on the vital prognosis. We thus recommend that otolaryngologists gain enough understanding of the close relationship between CVC insertion and cancer as risk factors for DVT. They must obtain a detailed history and perform careful clinical examination, keeping in mind the possibility of UEDVT, in cases with a CVC or cancer.

Disclosure

The authors disclose that this work has not been supported with any grants, drugs, or special equipment.

Competing Interests

All authors disclose no financial support or relationship that may pose a conflict of interests.

References

[1] S. M. Bleker, N. van Es, L. van Gils et al., "Clinical course of upper extremity deep vein thrombosis in patients with or without cancer: a systematic review," *Thrombosis Research*, vol. 140, supplement 1, pp. S81–S88, 2016.

[2] P. Prandoni, P. Polistena, E. Bernardi et al., "Upper-extremity deep vein thrombosis: risk factors, diagnosis, and complications," *Archives of Internal Medicine*, vol. 157, no. 1, pp. 57–62, 1997.

[3] A. Trousseau, "Phlegmasia alba dolens," *Clinique Médicale de l'Hôtel-Dieu de Paris. Paris*, vol. 3, pp. 654–712, 1865.

[4] A. Y. Lee, "Cancer and thromboembolic disease: pathogenic mechanisms," *Cancer Treatment Reviews*, vol. 28, no. 3, pp. 137–140, 2002.

[5] M. Levi, "Cancer and thrombosis," *Clinical Advances in Hematology & Oncology*, vol. 1, no. 11, pp. 668–671, 2003.

[6] G. L. Oktar, E. G. Ergul, and U. Kiziltepe, "Occult malignancy in patients with venous thromboembolism: risk indicators and a diagnostic screening strategy," *Phlebology*, vol. 22, no. 2, pp. 75–79, 2007.

[7] S. Ikushima, R. Ono, K. Fukuda, M. Sakayori, N. Awano, and K. Kondo, "Trousseau's syndrome: cancer-associated thrombosis," *Japanese Journal of Clinical Oncology*, vol. 46, no. 3, pp. 204–208, 2016.

[8] E. Bernardi, R. Pesavento, and P. Prandoni, "Upper extremity deep venous thrombosis," *Seminars in Thrombosis and Hemostasis*, vol. 32, no. 7, pp. 729–736, 2006.

[9] J. W. Blom, J. P. M. Vanderschoot, M. J. Oostindiër, S. Osanto, F. J. M. Van Der Meer, and F. R. Rosendaal, "Incidence of venous thrombosis in a large cohort of 66 329 cancer patients: results of a record linkage study," *Journal of Thrombosis and Haemostasis*, vol. 4, no. 3, pp. 529–535, 2006.

[10] A. Girolami, P. Prandoni, E. Zanon, P. Bagatella, and B. Girolami, "Venous thromboses of upper limbs are more frequently associated with occult cancer as compared with those of lower limbs," *Blood Coagulation and Fibrinolysis*, vol. 10, no. 8, pp. 455–457, 1999.

[11] J. A. Heit, M. D. Silverstein, D. N. Mohr, T. M. Petterson, W. M. O'Fallon, and L. J. Melton III, "Risk factors for deep vein thrombosis and pulmonary embolism: a population-based case-control study," *Archives of Internal Medicine*, vol. 160, no. 6, pp. 809–815, 2000.

[12] F. R. Rickles, "Mechanisms of cancer-induced thrombosis in cancer," *Pathophysiology of Haemostasis and Thrombosis*, vol. 35, no. 1-2, pp. 103–110, 2006.

[13] J. W. Blom, C. J. M. Doggen, S. Osanto, and F. R. Rosendaal, "Malignancies, prothrombotic mutations, and the risk of venous thrombosis," *Journal of the American Medical Association*, vol. 293, no. 6, pp. 715–722, 2005.

[14] F. J. Muñoz, P. Mismetti, R. Poggio et al., "Clinical outcome of patients with upper-extremity deep vein thrombosis: results from the RIETE registry," *Chest*, vol. 133, no. 1, pp. 143–148, 2008.

[15] A. Delluc, G. Le Gal, D. Scarvelis, and M. Carrier, "Outcome of central venous catheter associated upper extremity deep vein thrombosis in cancer patients," *Thrombosis Research*, vol. 135, no. 2, pp. 298–302, 2015.

[16] C. Kearon, E. A. Akl, A. J. Comerota et al., "Antithrombotic therapy for VTE disease: antithrombotic therapy and prevention of thrombosis, 9th ed: American College of Chest Physicians Evidence-Based Clinical Practice Guidelines," *Chest*, vol. 141, no. 2, supplement, pp. e419S–e496S, 2012.

[17] A. Tendas, L. Scaramucci, L. Cupelli et al., "International clinical practice guidelines for the treatment and prophylaxis of venous thromboembolism in patients with cancer: comment," *Journal of Thrombosis and Haemostasis*, vol. 12, no. 5, pp. 805–807, 2014.

[18] M. H. Prins, A. W. A. Lensing, R. Bauersachs et al., "Oral rivaroxaban versus standard therapy for the treatment of symptomatic venous thromboembolism: a pooled analysis of the EINSTEIN-DVT and PE randomized studies," *Thrombosis Journal*, vol. 11, no. 1, article 21, 2013.

[19] W. Ageno, L. G. Mantovani, S. Haas et al., "Safety and effectiveness of oral rivaroxaban versus standard anticoagulation for the treatment of symptomatic deep-vein thrombosis (XALIA): an international, prospective, non-interventional study," *The Lancet Haematology*, vol. 3, no. 1, pp. e12–e21, 2016.

25

Endoscopic Resection of Skull Base Teratoma in Klippel-Feil Syndrome through Use of Combined Ultrasonic and Bipolar Diathermy Platforms

Justin A. Edward,[1] **Alkis J. Psaltis,**[2] **Ryan A. Williams,**[1] **Gregory W. Charville,**[3] **Robert L. Dodd,**[4] **and Jayakar V. Nayak**[1]

[1]*Division of Rhinology, Department of Otolaryngology-Head and Neck Surgery, Stanford University School of Medicine, Stanford, CA 94305, USA*

[2]*Department of Surgery-Otorhinolaryngology, Head and Neck Surgery, University of Adelaide, Adelaide, SA, Australia*

[3]*Department of Pathology, Stanford University School of Medicine, Stanford, CA 94305, USA*

[4]*Department of Neurosurgery, Stanford University School of Medicine, Stanford, CA 94305, USA*

Correspondence should be addressed to Jayakar V. Nayak; jnayak@stanford.edu

Academic Editor: Rong-San Jiang

Klippel-Feil syndrome (KFS) is associated with numerous craniofacial abnormalities but rarely with skull base tumor formation. We report an unusual and dramatic case of a symptomatic, mature skull base teratoma in an adult patient with KFS, with extension through the basisphenoid to obstruct the nasopharynx. This benign lesion was associated with midline palatal and cerebral defects, most notably pituitary and vertebrobasilar arteriolar duplications. A multidisciplinary workup and a complete endoscopic, transnasal surgical approach between otolaryngology and neurosurgery were undertaken. Out of concern for vascular control of the fibrofatty dense tumor stalk at the skull base and need for complete teratoma resection, we successfully employed a tissue resection tool with combined ultrasonic and bipolar diathermy to the tumor pedicle at the sphenoid/clivus junction. No CSF leak or major hemorrhage was noted using this endonasal approach, and no concerning postoperative sequelae were encountered. The patient continues to do well now 3 years after tumor extirpation, with resolution of all preoperative symptoms and absence of teratoma recurrence. KFS, teratoma biology, endocrine gland duplication, and the complex considerations required for successfully addressing this type of advanced skull base pathology are all reviewed herein.

1. Introduction

Klippel-Feil syndrome (KFS) is a rare, skeletal bone disorder primarily associated with any form of congenital fusion anomaly of the cervical vertebrate. The classic triad in KFS consists of brevicollis, low posterior hairline, and severe restriction of neck motion due to congenital cervical vertebral fusion, recently linked to mutations in the GDF3 and GDF6 genes [1]. Though rare, selected cases of both posterior fossa dermoid tumors and teratomas have been reported in patients with KFS, with the majority of such masses being histologically benign [2].

Teratomas are germ cell neoplasms composed of tissues derived from all three embryological germ layers. Teratomas can be classified as either mature or immature, with mature teratomas considered benign tumors given low to absent mitotic activity, and characterized histologically by fully differentiated endoderm, mesoderm, and ectoderm. Immature teratomas, by contrast, constitute 10–50% of all teratomas and are commonly malignant [3, 4].

Teratomas of the head and neck are quite rare and generally present during the neonatal period, and while pediatric teratomas tend to be benign, in the adult these tumors are typically malignant [5]. Intracranial teratomas account for

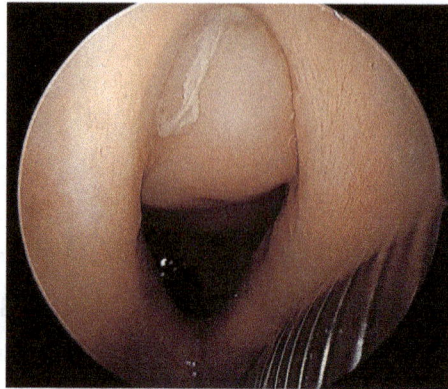

FIGURE 1: Endoscopic view of teratoma extending into the oropharynx. Transoral endoscopic view of a large mucosalized mass extending from the nasopharynx into the upper aspect of oral cavity and pharynx and occluding the cleft palate defect. The metal rings represent the reinforced endotracheal tube placed transorally following induction of anesthesia.

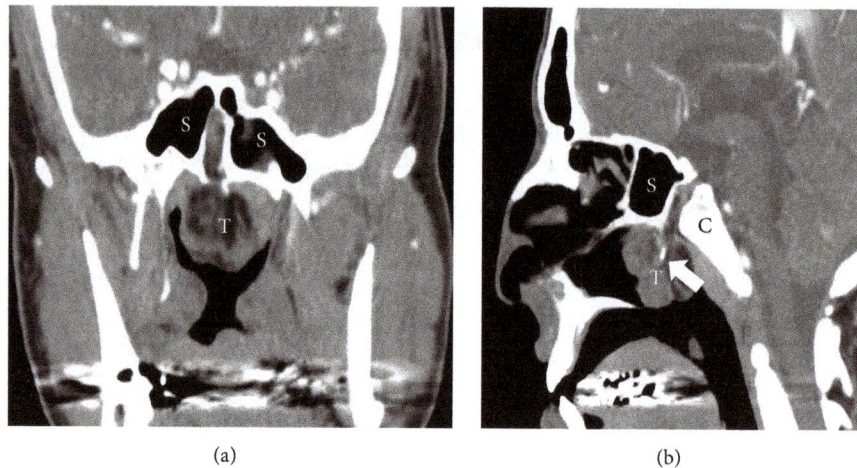

(a)   (b)

FIGURE 2: CT angiogram (CTA) imaging of pedunculated skull base lesion. (a) Coronal CT slice at level of the bilateral sphenoid sinuses (S), with tumor pedicle arising between sinus cavities, at typical site of intersinus septum. The 4×4 cm tumor (T) is composed of heterogeneously dense material, with suspected low-density (dark) fat seen. (b) CTA in sagittal view, showing relationship of tumor pedicle extending between anterior sphenoid sinus (S) and posterior clivus (C). Arrow shows the diminutive artery coursing through the pedicle, without direct communication with the ICA and vertebrobasilar system (not shown).

approximately 0.3–0.9% of all brain tumors and mimic other intracranial germ cell tumors in their tendency to present in midline sites, like the pineal gland and suprasellar regions [4, 6]. Benign teratomas arising from the midline nasal septum have been well described and resected endoscopically [4, 7]; however, a skull base teratoma on a neurovascular stalk arising from the craniopharyngeal duct, superimposed on a KFS background, presents a singular challenge. To resect a pedunculated mass with these features, combined ultrasonic and bipolar diathermy was used to cross-clamp and ligate the pedicle without concern for bleeding from, or retraction of, an uncontrolled skull base pedicle.

2. Case Report

A 38-year-old female presented with a large posterior cavity nasal mass that was being expectantly observed by outside physicians for years. However, on presentation, she endorsed worsening headaches, troublesome nasal obstruction affecting sleep, and intermittent nausea and vomiting without associated photophobia. Physical examination and neck radiograph imaging suggested a diagnosis of KFS with the patient exhibiting webbing of the neck, cleft lip and palate, and midline cranial and cervical anomalies including C2/C3 cervical fusion. Office endoscopy revealed a complex, mobile, midline mucosalized mass filling the entire posterior nasal airway with extension into the superior oropharynx through a cleft in the soft palate (Figure 1).

Computed tomography angiography (CTA) revealed a 4×4 cm multiloculated, nasal mass of the sphenoid skull base protruding through a "central corridor" in the sphenoid intersinus septum of the basisphenoid and anterosuperior to the clivus bone (Figures 2(a) and 2(b)). Magnetic resonance imaging (MRI) demonstrated a pedunculated, extradural heterogeneous mass extending into the nasopharynx, with high intensity fat signal seen within the tumor and its sizeable

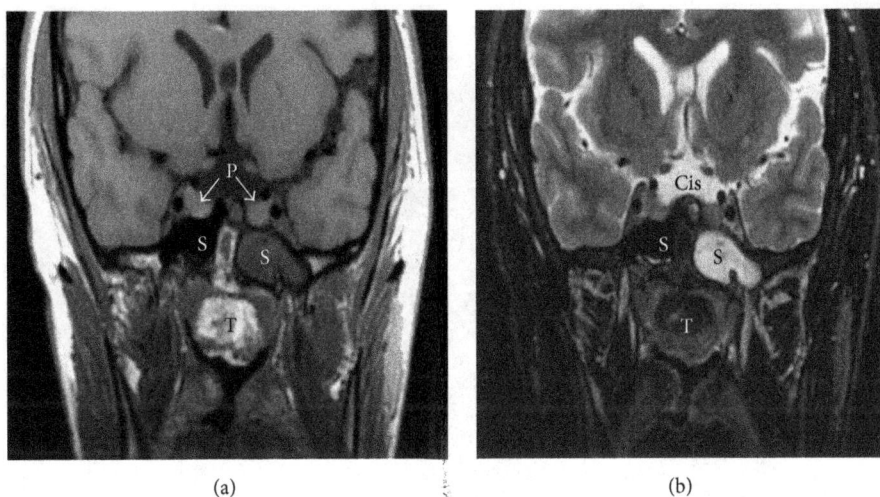

(a)　　　　　　　　　　　　　　　　　　　(b)

FIGURE 3: Magnetic resonance imaging (MRI) of pedunculated skull base lesion. (a) Coronal T1 MRI clearly demonstrates the tumor extending from intracranial midline defect into the nasopharynx. The bright intensity signal within the tumor (T) and stalk between the sphenoid sinuses (S) on T1 sequence represents fat, nearly pathognomonic of teratoma. Pituitary duplication (P with arrows) is best appreciated on T1 imaging as well. Of note, the left sphenoid sinus was noted to have mucosal thickening at the time of MRI compared to CT imaging (Figure 2). (b) Coronal T2 sequence at same slice location highlights the enlarged midline basilar cistern (Cis) with hyperintense signal representing cerebrospinal fluid.

stalk on T1 sequence (Figure 3(a)). Rare pituitary duplication (Figure 3(a)) and the enlarged intracranial basilar cistern with bright CSF fluid signal are readily noted on T2 sequence (Figure 3(b)). The tumor stalk was felt to represent a patent/persistent craniopharyngeal duct, and multiple other midline intracranial abnormalities including corpus callosum dysgenesis, midline lipoma, and dysmorphic hypothalamic and brainstem changes were also noted (not shown). CTA was also performed out of concern for large caliber vascular pedicle to the tumor, with only limited axial blood supply noted (Figure 2(b)). Given the patients' crescendo in symptoms and the collective imaging findings, an extended endonasal resection of this skull base teratoma was planned between otolaryngology and neurosurgery.

Access was obtained via inferior turbinate outfracture and limited posterior septectomy to permit binarial access. A two-surgeon, four-handed surgical approach, and intraoperative, computer-assisted image guidance confirmed unfettered access to the teratoma, with classic dentition seen in triplanar view (Figure 4). The main consideration was control of the midline stalk at the skull base without encountering a cerebrospinal fluid (CSF) leak from the basilar cistern or intracranial retraction of vascular feeders from the pedicle. The stalk, measuring approximately 1 cm laterally and 1.5 anteroposteriorly, was encased in a bony shell that extended through the midline floor of the sphenoid sinuses into the upper clivus. Using hand instruments and fine diamond drill bits, the ensconced stalk was liberated from the surrounding bone. This revealed a fibrovascular pedicle that was then cleanly truncated using the Thunderbeat™ device, for simultaneous ultrasonic wave (cutting) and bipolar diathermy (coagulation) action. The technique permitted transmural pedicle resection, precluding the need for awkward suture ligation of a thick pedicle adjacent to the skull base, while

allowing for the tumor to be delivered en bloc transorally (Figure 5). Microscopic analysis of the resected tumor using standard histology revealed a disordered arrangements of mature epithelial and mesenchymal tissues, including cartilage, adipose tissue, stratified squamous epithelium with cutaneous-type adnexal structures, ciliated respiratory-type epithelium, and striated muscle (Figure 6). No immature neural element was identified, consistent with a mature teratoma. No perioperative complications were noted, with resolution of all preoperative symptoms within 1 month. Postoperatively, in the absence of the obstructive mass, a palatal obturator was required to limit nasal regurgitation and hypernasal speech through coverage of the cleft palate defect. She continues to do well >3 years since surgery, with no untoward sequelae from the procedure.

3. Discussion

Teratomas are germ cell tumors that classically recapitulate all embryonic cell lines: endoderm, mesoderm, and ectoderm. They can be further classified as mature, immature, or malignant [8]. Mature teratomas are well-differentiated, generally benign masses possessing locally aggressive behavior (adhesion to/displacement of adjacent structures) [9]. Head and neck sites are rare and represent only 2% of all teratomas [5]. CT and MRI imaging are essential to determine lesion characteristics, such as the presence of mixed density tissues such as fat, muscle, bone, soft tissue, and cartilage. Suprasellar teratomas can be particularly challenging as the pituitary infundibulum can appear convoluted or elongated from local mass effect [9]. Such lesions that involve the skull base have been previously removed using an endoscopic endonasal approach [10]. Here, we report a striking case of a female patient with KFS with a longstanding, pendant skull base

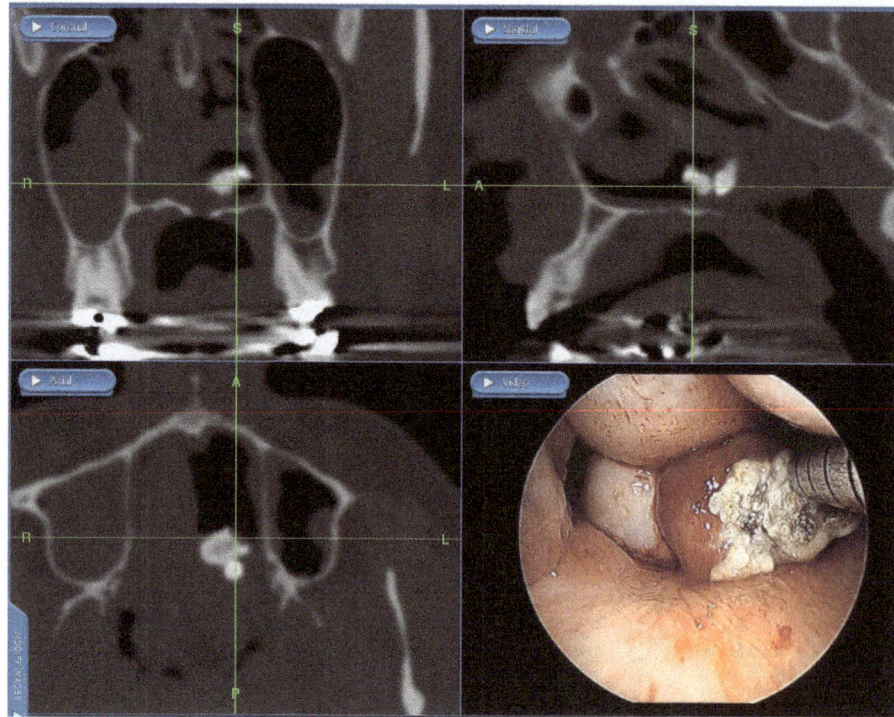

FIGURE 4: Use of intraoperative CT image guidance assistance during skull base approach. Computer-assisted navigation system (image guidance) highlighting intraoperative CT scan imaging in coronal, sagittal, and axial views. With the registered instrument tip contacting the anterior face of the lesion (endoscopic image at bottom right), the fine cut maxillofacial CT scan shows calcified material present within the skull base teratoma at this site of tumor contact (intersection point of green lines), representing intratumoral dentition.

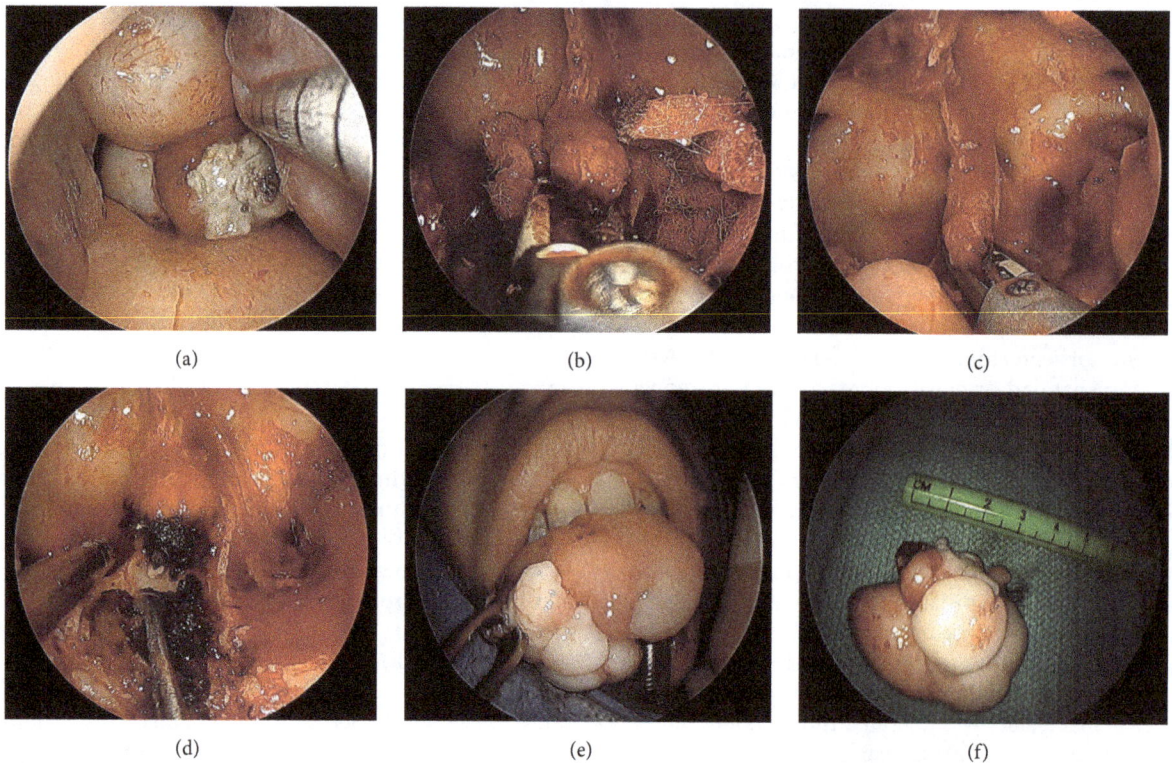

FIGURE 5: Surgical resection of skull base teratoma with ultrasonic bipolar diathermy. Endonasal view of the pedunculated skull base teratoma obstructing the posterior nasopharynx, with metal suction tip retracting the left inferior turbinate (a). Following sphenoidotomies, the tumor pedicle is approached (b), clamped in a full-thickness manner (c), and completely transected (d) using the vice-clamp tip and combined ultrasonic/bipolar platform energies. Teratoma passed into the oral cavity for transoral en bloc tumor removal (e), with lesion measuring approximately 4.0 cm in diameter (f).

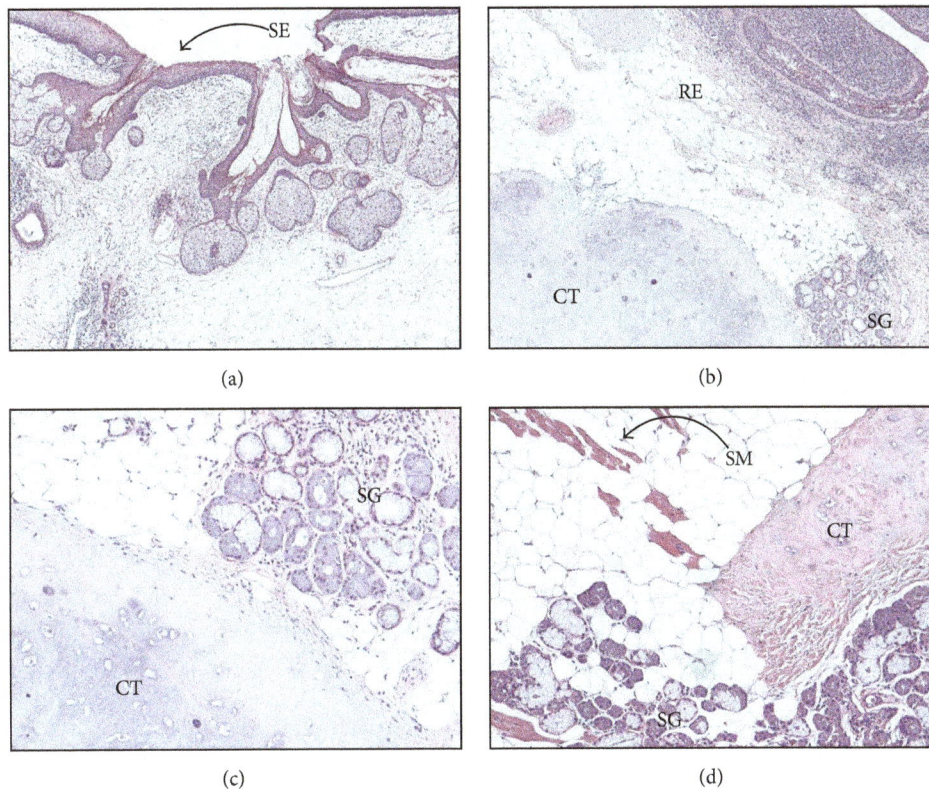

FIGURE 6: Representative histopathology photomicrographs of the skull base teratoma. (a) Stratified squamous epithelium (SE) with associated adnexal structures (4x magnification). (b) Ciliated respiratory epithelium- (RE-) lined cystic structure, salivary gland tissue (SG), and cartilage (CT) (4x magnification). (c) Scattered foci of SG adjacent to CT tissues (10x magnification). (d) Haphazard arrangements of CT, SG, and striated muscle (SM) (10x magnification). Mature adipose tissue is also present in the background (unlabeled clear cell bodies).

teratoma extending through a patent craniopharyngeal duct leading to obstruction of the nasopharynx and worsening headaches. While CT imaging showed a posterior nasal mass protruding through a defect in the clivus, MRI revealed an extradural mass containing admixed dentigerous and adipose pockets extending from the middle cranial fossa through the basisphenoid with associated dramatic duplication of the pituitary gland and vertebrobasilar feeders. This case highlights our experience with the workup and treatment of challenging skull base pathology and also the innovative intranasal utilization of the Thunderbeat device for management of the extradural stalk through an endoscopic approach. Postoperative examination of the mass revealed a benign, mature teratoma.

Patients with KFS can have anatomic abnormalities such as vertebral fusion, cleft palate, aortic arch anomalies, renal agenesis, spina bifida, and cerebral structural abnormalities [2]. This patient presented with cervical vertebral fusion, cleft lip and palate, webbed neck, anatomic duplication of the basilar artery and pituitary gland, midline developmental intracerebral dysmorphia, and patent craniopharyngeal duct. The association between posterior fossa dermoid tumors and KFS is well established, with approximately 24 reported cases in the literature [2, 3]. A teratoma arising from the

middle cranial fossa at the skull base, however, has not been reported. A patient with both KFS and a middle cranial fossa skull base teratoma presents a unique challenge in terms of both nonsurgical and surgical management due to anatomical variation and possible endocrine abnormalities. To our knowledge, this is the first case in the literature that highlights the management of both of these two rare disease processes.

The preoperative assessment of patients with either sellar or suprasellar teratomas includes otolaryngologic, endocrine, ophthalmologic, and neurological evaluations. Appropriate endocrine studies may suggest signs and symptoms of diabetes insipidus and anterior hypopituitarism [11], but lab studies of serum pituitary hormone levels and related functional studies were unremarkable in this patient, as were formal visual field and acuity testing. Although contrasted MRI assists in the evaluation of intracranial masses, this imaging confirmed intranasal extension through the skull base and strongly suggested the final diagnosis of teratoma. As in this case, treatment of mature teratomas is primarily surgical and affords a low recurrence rate following complete extirpation [11]. Endoscopic endonasal resection of skull base lesions is increasingly common, but to our knowledge, this is the first report of endoscopic resection of a skull base teratoma in the setting of pituitary duplication through use of combined ultrasonic bipolar diathermy.

The endonasal approach undertaken with neurosurgery allowed for complete, single stage tumor resection without CSF leak or pedicle hemorrhage or retraction. Given the unusual pendant teratoma on a dense fibrofatty stalk, complete pedicle control and transmural transection at this deep skull base site was mandatory, while avoiding suture ligation. Using the clamp on the Thunderbeat device to grasp the pedicle transnasally, the tumor stalk was able to be cleanly transected using the combined ultrasonic and bipolar energy sources transmitted through the "teeth" of the clamp, with minimal eschar and heat transmission [12, 13]. The dual modality ultrasonic bipolar instrument described allowed us to deftly manage the wide, thick, and potentially hemorrhagic tumor pedicle to this unusual skull base mass. In this case, single instrument ligation and hemostasis allowed for endoscopic resection with minimal blood loss and minimal risk of complications.

Skull base teratomas have been well associated with anatomic variants such as pituitary gland duplication, which typically warrants additional neuroendocrine workup. We identified approximately 41 documented cases of pituitary duplication in our literature analysis. Of these reports, less than half of cases are associated with the presence of a skull base teratoma [14–16]. Common anomalies associated with pituitary gland duplication include vertebral anomalies and cleft palate [16], both of which are present in this patient. Pituitary gland duplication is an exceedingly rare malformation that aligns with other midline craniofacial anomalies involving the skull base, midline developing notochord, and pharynx [15, 17], although the basis for this is not well understood. The cleft created by ultimate separation of the prechordal plate and notochordal process is theorized to lead to a potentially sizeable skull base defect as noted in this patient [15].

Surgical management of sinonasal teratomas is primary treatment, and naturally given the complex patient history and potential for comorbidities, a multidisciplinary team between otolaryngology, neurosurgery, and endocrinology was involved in the surgical and postoperative management of this patient. Benign, mature teratomas have been reported to have survival rates over 90% after 10 years [9]. However, tumor recurrence has been reported through a phenomenon known as "growing teratoma syndrome," which is extremely rare and refers to a relapse of malignancy due to partial response to surgical resection or chemotherapy [18]. In this syndrome, the recurrent tumor is often resistant to chemotherapy and radiation but generally only occurs in those with primary malignant tumors [18]. In this case, the patient had a benign, mature teratoma with no evidence of recurrence 3 years following removal. Contributing to the lack of tumor regrowth is likely near-total truncation of the skull base pedicle, which allowed for complete surgical resection of the teratoma mass. This could be achieved in a reassuringly atraumatic and hemostatic manner using the described combined cutting/coagulating technology in a novel application.

4. Conclusion

The typical treatment for benign, mature teratomas causing symptoms is surgical resection, which was successfully performed in this case involving a skull base teratoma extending from the skull base and middle cranial fossa. A multidisciplinary team approach is recommended in these cases due to the complexities of the disease process, aberrant anatomy, and potential for complications. In a patient with KFS and the presence of pituitary duplication and cleft palate, the use of ultrasonic bipolar diathermy allowed for complete and bloodless control and transection of the dense skull base pedicle and gratifying en bloc resection of the mass through the oral cavity. Future reports on the use of this dual modality technology in endonasal procedures and skull base surgery will help ascertain its broader utility and impact on outcomes.

Competing Interests

Jayakar V. Nayak is a consultant with Olympus America, which manufactures the Thunderbeat dual modality device employed in this report.

Acknowledgments

This work was supported in part by funds from the Stanford University Department of Otolaryngology.

References

[1] A. S. Sudhakar, V. T. Nguyen, and J. B. Chang, "Klippel-Feil syndrome and supra-aortic arch anomaly: a case report," *International Journal of Angiology*, vol. 17, no. 2, pp. 109–111, 2008.

[2] M. Turgut, "Klippel-Feil syndrome in association with posterior fossa dermoid tumour," *Acta Neurochirurgica*, vol. 151, no. 3, pp. 269–276, 2009.

[3] A. Adorno, C. Alafaci, F. Sanfilippo et al., "Malignant teratoma in Klippel-Feil syndrome: a case report and review of the literature," *Journal of Medical Case Reports*, vol. 9, no. 1, article no. 700, 2015.

[4] I. Cukurova, M. Gumussoy, A. Yaz, U. Bayol, and O. G. Yigitbasi, "A benign teratoma presenting as an obstruction of the nasal cavity: a case report," *Journal of Medical Case Reports*, vol. 6, article 147, 2012.

[5] M. M. April, R. F. Ward, and J. M. Garelick, "Diagnosis, management, and follow-up of congenital head and neck teratomas," *The Laryngoscope*, vol. 108, no. 9, pp. 1398–1401, 1998.

[6] M. Matsutani, K. Sano, K. Takakura et al., "Primary intracranial germ cell tumors: a clinical analysis of 153 histologically verified cases," *Journal of Neurosurgery*, vol. 86, no. 3, pp. 446–455, 1997.

[7] G. L. Coppit III, J. A. Perkins, and S. C. Manning, "Nasopharyngeal teratomas and dermoids: a review of the literature and case series," *International Journal of Pediatric Otorhinolaryngology*, vol. 52, no. 3, pp. 219–227, 2000.

[8] M. E. Huth, S. Heimgartner, I. Schnyder, and M. D. Caversaccio, "Teratoma of the nasal septum in a neonate: an endoscopic approach," *Journal of Pediatric Surgery*, vol. 43, no. 11, pp. 2102–2105, 2008.

[9] R. B. Sweiss, F. Shweikeh, F. B. Sweiss, S. Zyck, L. Dalvin, and J. Siddiqi, "Suprasellar mature cystic teratoma: an unusual

location for an uncommon tumor," *Case Reports in Neurological Medicine*, vol. 2013, Article ID 180497, 4 pages, 2013.

[10] D. Mistry and B. Figueroa, "An elongated pituitary stalk resembling the lining of a dermoid cyst during endoscopic endonasal approach," *Otolaryngology—Head and Neck Surgery*, vol. 153, no. 1, pp. 150–151, 2015.

[11] S. Chiloiro, A. Giampietro, A. Bianchi, and L. de Marinis, "Clinical management of teratoma, a rare hypothalamic-pituitary neoplasia," *Endocrine*, pp. 1–7, 2015.

[12] J. Milsom, K. Trencheva, S. Monette et al., "Evaluation of the safety, efficacy, and versatility of a new surgical energy device (THUNDERBEAT) in comparison with harmonic ACE, LigaSure V, and EnSeal devices in a porcine model," *Journal of Laparoendoscopic and Advanced Surgical Techniques*, vol. 22, no. 4, pp. 378–386, 2012.

[13] A. Shabbir and D. Dargan, "Advancement and benefit of energy sealing in minimally invasive surgery," *Asian journal of endoscopic surgery*, vol. 7, no. 2, pp. 95–101, 2014.

[14] S. Manjila, E. A. Miller, S. Vadera et al., "Duplication of the pituitary gland associated with multiple blastogenesis defects: duplication of the pituitary gland (DPG)-plus syndrome. Case report and review of literature," *Surgical Neurology International*, vol. 3, no. 1, Article ID 92939, 2012.

[15] M. Chariker, R. Ford, C. Morrison, A. Theile, K. Moeller, and T. Moriarty, "Pituitary duplication with nasopharyngeal teratoma and cleft palate," *Journal of Craniofacial Surgery*, vol. 22, no. 2, pp. 755–758, 2011.

[16] L. Azurara, M. Marcal, F. Vieira, and M. L. Tuna, "DPG-plus syndrome: new report of a rare entity," *BMJ Case Reports*, vol. 2015, 2015.

[17] T. A. G. M. Huisman, U. Fischer, E. Boltshauser, T. Straube, and C. Gysin, "Pituitary duplication and nasopharyngeal teratoma in a newborn: CT, MRI, US and correlative histopathological findings," *Neuroradiology*, vol. 47, no. 7, pp. 558–561, 2005.

[18] W. L. Bi, S. I. Bannykh, and J. Baehring, "The growing teratoma syndrome after subtotal resection of an intracranial nongerminomatous germ cell tumor in an adult: case report," *Neurosurgery*, vol. 56, no. 1, p. 188, 2005.

26

Bilateral Nasoalveolar Cyst Causing Nasal Obstruction

Uzeyir Yildizoglu,[1] Fatih Arslan,[2] Bahtiyar Polat,[3] and Abdullah Durmaz[4]

[1]*Department of Otorhinolaryngology Head and Neck Surgery, Beytepe Military Hospital, Ankara, Turkey*
[2]*Department of Otolaryngology, Head and Neck Surgery, Ankara Mevki Military Hospital, Ankara, Turkey*
[3]*Department of Otorhinolaryngology Head and Neck Surgery, Gelibolu Military Hospital, Çanakkale, Turkey*
[4]*Department of Otolaryngology, Head and Neck Surgery, Gulhane Military Medical Academy, Ankara, Turkey*

Correspondence should be addressed to Fatih Arslan; drfatiharslan@gmail.com

Academic Editor: Ricardo Alves Mesquita

Nasoalveolar cysts, which originate from epithelial remnants of nasolacrimal duct, are nonodontogenic soft tissue lesions of the upper jaw. These cysts are thought to be developmental and are presented with fullness in the upper lip and nose, swelling on the palate, and sometimes nasal obstruction. Because of cosmetic problems, they are often diagnosed at an early stage. These lesions are mostly revealed unilaterally but also can be seen on both sides. In this case report, a patient who complained of nasal obstruction and then diagnosed with bilateral nasoalveolar cysts and treated by sublabial excision is presented and clinical features and treatment approaches are discussed with the review of literature.

1. Introduction

Nasoalveolar cyst (NAC) is called nasolabial cyst or Klestadt's cyst. This developmental disorder which is defined as a nonodontogenic cyst of the upper jaw is seen four times more in women than men. It is mostly located unilaterally and left sided but rarely can be seen bilaterally. The patients are presented mainly in the fourth or fifth decade [1]. These lesions constitute about 0.7% of all jaw cysts. Typically, complaints of the patients are nasal obstruction and facial deformity. NACs, located in the hard palate and nasal vestibule, are presented with fullness of alar and nasolabial sulcus, submucosal mass with smooth surface on the hard palate, and bulging at the base of the nasal vestibule [2]. These cysts are usually painless but if infected, may cause pain and purulent discharge in nasal passages or in oral cavity. In this paper, due to rarity, a case of bilaterally located NAC is presented. The etiology, clinical features, and treatment approaches are discussed with the review of literature.

2. Case Presentation

A thirty-two-year-old female patient was admitted to our otolaryngology department with the complaints of having difficulty in breathing and rapidly growing painful swelling on the right side of the nose which has been existing for a few days and then caused purulent discharge by bursting. Anterior rhinoscopic examination revealed an infected cystic lesion at the base of the right nasal vestibule, towards the inferior turbinate by narrowing right nasal passage. A similar cystic lesion in the left nasal cavity was also observed, but it was painless and did not show signs of infection. Antibiotherapy (amoxicillin + clavulanate 1000 mg, 2 × 1, 7 d) and anti-inflammatory therapy were begun. In computed tomography (CT) images were obtained with the following parameters: field of view: 150 mm; section thickness: 1 mm; 200 mA 120 kV (Aquilion ONE 320, Toshiba Medical Systems Corporation, Japan). The CT scan showed well-bordered hypodense cystic lesions in both sides of the nasal vestibule floor which is about 2 cm in diameter on the left and about 1 cm in diameter on the right side (Figures 1(a) and 1(b)). The magnetic resonance (MR) imaging was made using Ingenia 3.0 T (Philips Healthcare, Netherlands) after the antibiotherapy. The MR imaging showed the well-circumscribed cystic lesions that did not show contrasting and looked hypointense at T1 display and hyperintense at T2 display at the same location (Figures 1(c) and 1(d)). The cysts were excised by sublabial approach (Figure 2). The right cyst

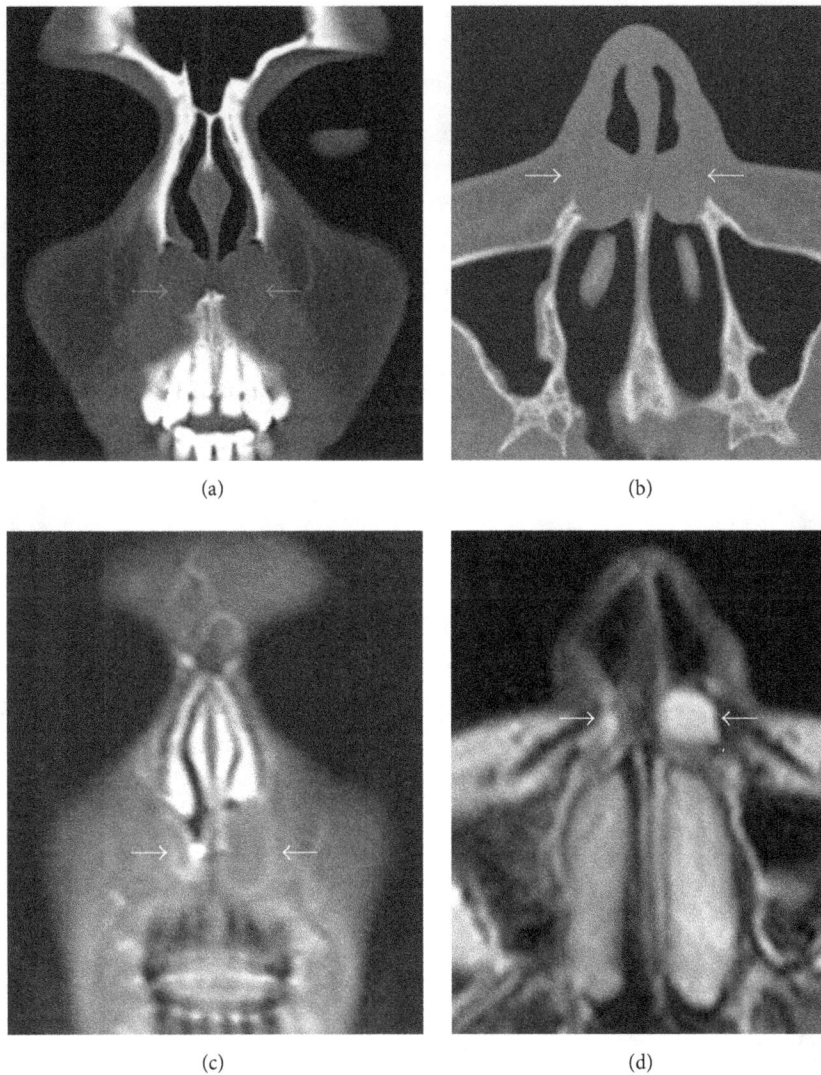

(a)

(b)

(c)

(d)

FIGURE 1: In the CT imaging of the maxillary bone, in both nasal vestibule floors, properly limited hypodense cystic lesions were observed, which were measured to be approximately 2 cm in the left and 1 cm in the right ((a) coronal view, (b) axial view). In the MR imaging performed after the antibiotherapy, at the same location, there were observed properly limited cystic lesions that did not show contrasting and looked hypointense at T1 display and hyperintense at T2 display ((c) coronal view, (d) axial view).

has fibrotic adhesions due to previous infection, while the boundaries of the cyst in the left could easily be separated from the surrounding structures. Light microscopy of the cystic wall showed a connective tissue with few cells, lined with a flattened squamous epithelium. Microscopically, this cyst wall showed foci of chronic inflammatory cells and the wall was lined with two layers of squamous epithelium. The wall of the second cyst was lined with pseudostratified columnar epithelium (Figure 3). Both lesions were verified to be nasoalveolar cysts by histopathological examination. After the surgery no complications were observed and no recurrence was detected in the 6-month follow-up.

3. Discussion

Nasoalveolar cyst (NAC) is a congenital pathology and two theories have been developed about its etiology. The first theory is about cysts developing as nasolacrimal canal residues and the other is about the cysts being embryonic fissure cysts. When first described they were thought to develop from the retention of the mucosal glands [3]. Later, Kleinstadt suggested that these lesions developed from the tissue remaining in between during the merging of embryonic nasal mucosa, the maxillary process, and lateral-medial nasal process [4].

NAC usually is asymptomatic and is located next to the nasal wing. As the size of cyst increases it becomes symptomatic and usually causes swelling in the face and hard palate. The most common complaint is nasal congestion [2]. Fluid-containing serous-character NAC can become infected and drain into the nasal or oral cavity causing foul smell and pain in the mouth and nose. Although nasoalveolar cyst is a benign disease, it has been reported to be associated with malignant degeneration [3].

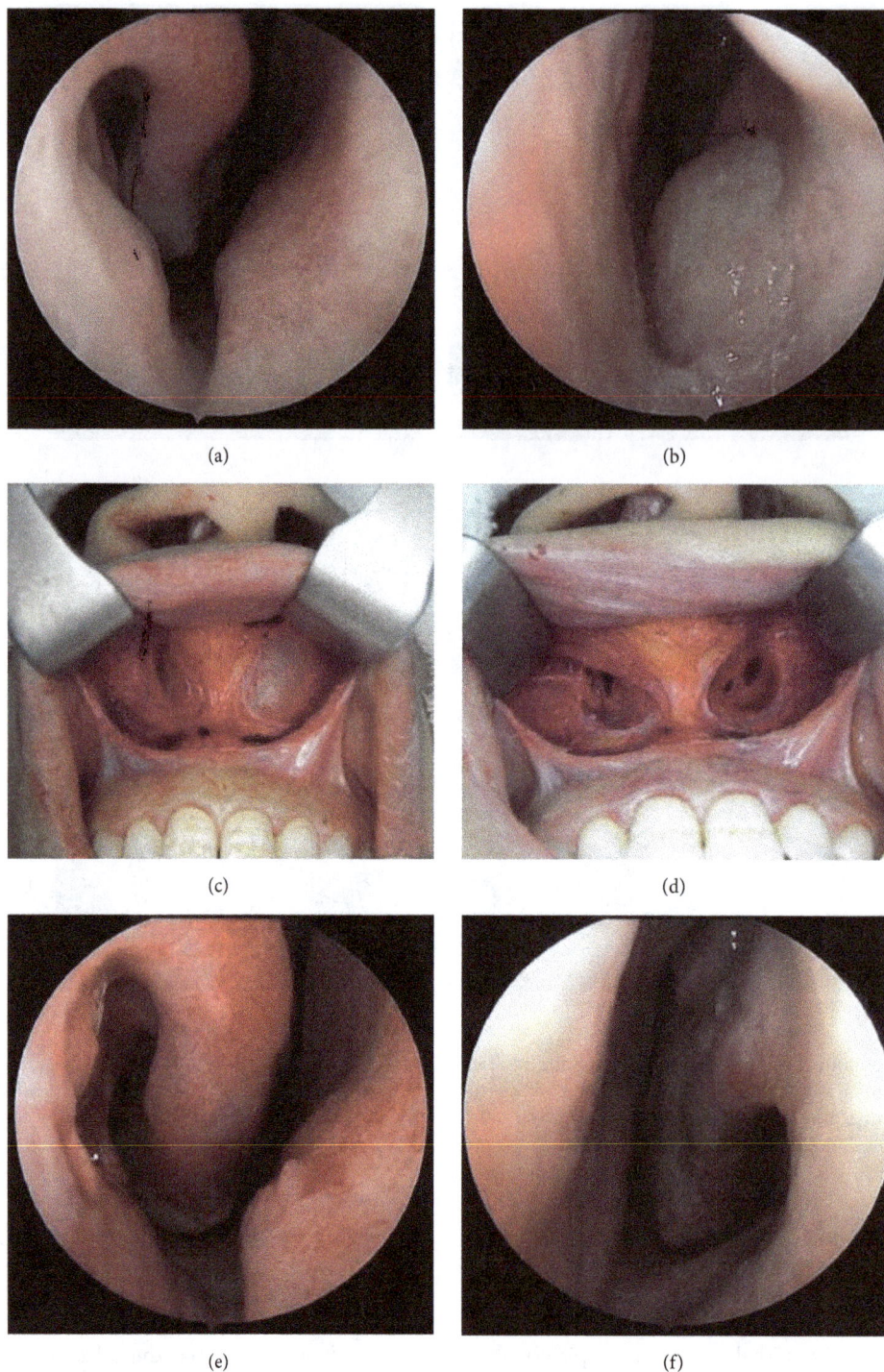

FIGURE 2: Intraoperative image of the cysts that were excised by sublabial approach. The cyst on the right was reduced in size because it ruptured due to an infection, but the cyst on the left kept narrowing the inferior meatus in the vestibule floor (a, b). In the intraoperative assessment fibrotic adhesions of the cyst on the right due to infection were seen, while the left cyst's borders were seen to be easily separated from the surrounding structures (c, d). After the cysts were totally excised nasal obstruction also passed (e, f).

NAC is a soft tissue lesion which usually is placed inside the maxillary bone. Therefore CT imaging is the preferred method of viewing since it shows the location of the cyst and its relationship with the nasal and oral cavity and the status of the bone structure in a detailed way [5]. MR imaging has an advantage over CT imaging since it can show the content of the cyst and should be preferred as an additional survey in cases where malignancy is suspected. NAC does not cause destruction in the adjacent bone structures. However, the long term compression effect of the cyst can cause

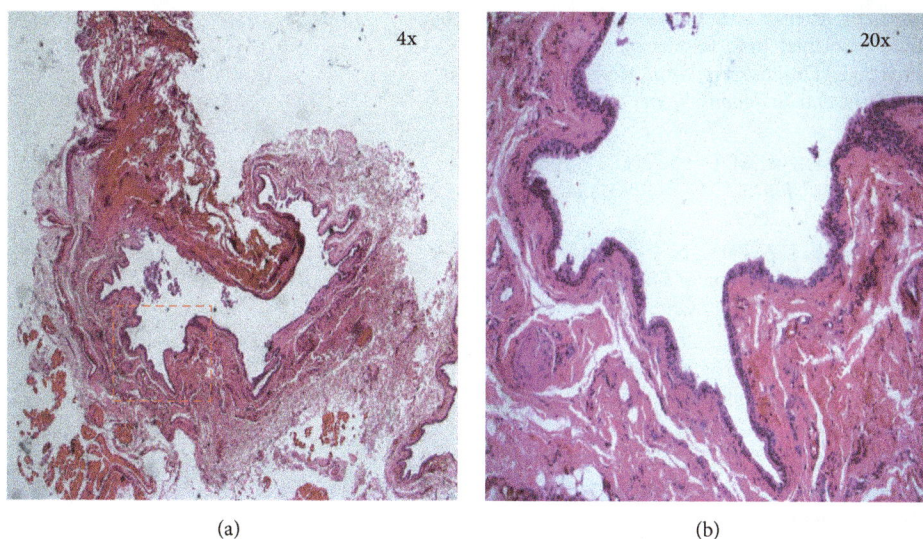

FIGURE 3: Light microscopy appearances of the cyst at 4x (a) and 20x (b) magnification. The cystic wall was lined with pseudostratified columnar epithelium.

bone tissue erosion and even defects. In CT imaging, apart from these findings, sclerosing density increase around the lesion can be observed [3]. In our case the CT imaging examination showed a well-circumscribed cystic lesion. Due to compression in the surrounding bone structures, a smooth surface erosion was observed. In the differential diagnosis of the well-circumscribed cysts related to the anterior maxillary region, the nasal vestibule, and the hard palate, apart from the nasoalveolar cyst, the odontogenic cysts and the neoplastic lesions should also come to mind as well [6].

NAC is treated with surgical excision by sublabial approach [2, 3]. Other optional treatments include aspiration of the contents of the cyst, endoscopic cyst marsupialization by transnasal approach, and injection of sclerosing agents [2]. Lee et al. compared both groups of NAC patients, the ones who they treated by sublabial approach with the ones they treated by transnasal endoscopic marsupialization [7, 8]. According to these studies the transnasal endoscopic marsupialization was reported to be more advantageous when compared to sublabial excision since it shortened the surgery time, decreased the cost, and shortened the time of the postoperative pain. After the surgery no recurrence was reported in either groups. As a conclusion, transnasal endoscopic marsupialization was stated to be an advantageous and effective method in the treatment of NAC. Özer et al. reported a nasoalveolar cyst case that was treated by transnasal endoscopic approach and complete cyst excision was performed [9]. In our case, we aimed to remove the entire cyst wall instead of marsupialization and did excision by sublabial approach because of the localization, size, and infection history of the cysts. The part of the cystic wall which was adherent to the bone was delineated easily whereas the part of the cyst wall in the soft tissue of sublabial region was separated with difficulty especially in the infected cyst side. Thin cyst wall required slow dissection and sublabial approach permits good access to the pyriform aperture and wide exposure to the complete cyst.

Clinical and radiological findings are sufficient for the diagnosis of NAC but the definitive diagnosis is set by histopathological examination. Histopathological examination of NAC reveals cystic structure with fibrous capsule, which may contain goblet cells and is paved with pseudostratified columnar epithelium. As the size of the cyst grows, the intraluminal pressure increases and the columnar epithelium is replaced with stratified squamous epithelium. In our case, histopathological examination corrected the preoperative diagnosis compatible with NAC.

4. Conclusion

Bilateral NAC seems very rare and may cause nasal obstruction. When assessing breathing difficulties NAC should be kept in mind.

Competing Interests

The authors declare that they have no competing interests.

Authors' Contributions

Patient follow-up and writing were done by Uzeyir Yildizoglu and Fatih Arslan. Literature review was done by Bahtiyar Polat. Consultant Dr. Abdullah Durmaz performed the final check.

References

[1] K. el-Din and A. A. el-Hamd, "Nasolabial cyst: a report of eight cases and a review of the literature," *The Journal of Laryngology and Otology*, vol. 113, no. 8, pp. 747–749, 1999.

[2] H.-W. Yuen, C.-Y. L. Julian, and C.-L. Y. Samuel, "Nasolabial cysts: clinical features, diagnosis, and treatment," *British Journal of Oral and Maxillofacial Surgery*, vol. 45, no. 4, pp. 293–297, 2007.

[3] F. López-Ríos, L. Lassaletta-Atienza, C. Domingo-Carrasco, and F. J. Martinez-Tello, "Nasolabial cyst. Report of a case with extensive apocrine change," *Oral Surgery, Oral Medicine, Oral Pathology, Oral Radiology, and Endodontics*, vol. 84, no. 4, pp. 404–406, 1997.

[4] M. P. Marcoviceanu, M. C. Metzger, H. Deppe et al., "Report of rare bilateral nasolabial cysts," *Journal of Cranio-Maxillofacial Surgery*, vol. 37, no. 2, pp. 83–86, 2009.

[5] R. N. Aquilino, V. J. Bazzo, R. J. A. Faria, N. L. M. Eid, and F. N. Bóscolo, "Nasolabial cyst: presentation of a clinical case with CT and MR images," *Brazilian Journal of Otorhinolaryngology*, vol. 74, no. 3, pp. 467–471, 2008.

[6] L. Van Gerven, V. Vander Poorten, and M. Jorissen, "Adenocarcinomas of the sinonasal tract: current opinion," *B-ENT*, vol. 7, supplement 17, pp. 15–20, 2011.

[7] J. Y. Lee, B. J. Baek, J. Y. Byun, H. S. Chang, B. D. Lee, and D. W. Kim, "Comparison of conventional excision via a sublabial approach and transnasal marsupialization for the treatment of nasolabial cysts: a prospective randomized study," *Clinical and Experimental Otorhinolaryngology*, vol. 2, no. 2, pp. 85–89, 2009.

[8] W.-C. Chao, C.-C. Huang, P.-H. Chang, Y.-L. Chen, C.-W. Chen, and T.-J. Lee, "Management of nasolabial cysts by transnasal endoscopic marsupialization," *Archives of Otolaryngology—Head and Neck Surgery*, vol. 135, no. 9, pp. 932–935, 2009.

[9] S. Özer, C. Cabbarzade, and O. Ögretmenoglu, "A new transnasal approach to nasolabial cyst: endoscopic excision of nasolabial cyst," *Journal of Craniofacial Surgery*, vol. 24, no. 5, pp. 1748–1749, 2013.

27

Functional and Aesthetic Tragal Reconstruction in the Age of Mobile Electronic Devices

Colleen F. Perez and Curtis W. Gaball

Naval Medical Center San Diego, San Diego, CA, USA

Correspondence should be addressed to Colleen F. Perez; col.perez@gmail.com

Academic Editor: I. Todt

We present a method to create a tragus using the patient's conchal cartilage. It is a simplified, single-stage technique with well-hidden incisions, yet it maintains the rigidity of a natural tragus. This patient did not have a history of radiation to the area, which may compromise healing with this technique. The cosmetic importance of the tragus has been described, but its functionality in accommodating modern technology has not been previously discussed. The main treatment goal for this patient was to gain the ability to wear earphones (clinical question/level of evidence: therapeutic, V).

1. Introduction

Various techniques for tragal reconstruction have been described primarily in the setting of microtia repair. Methods for reconstruction after tumor excision have been reported using the concha, lobule, costal cartilage, and various flaps [1–4]. The goals of tragus reconstruction in the past were only to create a pretragal depression and good tragus projection, hide the external meatus, and leave an inconspicuous scar [5].

2. Case Report

A 43-year-old female presented with a surgically absent left tragus several years after Mohs excision for basal cell carcinoma. The original defect was closed primarily. A small remnant of the tragus remained after the original excision. She was having difficulty wearing earphones and earplugs and desired an improved appearance. She brought examples of the types of earphones she hoped to wear for surgical planning. Her preoperative photo is shown in Figure 1.

A single-stage reconstructive procedure was performed. A preauricular incision was made in a standard rhytidectomy-type configuration. The residual tragal cartilage was exposed and dissection was made on both surfaces, exposing approximately 7 mm on either side. This involved elevating off the canal skin posteriorly and the pretragal soft tissue anteriorly.

Care was taken not to dissect past the tragal pointer in order to avoid facial nerve injury. The anticipated size of the new tragal cartilage and its shape were designed using the opposite ear as a guide. An area with a cartilaginous contour similar to that required was identified in the ipsilateral conchal bowl, and this segment of cartilage was harvested through a postauricular incision (Figure 2). Key landmarks of the concha were left intact, including the rim and helical root, in order to avoid any stigmata of surgery. The graft was trimmed and placed in the pretragal pocket adjacent to the residual tragal cartilage (Figure 3).

It was sutured to this residual cartilage with horizontal mattress sutures of 4-0 polydioxanone (PDS). The pretragal skin was then undermined in the subcutaneous fat plane for a distance of approximately 3 cm. The skin flap was advanced posteriorly, and the advanced skin was sutured into this new position with 4-0 PDS deep sutures to the platysma auricular fascia (PAF) to take any tension off the neotragus upon closure. The new tragal and pretragal skin was defatted as is commonly performed in facelift surgery and wrapped around the lateral surface where it met with the canal skin. Cotton soaked in mineral oil can be used as packing to coapt the overlying skin to the cartilage if skin tenting occurs. This resulted

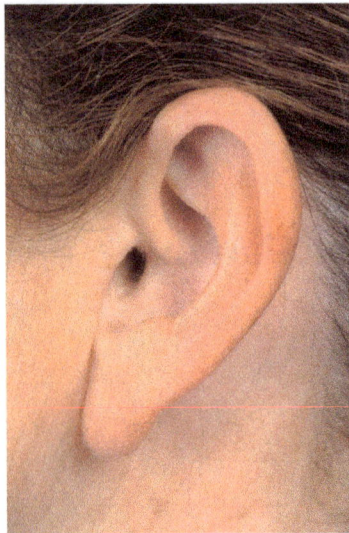

FIGURE 1: Preoperative photograph of a left tragus defect several years after excision for basal cell carcinoma.

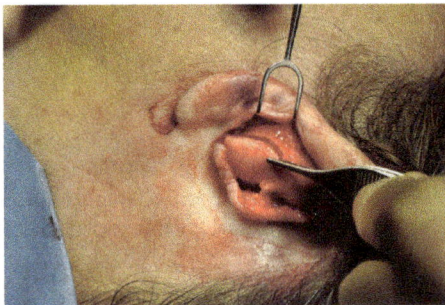

FIGURE 2: Intraoperative photograph showing conchal cartilage harvest through a postauricular incision.

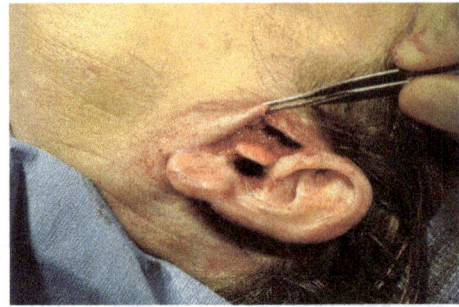

FIGURE 3: Intraoperative photograph showing the cartilage graft placement into the pretragal pocket.

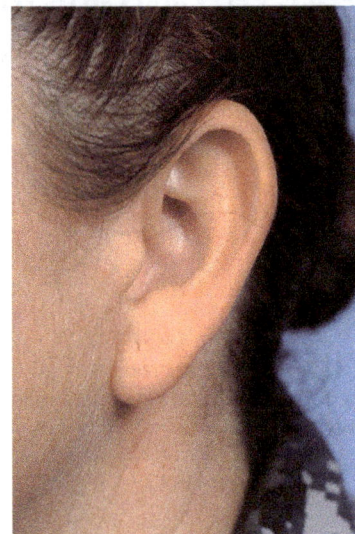

FIGURE 4: Postoperative photograph of the patient after 9 months.

in a natural appearing pretragal depression. The closure to the canal skin was approximated with 4-0 plain gut suture. Residual skin from the advancement in the preauricular area anterior to the lobule and helix was excised away, and the remaining incision was closed with 5-0 monofilament polypropylene (Prolene) suture. The site was dressed with antibiotic ointment-soaked cotton placed in the ear canal, and a standard dental roll bolster dressing was applied to the concha and secured with a transauricular Prolene suture.

The patient returned for follow-up and postoperative photos at 1 week and again at 1, 9 (Figure 4), and 13 months. At the last follow-up she reported being very pleased with her appearance and with her ability to wear earphones.

3. Discussion

Few reports exist describing isolated tragus reconstruction after excision of tumor in a nonirradiated field. Martínez et al. [6] reported a single-stage method using a transposition flap rotated 180 degrees based on the earlobe to reconstruct the tragus, creating projection and hiding the auricular canal. Adler et al. [5] also described a single-stage transposition flap

from the preauricular area, taking care to restore the pretragus depression and create good projection. Coombs and Lin [7] used a two-stage procedure with a chondrocutaneous transposition flap from the posterior aspect of the conchal bowl. The flap is based inferiorly and transposed anteriorly as an interpolation flap. It is then divided 10 weeks later with inset of the pedicle. Scars are hidden in the postauricular sulcus, and tragal projection is maintained. No other reports of a similar single-stage conchal cartilage reconstruction for isolated tragus defect have been described. Regardless of the surgical techniques previously reported, complications related to contraction of the skin flap or distortion of the repair with time are not described.

We describe a method of a lasting, sturdy reconstruction of the tragus using ipsilateral conchal cartilage, harvested through a postauricular incision. It is a simplified, single-stage technique with well-hidden incisions and a functional result. The various techniques that have previously been described may also create excellent cosmetic results; however, more complicated or multistage methods are not always necessary. The stronger and thicker rib cartilage is most often used for microtia repair; however, for isolated tragus reconstruction, conchal cartilage has the advantages of similar character, less harvest morbidity, and faster harvest. The preauricular skin quality and laxity can be assessed by palpation, especially in those patients where there is concern for preauricular scarring or radiation damage, which may preclude them from this technique. Older individuals, who are the most common patients for Mohs, often have a large degree of excess thin skin in the preauricular area that is adequate for graft coverage. This feature makes folding the pretragal skin over the cartilage an excellent option for repair as well as for creating a tension-free closure. There should be no tension on the repair in order to prevent the reconstructed tragus from becoming distorted. The ease of using the ipsilateral ear for graft material without a distant harvest site is another advantage of this technique.

Care was taken to ensure preservation of the pretragal depression to avoid blunting of the tragus, a well-known complication after rhytidectomy [8]. Tanzer [2] described a method of creating a tragal prominence by placing a disc of cartilage through an incision behind the lobule into a tragal pocket and affixing it with compression suture. Addressing the aesthetic importance of the tragus has also been described such as the method by Chin et al. [9] in microtia repair that used a cartilage cube under the tragus for better projection and to enhance the conchal depth.

The tragus has gained a new functional importance in the modern age, since earphones are generally engineered to be reliant on it in order to maintain position. The inability to wear earphones and earplugs was the patient's biggest complaint regarding the defect after Mohs excision. With the common and growing reliance on mobile devices and technologies, which are used with earphones, this type of defect could be considered a disability. This method is a simple way to reconstruct the tragus and restore a patient's ability to wear earphones, earplugs, or hearing aids with minimal morbidity and well-hidden scars.

Disclosure

The views expressed in this article are those of the authors and do not necessarily reflect the official policy or position of the Department of the Navy, the Department of Defense, or the US Government.

Competing Interests

The authors declare no competing interests.

Authors' Contributions

Colleen Perez was responsible for conception, analysis, drafting, and revision of the manuscript. Curtis Gaball was responsible for conception, analysis, and revision of manuscript.

References

[1] H. L. Kirkham, "The use of preserved cartilage in ear reconstruction," *Annals of Surgery*, vol. 111, no. 5, pp. 896–902, 1940.

[2] R. C. Tanzer, "An analysis of ear reconstruction," *Plastic and Reconstructive Surgery*, vol. 31, no. 1, pp. 16–30, 1963.

[3] B. Brent, "The correction of microtia with autogenous cartilage grafts: I. The classic deformity," *Plastic and Reconstructive Surgery*, vol. 66, no. 1, pp. 1–12, 1980.

[4] Q. Xiao, W. Shujie, Z. Hongxing, J. Haiyue, Y. Qinghua, and Y. Dashan, "Using a remnant ear to reconstruct the tragus in total ear reconstruction," *Journal of Plastic, Reconstructive and Aesthetic Surgery*, vol. 62, no. 11, pp. 1411–1417, 2009.

[5] N. Adler, R. Azaria, and D. Ad-El, "Tragus reconstruction after tumor excision with preauricular folded flap," *Dermatologic Surgery*, vol. 33, no. 6, pp. 723–726, 2007.

[6] J. M. Martínez, M. D. Alconchel, C. Olivares, and G. A. Cimorra, "Reconstruction of the tragus after tumour excision," *British Journal of Plastic Surgery*, vol. 50, no. 7, pp. 552–554, 1997.

[7] C. J. Coombs and F. Lin, "Tragal reconstruction after tumor excision," *Annals of Plastic Surgery*, vol. 74, no. 2, pp. 191–194, 2015.

[8] O. M. Ramirez and L. Heller, "The anchor tragal flap: a method of preserving the natural pretragal depression during rhytidectomy," *Plastic and Reconstructive Surgery*, vol. 116, no. 4, pp. 1115–1121, 2005.

[9] W.-S. Chin, R. Zhang, Q. Zhang et al., "Techniques for improving tragus definition in auricular reconstruction with autogenous costal cartilage," *Journal of Plastic, Reconstructive and Aesthetic Surgery*, vol. 64, no. 4, pp. 541–544, 2011.

28

A Case of Periodontal Necrosis following Embolization of Maxillary Artery for Epistaxis

Kohei Nishimoto,[1] Ryosei Minoda,[1] Ryoji Yoshida,[2] Toshinori Hirai,[3] and Eiji Yumoto[1]

[1]Department of Otolaryngology Head and Neck Surgery, Graduate School of Medicine, Kumamoto University, Kumamoto, Japan
[2]Department of Oral and Maxillofacial Surgery, Graduate School of Medicine, Kumamoto University, Kumamoto, Japan
[3]Department of Diagnostic Radiology, Graduate School of Medicine, Kumamoto University, Kumamoto, Japan

Correspondence should be addressed to Kohei Nishimoto; koheihei@hotmail.co.jp

Academic Editor: M. Tayyar Kalcioglu

Embolization of the maxillary artery (MA) is a common treatment modality for refractory epistaxis. Tissue necrosis after embolization of the MA is a rare complication. Here, we reported the first case of the development of necrosis of soft tissue and alveolar bone in the periodontium after embolization. A 48-year-old man with poor oral hygiene and a heavy smoking habit was referred to our clinic due to intractable epistaxis. After treatment with anterior-posterior nasal packing (AP nasal packing), the epistaxis relapsed. Therefore, he underwent embolization of the MA. Although he did not experience epistaxis after embolization, periodontal necrosis developed gradually. The wound healed with necrotomy, administration of antibiotics and prostaglandin, and hyperbaric oxygen therapy. We speculated that the periodontal necrosis was provoked by reduction of blood supply due to embolization and AP nasal packing based on this preexisting morbid state in the periodontium. Poor condition of the oral cavity and smoking may increase the risk of periodontal necrosis after embolization.

1. Introduction

Epistaxis is a common medical problem, occurring in approximately 60% of the population at some time in their life [1–3]. Only 6% of patients with epistaxis require professional medical attention [4]. However, posterior or superior bleeding can often result in intractable epistaxis. Since Sokoloff et al. first reported selective angiography with embolization of the maxillary artery (MA) for treatment of intractable epistaxis in 1974 [5], this technique has gained increased acceptance as a safe and effective treatment for posterior nasal bleeding, with reported success rates of 77.3–94.6%, taking early rebleeding into account [1]. The incidence rate of major complications was reported to be 0–2% [1–3, 6–10]. The reported complications include necrosis of facial skin, nasal alar cartilage, and hard palate mucosa, ischemic sialadenitis of the parotid and submandibular glands, facial scarring following ischemia, temporary hemiparesis, monocular visual field loss and blindness, peripheral facial nerve paralysis, and

cerebral infarction. However, necrosis in the alveolar bone and the surrounding soft tissue in the periodontium after embolization of the MA have not been reported. Here, we report on the first case of necrosis developing in the soft tissue and alveolar bone in the periodontium after embolization.

2. Case Report

A 48-year-old man was referred to our clinic due to intractable epistaxis on the left side. Although the patient had no remarkable medical history, he had been smoking 20 cigarettes per day for 30 years and had received no medical checkups or dental care for many years. On arrival, the source of bleeding was not visible due to continuous bleeding, and his blood pressure was significantly high (194/125 mmHg). Upon intraoral examination, marked accumulation of plaque and calculus was observed at the gingival margin of his maxillary left premolar and molar teeth (Figure 1(a)). Blood

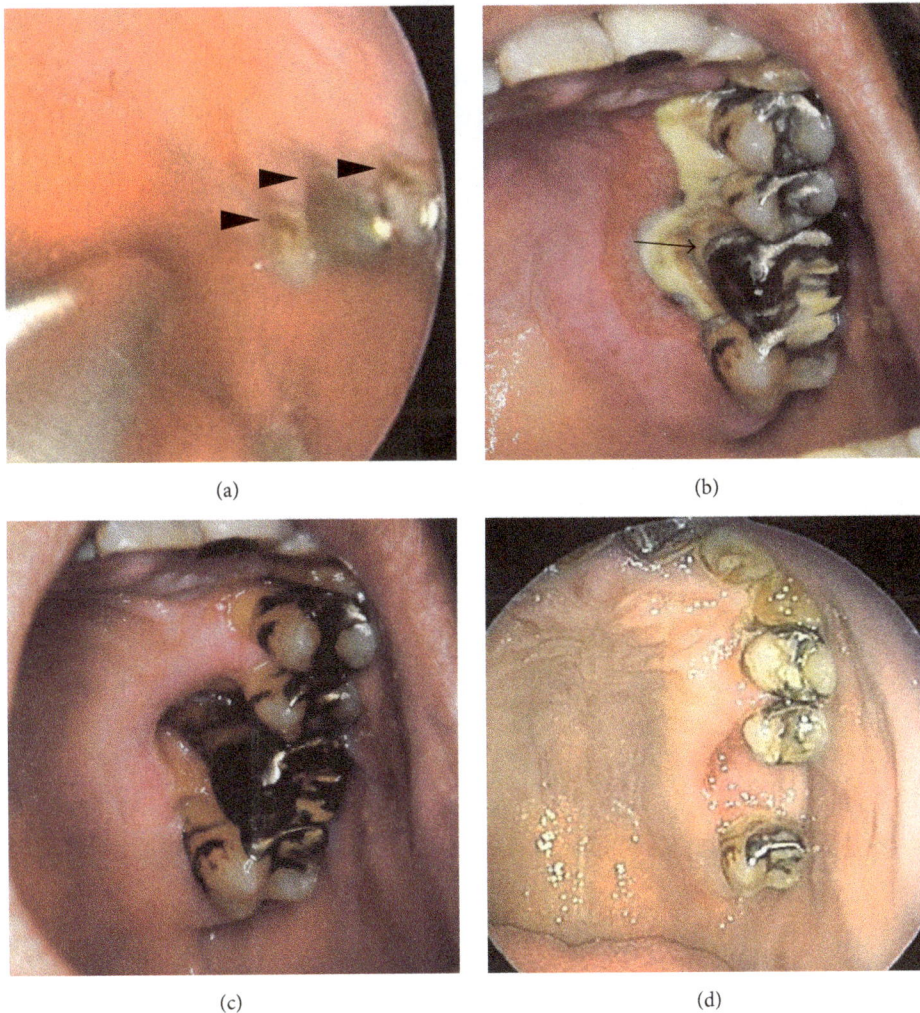

FIGURE 1: Temporal changes in the gingiva around the left upper teeth. (a) At the initial visit, plaque and calculus were observed on the tooth surface (arrowhead), and pockets had developed especially around his maxillary left first molar, which had been capped in silver. (b) Nine days after embolization, necrotizing ulcer formation was observed on the gingiva on the palatal side of the maxillary left premolar and molar teeth. The alveolar bone was exposed due to loss of gingiva (arrow). (c) At 2 weeks after treatment, resorption of the alveolar bone had occurred, and the palatal side of the first molar was fully exposed. Granulation tissue proliferated around the edge of the defect. (d) At 2 months after treatment, the wound was replaced by granulation tissue and epithelialized almost completely, with the exception of the deep socket on the palatal side.

test revealed no significant abnormalities, including diabetes. The bleeding was stopped by nasal packing and nasopharyngeal balloon (hereafter referred to as anterior-posterior nasal packing: AP nasal packing). After hospitalization, a cardiologist started treatment for hypertension and his systolic blood pressure (SBP) decreased to 140–160 mmHg with 40 mg of nifedipine and 1.25 mg of bisoprolol fumarate, and then the pack was removed 5 days after packing. However, 2 days later, epistaxis relapsed, and he was referred to the interventional radiology division for angiography on the same day.

Angiography of the external carotid artery revealed a well-developed left sphenopalatine artery (SPA) and retained contrast medium in the nose, but there was no extravasation. The left MA was selectively embolized using porous cellulose beads (PCBs; Asahi-Kasei, Tokyo, Japan) 230 and 400 μm

in diameter. After embolization, the SPA and descending palatine artery (DPA) disappeared (Figure 2). There was no bleeding after the procedure, although the patient reported slight pain in the left upper teeth, which increased gradually. On the day after removal of the AP nasal packing, the SBP was well controlled to around 120 mmHg by adding 80 mg of valsartan. He was discharged from the hospital 5 days after embolization because of no further epistaxis.

Nine days after embolization, he visited the dental clinic in our hospital because of increasing tooth pain. Marked gingival necrosis was observed on the palatal side of the left maxillary premolar and molar, and the alveolar bone was exposed due to the loss of gingiva (Figure 1(b)). The buccal side was intact and there was no tooth mobility. Panoramic and dental radiographic images detected

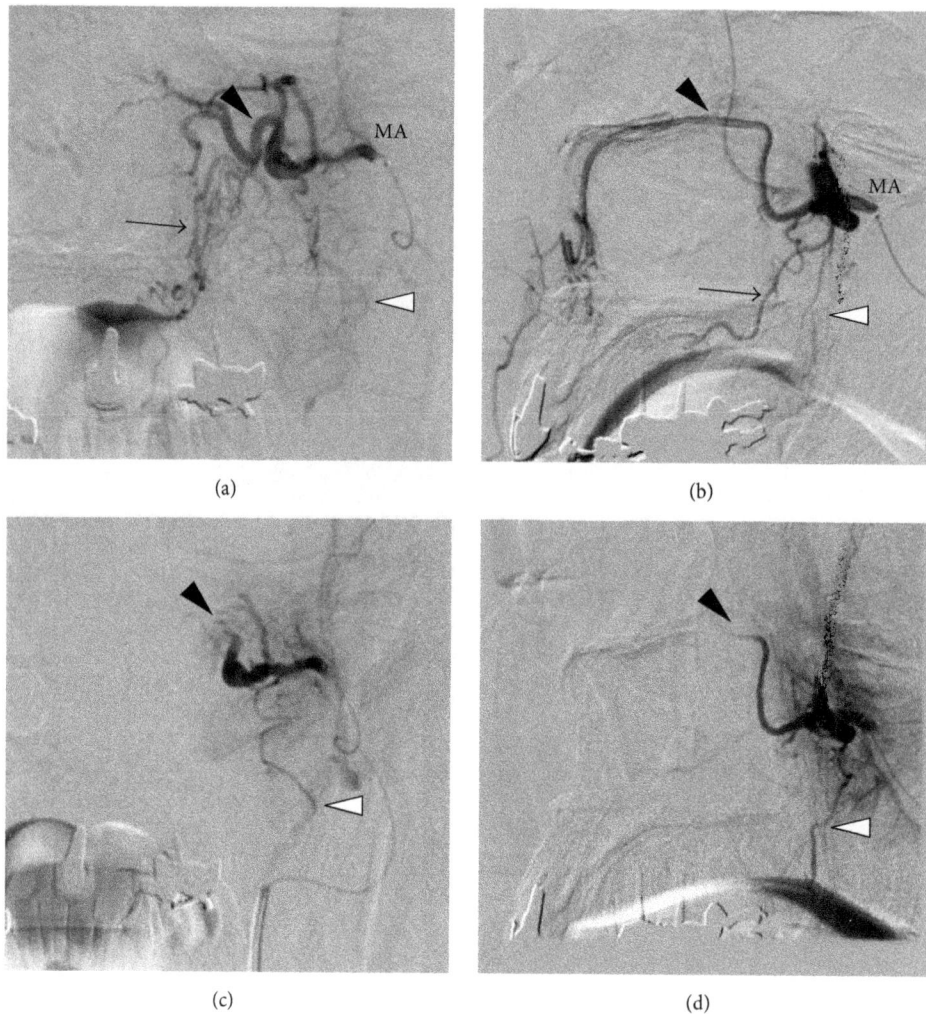

(a)

(b)

(c)

(d)

FIGURE 2: Digital subtraction angiography of the left maxillary artery (MA) in AP view (a, c) and lateral view (b, d). (a, b) Before embolization, well-developed sphenopalatine artery (SPA, black arrowhead) and descending palatine artery (DPA, arrow) were detected. (c, d) After embolization, the SPA and DPA disappeared, while the posterior superior alveolar artery (white arrowhead) was preserved.

a carious cavity, but no defects in the alveolar bone (Figures 3(a) and 3(b)). He was hospitalized again and treated with necrotomy of the gingiva under local anesthesia preserving the alveolar bone, intravenous injection of ceftriaxone sodium (2 g/day), clindamycin (1200 mg/day), and prostaglandin E1 (120 μg/day) and hyperbaric oxygen therapy for 2 weeks. The severe pain was controlled well by oral tramadol hydrochloride/acetaminophen. While granulation occurred gradually around the wound, resorption of the alveolar bone occurred, and the palatal side of the first molar was fully exposed (Figure 1(c)). At 3 weeks after admission, the maxillary left first molar showed mobility, and the tooth was extracted. The extracted tooth had cavities and marked calculus accumulation on the root surface (Figures 3(c) and 3(d)), indicating periodontitis that may have developed for several years. Two months after embolization, the wound was covered by granulation tissue and had epithelialized almost completely, with the exception of the deep socket on the palatal side (Figure 1(d)).

3. Discussion

The MA, which branches from the external carotid artery, is divided into three parts; the portion in the pterygopalatine fossa is called the "third portion" or pterygopalatine portion [11]. In this section, the MA enters through the pterygomaxillary fissure and branches into five arteries; in order before entering the sphenopalatine foramen, these are the posterior superior alveolar artery (PSAA) and the infraorbital artery branch off first and then the DPA, the artery of the pterygoid canal, and the SPA rise [11, 12]. The DPA branches into the greater and lesser palatine arteries and receives branches from the ascending palatal artery originating from the facial artery and the ascending pharyngeal artery [13, 14] and the greater palatine artery anastomoses with SPA at the nasal septum [15]. The palatal side of the upper periodontium is supplied by branches from the SPA (incisor and canine teeth) and greater palatine (premolar and molar teeth) arteries, while the premolar and molar teeth are supplied by the PSAA

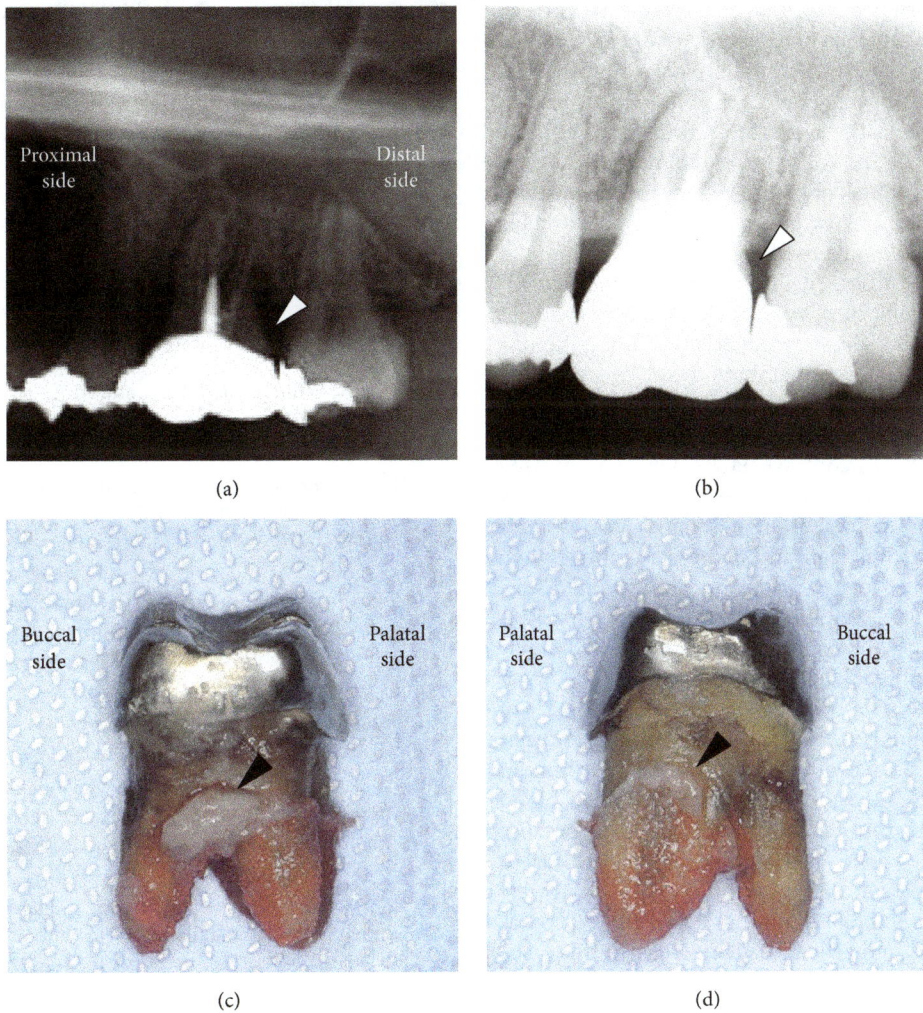

FIGURE 3: (a, b) Panoramic and dental radiographic images after embolization. The maxillary left first molar with crown and root filling material had a carious cavity on the distal side (white arrowhead). There was no defect in the alveolar bone. (c) The proximal and (d) distal sides of the extracted tooth. Cavities, remarkable calculus accumulation on the root surface, and infectious granuloma (arrowhead) were found.

[15]. In our case, the third portion of MA was embolized, and consequently the SPA and the DPA disappeared on angiography while the PSAA remained. The feeding vessel of the molar tooth had been extirpated in previous root canal therapy and the simple loss of blood supply did not cause tooth loss. Embolization of the SPA and the DPA, which are feeding arteries of the palatal side of the upper periodontium, should cause loss of blood supply and/or tissue necrosis in the palatal side of the upper periodontium. Nevertheless, Pearson et al. reported that epistaxis patients did not show any tissue necrosis after ligation of the DPA and the proximal portion of the MA [16], and there have been no previous reports of periodontal necrosis after simple ligation or embolization of the MA and its branches. The blood supply in the palatal side of the periodontium should be maintained through the collateral blood supply from the ascending palatal artery and the ascending pharyngeal artery and through anastomosis between the greater palatine artery and the SPA, as mentioned above.

Guss et al. suggested that AP nasal packing likely exerts pressure on the soft palate and may cause reduction of blood flow to the greater palatine artery by compression of the ascending palatine artery and the ascending pharyngeal artery at the soft palate level [6]. This compression probably reduces the blood supply to the palatal side of the periodontium from the greater palatine artery and the SPA due to reduction of collateral blood supply from the ascending palatine artery and the ascending pharyngeal artery. The effect of reduction of blood supply to the palatal side of the periodontium by AP nasal packing may be more significant in cases where the proximal portions of the DPA and the SPA have been embolized or ligated. Indeed, Guss et al. reported one case in which intravascular embolization of the MA was performed along with AP nasal packing for 2 days [6], and the patient subsequently developed necrosis of the hard palate, which is also fed by the greater palatine artery [15]. Simultaneous embolization and AP nasal packing may also increase the risk of tissue necrosis in the periodontium, but not in the molar teeth, via a similar mechanism. Because of the patient's significantly high blood pressure, we maintained the AP packing for 5 days to decrease the risk of rebleeding. If we removed the AP packing before his blood pressure was normalized with medications, the rebleeding risk could be problematic. Changing the AP packing regimen might have resulted with a reduced risk of tissue necrosis in this case.

Polyvinyl alcohol (PVA), which is a nonabsorbable agent, is the most commonly used material for intravascular embolization [17]. PVA particles have a high friction coefficient due to the irregular surface, which permits the particles to rest against the wall without completely occluding the vessel, and sometimes they agglomerate in the delivery system itself [17]. This characteristic of PVA may cause incomplete filling of the vessel and may increase the probability of recanalization [17, 18]. In contrast, PCBs, which were used in our patient, are also nonabsorbable and exceptionally uniform in size. The nature of PCBs contributes to their smooth intravascular injection and complete embolization. Therefore, PCBs have longer occlusion ability and a low recanalization rate after embolization compared with PVA [17, 18]. Although the low recanalization rate of PCBs may decrease the possibility of relapse of epistaxis, the longer complete embolization by PCBs may increase the risk of tissue necrosis. Although we could not determine the precise locations of embolization in our patient, the distal portions of the SPA and the DPA appeared to be patent, and their blood flow was maintained from the collateral blood flow because the palatal side of the upper periodontium around the incisor and canine teeth, which are fed by branches of the SPA, were unaffected even after embolization. Thus, the use of PCBs was unlikely to be related to the local tissue necrosis in this case.

On the patient's first visit to our clinic, we found marked accumulation of plaque and calculus at the gingival margin of the patient's maxillary left premolar and molar teeth. These findings suggest that he had poor oral hygiene and had periodontitis for many years. Although he underwent dental treatment for these conditions after embolization, his periodontitis and tissue necrosis in the periodontium deteriorated, and he finally lost a tooth. Additionally, our patient had been smoking 20 cigarettes per day for 30 years. Smoking is known to reduce gingival blood flow and is a well-known aggravating factor for the development of periodontitis [19, 20]. His preexisting periodontitis and smoking habit would be major exacerbating factors for the progression of tissue necrosis in the periodontium and loss of the molar tooth. This preexisting morbid state in the periodontium of the premolar and molar teeth likely deeply affected the onset of tissue necrosis in our patient.

4. Conclusions

A side effect to embolization is necrosis of otherwise healthy tissue. This risk is increased if the patient has other vascular risks, as smoking, diabetes, or as in this case poor dental hygiene. We presented an epistaxis patient that developed tissue necrosis in the periodontium and loss of a molar tooth after intravascular embolization of the SPA and the DPA.

Poor oral hygiene and smoking may increase the risk of periodontal necrosis after embolization. Furthermore, the period of AP nasal packing after embolization should be minimized to avoid reduction of blood supply in other areas.

Competing Interests

The authors declare that there is no conflict of interests regarding the publication of this paper.

References

[1] P. W. A. Willems, R. I. Farb, and R. Agid, "Endovascular treatment of epistaxis," *American Journal of Neuroradiology*, vol. 30, no. 9, pp. 1637–1645, 2009.

[2] P. J. Andersen, A. D. Kjeldsen, and J. Nepper-Rasmussen, "Selective embolization in the treatment of intractable epistaxis," *Acta Oto-Laryngologica*, vol. 125, no. 3, pp. 293–297, 2005.

[3] M. Sadri, K. Midwinter, A. Ahmed, and A. Parker, "Assessment of safety and efficacy of arterial embolisation in the management of intractable epistaxis," *European Archives of Oto-Rhino-Laryngology*, vol. 263, no. 6, pp. 560–566, 2006.

[4] M. Small, J. A. Murray, and A. G. Maran, "A study of patients with epistaxis requiring admission to hospital," *Health Bulletin*, vol. 40, no. 1, pp. 20–29, 1982.

[5] J. Sokoloff, I. Wickbom, D. McDonald, F. Brahme, T. C. Goergen, and L. E. Goldberger, "Therapeutic percutaneous embolization in intractable epistaxis," *Radiology*, vol. 111, no. 2, pp. 285–287, 1974.

[6] J. Guss, M. A. Cohen, and N. Mirza, "Hard palate necrosis after bilateral internal maxillary artery embolization for epistaxis," *Laryngoscope*, vol. 117, no. 9, pp. 1683–1684, 2007.

[7] L. Elden, W. Montanera, K. Terbrugge, R. Willinsky, P. Lasjaunias, and D. Charles, "Angiographic embolization for the treatment of epistaxis: a review of 108 cases," *Otolaryngology—Head and Neck Surgery*, vol. 111, no. 1, pp. 44–50, 1994.

[8] M. Yilmaz, M. Mamanov, M. Yener, F. Aydin, O. Kizilkilic, and A. Eren, "Acute ischemia of the parotid gland and auricle following embolization for epistaxis," *Laryngoscope*, vol. 123, no. 2, pp. 366–368, 2013.

[9] A. Ntomouchtsis, G. Venetis, L. Zouloumis, and N. Lazaridis, "Ischemic necrosis of nose and palate after embolization for epistaxis. A case report," *Oral and Maxillofacial Surgery*, vol. 14, no. 2, pp. 123–127, 2010.

[10] M. Wehrli, U. Lieberherr, and A. Valavanis, "Superselective embolization for intractable epistaxis: experiences with 19 patients," *Clinical Otolaryngology and Allied Sciences*, vol. 13, no. 6, pp. 415–420, 1988.

[11] J. Choi and H.-S. Park, "The clinical anatomy of the maxillary artery in the pterygopalatine fossa," *Journal of Oral and Maxillofacial Surgery*, vol. 61, no. 1, pp. 72–78, 2003.

[12] J.-K. Kim, J. H. Cho, Y.-J. Lee et al., "Anatomical variability of the maxillary artery: findings from 100 Asian cadaveric dissections," *Archives of Otolaryngology—Head and Neck Surgery*, vol. 138, no. 5, p. 525, 2012.

[13] J. W. Siebert, C. Angrigiani, J. G. McCarthy, and M. T. Longaker, "Blood supply of the Le Fort I maxillary segment: An Anatomic Study," *Plastic and Reconstructive Surgery*, vol. 100, no. 4, pp. 843–850, 1997.

[14] L. Hacein-Bey, D. L. Daniels, J. L. Ulmer et al., "The ascending pharyngeal artery: branches, anastomoses, and clinical significance," *American Journal of Neuroradiology*, vol. 23, no. 7, pp. 1246–1256, 2002.

[15] R. L. Drake, W. Vogl, and A. W. M. Mitchell, *Gray's Anatomy for Students*, Churchill Livingstone, Edinburgh, Scotland, 3rd edition, 2015.

[16] B. W. Pearson, R. G. Mac Kenzie, and W. S. Goodman, "The anatomical basis of transantral ligation of the maxillary artery in severe epistaxis," *Laryngoscope*, vol. 79, no. 5, pp. 969–984, 1969.

[17] J.-I. Hamada, Y. Ushio, K. Kazekawa, T. Tsukahara, N. Hashimoto, and H. Iwata, "Embolization with cellulose porous beads, I: An Experimental Study," *American Journal of Neuroradiology*, vol. 17, no. 10, pp. 1895–1899, 1996.

[18] J.-I. Hamada, Y. Kai, S. Nagahiro, N. Hashimoto, H. Iwata, and Y. Ushio, "Embolization with cellulose porous beads, II: clinical trial," *American Journal of Neuroradiology*, vol. 17, no. 10, pp. 1901–1906, 1996.

[19] D. A. Baab and P. Å. Öberg, "The effect of cigarette smoking on gingival blood flow in humans," *Journal of Clinical Periodontology*, vol. 14, no. 7, pp. 418–424, 1987.

[20] M. Petrovic, L. Kesic, R. Obradovic et al., "Comparative analysis of smoking influence on periodontal tissue in subjects with periodontal disease," *Materia Sociomedica*, vol. 25, no. 3, pp. 196–198, 2013.

29

Refractory Obstructive Sleep Apnea in a Patient with Diffuse Idiopathic Skeletal Hyperostosis

Ara Darakjian,[1] Ani B. Darakjian,[2] Edward T. Chang,[3] and Macario Camacho[3,4]

[1]Department of Psychiatry and Behavioral Sciences, Keck School of Medicine, 1975 Zonal Ave, Los Angeles, CA 90033, USA
[2]Department of Radiology, Southern California Permanente Medical Group, 4867 W. Sunset Blvd, Los Angeles, CA 90027, USA
[3]Division of Otolaryngology-Head and Neck Surgery, Tripler Army Medical Center, 1 Jarrett White Rd, Honolulu, HI 96859, USA
[4]Department of Psychiatry and Behavioral Sciences, Sleep Medicine Division, Stanford Hospital and Clinics, 450 Broadway St,
 Pavillion B., Redwood City, CA 94063, USA

Correspondence should be addressed to Macario Camacho; drcamachoent@yahoo.com

Academic Editor: Rong-San Jiang

Diffuse Idiopathic Skeletal Hyperostosis (DISH) can cause ossification of ligaments and may affect the spine. We report a case of obstructive sleep apnea in a patient with significant upper airway narrowing secondary to cervical DISH. This patient had an initial apnea-hypopnea index (AHI) of 145 events/hour and was treated with uvulopalatopharyngoplasty, genial tubercle advancement, hyoid suspension, septoplasty, inferior turbinoplasties, and radiofrequency ablations to the tongue base which reduced his AHI to 40 events/hour. He redeveloped symptoms, was started on positive airway pressure (PAP) therapy, and later underwent a maxillomandibular advancement which improved his AHI to 16.3 events/hour. A few years later his AHI was 100.4 events/hour. His disease has gradually progressed over time and he was restarted on PAP therapy. Despite PAP titration, years of using PAP therapy, and being 100 percent compliant for the past three months (average daily use of 7.6 hours/night), he has an AHI of 5.1 events/hour and has persistent hypersomnia with an Epworth Sleep Scale questionnaire score of 18/24. At this time he is pending further hypersomnia work-up. DISH patients require prolonged follow-up to monitor the progression of disease, and they may require unconventional measures for adequate treatment of obstructive sleep apnea.

1. Introduction

Diffuse Idiopathic Skeletal Hyperostosis (DISH) is an idiopathic noninflammatory disease that is characterized by calcification and ossification of spinal ligaments and enthuses [1]. It is a surprisingly common condition, being found in 6–12% of a population that underwent an autopsy for other reasons [1]. DISH can be asymptomatic; however, in those who are symptomatic, the most common manifestations include a decreased range of motion in the thoracic spine, shoulder pain, and neck pain. Most cases are sufficiently managed with NSAIDs and supportive therapies. Less commonly, DISH has been reported to cause dysphagia and obstructive sleep apnea secondary to narrowing of the upper airway [2], but few cases are severe enough to manifest in this way. Previous reports in the literature of obstructive sleep apnea secondary to DISH have shown successful treatment with continuous positive airway pressure (CPAP) therapy [2–4]. We describe the complicated treatment course of a patient with DISH, whose large anterior cervical osteophytes caused significant narrowing of his upper airway and subsequent sleep apnea. While sleep surgeries initially led to resolution of symptoms, the patient continued to have an elevated apnea-hypopnea index and required further surgery as well as positive airway pressure therapy due to recurrence of obstructive sleep apnea.

2. Case Presentation

A 38-year-old man presented to the sleep medicine clinic with hypersomnia. A polysomnogram demonstrated obstructive sleep apnea (OSA) with an apnea-hypopnea index (AHI) of 145 events/hour. The patient was treated with CPAP therapy at 9 cm of water pressure (cwp). He was unable to tolerate CPAP and had significant symptoms, and therefore he was referred to a sleep surgeon for evaluation. The patient underwent sleep surgery in 1996, consisting of uvulopalatopharyngoplasty (UPPP), genial tubercle advancement, hyoid suspension, septoplasty, and bilateral inferior turbinate reduction. The patient had such significant improvement in his symptoms that he did not use CPAP therapy after surgery (however, it is unknown to what extent his AHI improved, if at all, since no sleep study was performed after surgery). Two years after the sleep surgery, the patient subsequently complained of dysphagia, neck stiffness, headache, and tingling in his left hand. After various forms of imaging he was diagnosed with DISH with significant anterior cervical osteophytes at the C5-C6 level.

Over the next three years, he developed hypersomnia and was treated with five radiofrequency ablations of the tongue base. After the treatment, he noted significant improvement in symptoms. However, his neck pain worsened to the point where he required a C5-C6 discectomy. The patient subsequently redeveloped hypersomnia in 2002 and a repeat polysomnogram demonstrated an AHI of 40 events/hour. The patient again attempted CPAP but was intolerant to the therapy and underwent an advancement of the maxillo-mandibular complex by 10 mm. Despite a reduction of the AHI to 16.3 events/hour, the patient's hypersomnia persisted. The patient was then counseled to reattempt treatment with CPAP. In 2006, the patient underwent a split night study which demonstrated an AHI of 100.4 events/hour and a positive airway pressure titration study recommending bilevel positive airway pressure (bilevel) therapy, set to an inspiratory positive airway pressure (IPAP) of 10 centimeters of water pressure (cwp) and expiratory positive airway pressure (EPAP) of 6 cwp. Over the years his hypersomnia progressively worsened, requiring bilevel titration, and his new pressures were an IPAP of 22 cwp and an EPAP of 14 cwp.

Today, the patient is 57 years old and has continued to use positive airway pressure therapy. The bilevel data download demonstrates 100% compliance for the past three months and an average daily use of 7.6 hours/night. Despite the higher pressures, there was a residual device downloaded AHI of 5.1/h and the patient had persistent hypersomnia with an Epworth Sleep Scale (ESS) questionnaire score of 18/24 (≥11 being the cutoff for hypersomnia). Physical examination reveals that the patient is 71 inches and 240 lbs (body mass index of 33.5 kg/m^2) with a blood pressure of 143/76. His nasal septum is straight and his inferior turbinates are nonobstructing bilaterally (grades 1 or 2) [5]. He has a high-arched and narrow hard palate, an overjet of 3 mm, tongue scalloping, and a Grade 3 Friedman Palate Position [6]. A plain neck radiograph (Figure 1) demonstrates large anterior cervical spine osteophytes involving C2 through C4, with sparing of the disc space and clear obstruction of the upper airway. The osteophytes are so large that they abut against the epiglottis. Potential causes for the patient's hypersomnia that were explored include (1) insomnia secondary to pain where he awakens several times throughout the night secondary to neck pain, currently treated with gabapentin 900 mg three times a day, and sometimes takes hydrocodone when the pain

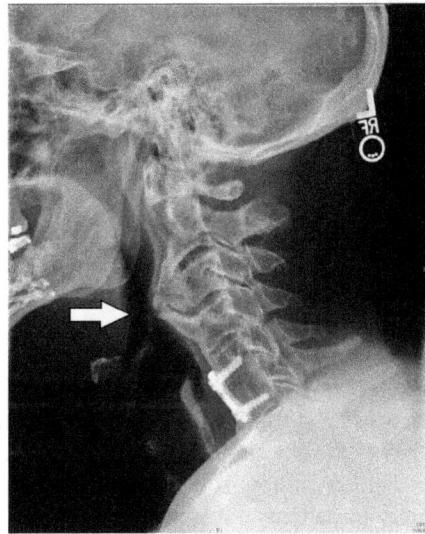

FIGURE 1: Large anterior osteophytes involving C2–4 (white arrow). Note there is sparing of the disc spaces. The bulge narrows the upper airway, abutting the epiglottis.

is significant, (2) history of prostate hypertrophy with nocturnal awakenings treated with tamsulosin 0.4 mg daily, (3) higher bilevel pressures awaken him because of "the sensation of strong airflow," and (4) restless leg syndrome treated with pramipexole 0.5 mg daily. Despite the appropriate medical management, the patient's hypersomnia has persisted, so he was prescribed modafinil 200 mg each morning. The patient states that the modafinil helps somewhat during the day, but it does not help him enough. In order to further assist the patient in reducing his hypersomnia, we are considering the following: (1) a new bilevel titration study to improve his experience with positive airway pressure therapy, (2) a multiple sleep latency test (MSLT) to help rule out narcolepsy, and (3) blood testing for other sources that can cause fatigue, sleepiness, and tiredness to include testosterone levels and iron levels.

3. Discussion

This case study patient presents with classic clinical manifestations and radiographic findings of DISH. He describes dysphagia and a stiff neck with a decreased range of motion in addition to neck and shoulder pain. The radiographic findings are consistent with DISH, which is described as "flowing mantles" of ossification most commonly involving the anterior longitudinal ligament, without significant narrowing of the disc space [7, 8]. Given that the upper airway can narrow significantly (33%) in OSA patients by the simple act of changing from the upright to the supine positions [9], it is not surprising that, with such large osteophytes, the patient is experiencing upper airway obstruction during sleep.

OSA is a common disorder, and CPAP is a highly efficacious treatment [10]. However, as in this patient, the effectiveness is limited by compliance, which is estimated to be 46–83% when adherence is defined as greater than 4 hours of nightly use [11]. In addition to CPAP or bilevel, other medical options include mandibular advancement devices, weight loss, positional therapy, and wedge pillows; however, the efficacy and effectiveness of each of these are variable. After exhausting medical management, soft tissue sleep surgery or maxillomandibular advancement surgeries are commonly used to relieve upper airway obstruction. When performing soft tissue sleep surgery, the most effective technique has been demonstrated to be multilevel surgeries that target the sites of obstruction, including nasal surgeries, tongue reduction/stabilization or advancement surgeries, oropharyngeal surgeries, and hypopharyngeal surgeries. A systematic review of multilevel surgeries has demonstrated a 66.4% success rate [12]. Maxillomandibular advancement, one of the most effective surgeries for sleep apnea [13], can be performed either without soft tissue sleep surgery or as a second surgery in patients not successfully treated with soft tissue sleep surgery. In this patient, it is unclear why there was a sixfold increase in the AHI after the maxillomandibular advancement (from 16.3 events/hour to 100.4 events/hour) over a matter of four years.

This patient currently uses a bilevel positive airway pressure (bilevel) machine, which is used for patients that have a persistently elevated AHI despite use of CPAP. According to the 2013 Official American Thoracic Society Statement for CPAP adherence and tracking, an AHI < 10 events/hour is considered effective treatment. Therefore, we consider our patient, with residual AHI of 5.1, to be effectively treated and are considering other sources for his hypersomnia [14]. However, given his persistent hypersomnia and residual AHI, there is an argument for another BiPAP titration study with a goal of further reducing his AHI, especially if other causes for his hypersomnia are ruled out.

4. Conclusion

DISH is a common disorder that can cause obstructive sleep apnea secondary to large anterior cervical osteophyte formation in severe cases. This case study demonstrates the need to follow the patients in the long term as they may initially do well with soft tissue sleep surgery or maxillomandibular advancement surgeries but may require positive airway pressure via CPAP or bilevel in the long term.

Disclosure

The work was primarily performed in Stanford Hospital and Clinics. The views expressed in this manuscript are those of the authors and do not reflect the official policy or position of the Department of the Army, Department of Defense, or the US Government.

Competing Interests

The authors declare that there is no conflict of interest regarding the publication of this paper.

References

[1] D. Resnick, R. F. Shapiro, K. B. Wiesner, G. Niwayama, P. D. Utsinger, and S. R. Shaul, "Diffuse idiopathic skeletal hyperostosis (DISH)," *Seminars in Arthritis and Rheumatism*, vol. 7, no. 3, pp. 153–187, 1978.

[2] B. Naik, E. B. Lobato, and C. A. Sulek, "Dysphagia, obstructive sleep apnea, and difficult fiberoptic intubation secondary to diffuse idiopathic skeletal hyperostosis," *Anesthesiology*, vol. 100, no. 5, pp. 1311–1312, 2004.

[3] T. A. T. Hughes, C. M. Wiles, B. W. Lawrie, and A. P. Smith, "Case report: dysphagia and sleep apnoea associated with cervical osteophytes due to diffuse idiopathic skeletal hyperostosis (DISH)," *Journal of Neurology, Neurosurgery & Psychiatry*, vol. 57, no. 3, p. 384, 1994.

[4] E. Kawauchi, T. Yamagata, and Y. Tohda, "A case of Forestier disease with obstructive sleep apnea syndrome," *Sleep & Breathing*, vol. 16, no. 3, pp. 603–605, 2012.

[5] M. Camacho, S. Zaghi, V. Certal et al., "Inferior turbinate classification system, grades 1 to 4: development and validation study," *The Laryngoscope*, vol. 125, no. 2, pp. 296–302, 2015.

[6] M. Friedman, H. Tanyeri, M. La Rosa et al., "Clinical predictors of obstructive sleep apnea," *The Laryngoscope*, vol. 109, no. 12, pp. 1901–1907, 1999.

[7] D. Resnick and G. Niwayama, "Radiographic and pathologic features of spinal involvement in diffuse idiopathic skeletal hyperostosis (DISH)," *Radiology*, vol. 119, no. 3, pp. 559–568, 1976.

[8] B. Vernon-Roberts, C. J. Pirie, and V. Trenwith, "Pathology of the dorsal spine in ankylosing hyperostosis," *Annals of the Rheumatic Diseases*, vol. 33, no. 4, pp. 281–288, 1974.

[9] M. Camacho, R. Capasso, and S. Schendel, "Airway changes in obstructive sleep apnoea patients associated with a supine versus an upright position examined using cone beam computed tomography," *The Journal of Laryngology and Otology*, vol. 128, no. 9, pp. 824–830, 2014.

[10] T. L. Giles, T. J. Lasserson, B. H. Smith, J. White, J. Wright, and C. J. Cates, "Continuous positive airways pressure for obstructive sleep apnoea in adults," *Cochrane Database of Systematic Reviews*, vol. 3, Article ID CD001106, 2006.

[11] T. E. Weaver and R. R. Grunstein, "Adherence to continuous positive airway pressure therapy: the challenge to effective treatment," *Proceedings of the American Thoracic Society*, vol. 5, no. 2, pp. 173–178, 2008.

[12] S. M. Caples, J. A. Rowley, J. R. Prinsell et al., "Surgical modifications of the upper airway for obstructive sleep apnea in adults: a systematic review and meta-analysis," *Sleep*, vol. 33, no. 10, pp. 1396–1407, 2010.

[13] S. Zaghi, J.-E. C. Holty, V. Certal et al., "Maxillomandibular advancement for treatment of obstructive sleep apnea: a meta-analysis," *JAMA Otolaryngology—Head and Neck Surgery*, vol. 142, no. 1, pp. 58–66, 2016.

[14] R. J. Schwab, S. M. Badr, L. J. Epstein et al., "An official american thoracic society statement: continuous positive airway pressure adherence tracking systems the optimal monitoring strategies and outcome measures in adults," *American Journal of Respiratory and Critical Care Medicine*, vol. 188, no. 5, pp. 613–620, 2013.

30

Bilateral Vocal Cord Paralysis and Cervicolumbar Radiculopathy as the Presenting Paraneoplastic Manifestations of Small Cell Lung Cancer: A Case Report and Literature Review

Jeffrey C. Yeung,[1] C. Elizabeth Pringle,[2] Harmanjatinder S. Sekhon,[3] Shaun J. Kilty,[1] and Kristian Macdonald[1]

[1]*Department of Otolaryngology-Head & Neck Surgery, University of Ottawa, Ottawa, ON, Canada*
[2]*Division of Neurology, Department of Medicine, University of Ottawa, Ottawa, ON, Canada*
[3]*Department of Pathology & Laboratory Medicine, University of Ottawa, Ottawa, ON, Canada*

Correspondence should be addressed to Jeffrey C. Yeung; jeffrey.yeung@childrens.harvard.edu

Academic Editor: Tamás Karosi

Introduction. Bilateral vocal cord paralysis (BVCP) is a potential medical emergency. The Otolaryngologist plays a crucial role in the diagnosis and management of BVCP and must consider a broad differential diagnosis. We present a rare case of BVCP secondary to anti-Hu paraneoplastic syndrome. *Case Presentation.* A 58-year-old female presented to an Otolaryngology clinic with a history of progressive hoarseness and dysphagia. Flexible nasolaryngoscopy demonstrated BVCP. Cross-sectional imaging of the brain and vagus nerves was negative. An antiparaneoplastic antibody panel was positive for anti-Hu antibodies. This led to an endobronchial biopsy of a paratracheal lymph node, which confirmed the diagnosis of small cell lung cancer. *Conclusion.* Paraneoplastic neuropathy is a rare cause of BVCP and should be considered when more common pathologies are ruled out. This is the second reported case of BVCP as a presenting symptom of paraneoplastic syndrome secondary to small cell lung cancer.

1. Introduction

Bilateral vocal cord paralysis (BVCP) is a potentially life-threatening emergency and the presenting symptoms include upper airway obstruction, dyspnea, and stridor. The Otolaryngologist-Head and Neck Surgeon has an integral role in the evaluation, diagnosis, and management of patients with such symptoms. In adults, the most common etiologies of BVCP include iatrogenic injury, direct tumour compression, neurologic disease, and idiopathic etiologies [1]. In the event that imaging of the brain and recurrent laryngeal nerve is normal, the Otolaryngologist must broaden his/her differential diagnosis and consider more infrequent causes before concluding that BVCP is idiopathic. We present a rare case of BVCP secondary to anti-Hu paraneoplastic syndrome.

2. Case Report

A 58-year-old female was referred to an Otolaryngology outpatient clinic with a 6-month history of progressive hoarseness and dysphagia, associated with a 20-pound weight loss.

On further history examination, she had several seemingly unassociated medical symptoms over the previous year, including right hand and lower limb pain and weakness. She was subsequently diagnosed with carpal tunnel syndrome and right C6, left C7, and right L5 radiculopathy.

Four months prior to the current presentation, she was diagnosed with right middle lobe pneumonia and treated with a course of antibiotics. Despite medical management, she had persistent symptoms and consequently a computed tomography (CT) scan of the thorax was ordered. This scan demonstrated right middle lobe consolidation and atelectasis with mediastinal and hilar lymphadenopathy. Flexible bronchoscopy was performed at the time, and bronchoalveolar lavage of the right middle lobe, brush biopsies, and endobronchial biopsies were negative for malignancy. At that time, her vocal cords were documented to be normal.

A follow-up CT scan demonstrated moderate resolution of the pneumonia.

The patient's relevant past medical history included a 40-pack-year smoking history and chronic obstructive pulmonary disease. She had no known medication allergies. There was no previous history of head and neck surgery.

On physical examination, she was cachectic in appearance. She had audible inspiratory stridor and increased work of breathing. Flexible nasolaryngoscopy revealed bilateral vocal cord paralysis. There was no palpable neck mass. The remainder of the cranial nerve examination was normal, as was the remainder of the head and neck examination.

Informed consent was obtained and the patient was taken to the operating room for a tracheostomy. Postoperatively, a CT scan of the skull base to the aortic arch was ordered and no lesion along the course of either vagus nerve was found. A modified barium swallow demonstrated mild oral and moderate pharyngeal phase dysphagia with frank aspiration, and, as a result, enteral feeding was initiated.

The patient went on to develop polyradiculoneuropathy, bilateral facial weakness, and recurrent tachyarrhythmias. Electrophysiologic studies were repeated and revealed length-dependent axonal sensorimotor polyneuropathy, progressive compared to her previous study. The study did not demonstrate hallmarks of acute inflammatory demyelinating polyradiculoneuropathy (namely, conduction block or temporal dispersion). Pending further investigations, a trial of intravenous immunoglobulin was initiated. A full workup, including magnetic resonance imaging of the brain, lumbar puncture, vasculitic markers, and serum/urine protein electrophoresis, was ordered. Cerebrospinal fluid analysis demonstrated mild pleiocytosis and elevated protein levels but no malignant cells. An anti-paraneoplastic antibody panel was positive for anti-Hu antibodies. A repeat CT scan of the thorax was performed, which demonstrated a new necrotic level 4R paratracheal lymph node (Figure 1). An endobronchial ultrasound guided biopsy of this node confirmed the diagnosis of small cell lung cancer (SCLC) (Figure 2). A complete oncologic workup was subsequently performed and no primary tumour or distant metastases were identified.

The patient's symptoms did not respond to therapeutic trials of intravenous immunoglobulin, plasmapheresis, or chemotherapy (carboplatin, etoposide, and dexamethasone). She unfortunately developed febrile neutropenia and acute hypoxemic respiratory failure and was admitted to the intensive care unit for positive pressure ventilation. Her condition continued to worsen and she unfortunately passed away following withdrawal of ventilatory support.

3. Discussion

We used the search query ("vocal cord paralysis" OR ("vocal" AND "cord" AND "paralysis") OR "vocal cord paralysis") AND (anti-Hu OR paraneoplastic) in Pubmed until October 1st, 2015. We identified one other reported case of bilateral vocal cord paralysis as a paraneoplastic manifestation of SCLC [2, 3]. Similar to the patient described in our case

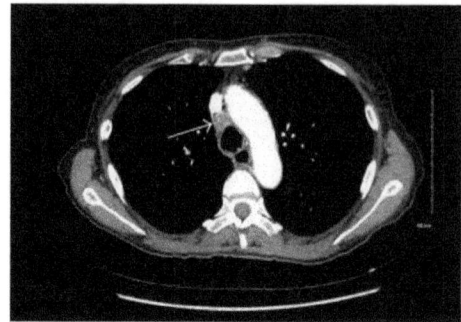

FIGURE 1: CT scan of the thorax demonstrating necrotic paratracheal node. Enhanced axial CT scan of the thorax, mediastinal window, in a 58-year-old female who presented with bilateral vocal cord immobility of unknown etiology. The positive serum anti-Hu antibody, which is highly associated with small cell lung carcinoma, led to this repeat CT scan. The arrow demonstrates an enlarged level 4R paratracheal lymph node with central necrosis. See Figure 2 for the pathologic description of a biopsy from this node.

report, this patient had also developed several somatic complaints before BVCP was diagnosed, including psychiatric symptoms, paresthesias, vertigo, anxiety, and depression. The patient had also recently been diagnosed with fibromyalgia and systemic lupus erythematosus. Years after these initial symptoms manifested, she was referred to an Otolaryngologist for progressive weight loss, dysphagia, and dysphonia and was then diagnosed with BVCP.

3.1. Paraneoplastic Neuropathy. Several malignancies have a higher propensity to cause paraneoplastic neuropathies, including SCLC, lymphoma, adenocarcinoma, and thymic carcinoma [4]. Paraneoplastic neuropathy associated with anti-Hu antibodies (or anti-Hu syndrome) commonly presents as encephalomyelitis, sensory neuronopathy, cerebellar degeneration, and autonomic neuropathy [5]. The diagnosis can typically be confirmed by the presence of autoantibodies in serum. In the case of anti-Hu syndrome, the majority of patients with paraneoplastic sensory neuronopathy are seropositive, though up to 16% of patients can be seronegative [4].

3.2. Hu Antigens and Anti-Hu Antibodies. The Hu antigens are a family of intranuclear and intracytoplasmic proteins that are expressed by all neurons of central and peripheral nervous systems. These antigens are also present in almost all SCLC tumour cells but are characteristically absent in most normal nonneuronal cells [6]. The function of these proteins is not currently known, but it is postulated that they promote differentiation and maintenance of the neuronal phenotype. The anti-Hu IgG antibodies were discovered in 1985, identified in the CSF of a patient with SCLC [7]. The antibody and antigen now bear the name of this index patient.

The presence of anti-Hu antibodies in serum carries a 99% specificity for SCLC [8]. Consequently, the prospect of anti-Hu antibodies as an early marker and prognostic indicator for SCLC has been proposed [9]. However, anti-Hu antibodies have also been identified in patients with various

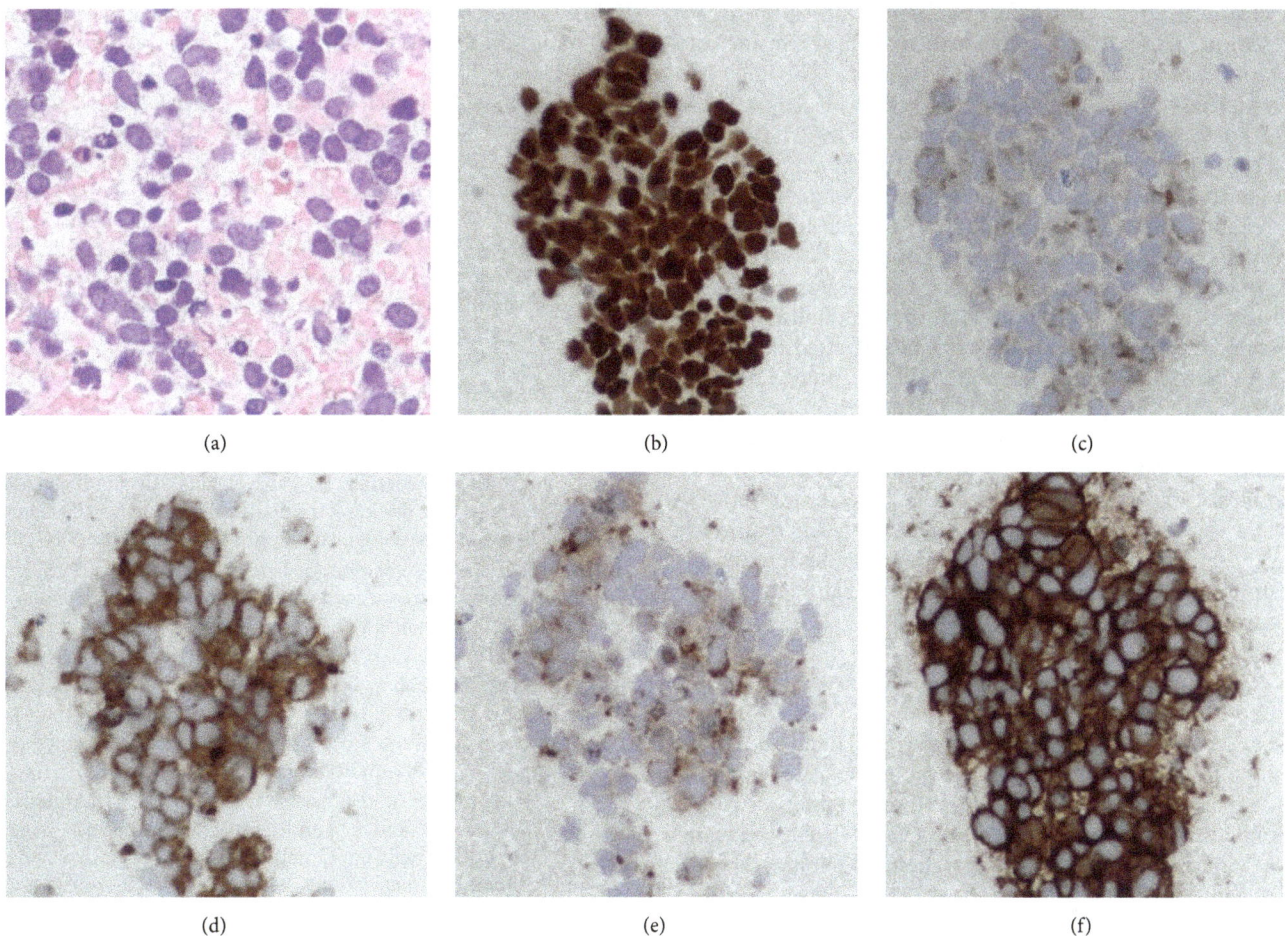

FIGURE 2: Representative cytology slides of paratracheal lymph node. Cytology of endobronchial ultrasound guided fine needle biopsy from the necrotic mediastinal lymph node in Figure 1. Hematoxylin and eosin stain of cell block section (a) demonstrated crowded, overlapping groups of malignant cells in a background of necrosis. Immunohistochemistry was positive for TTF-1 (b), AE-1/AE-3, perinuclear dot-like positivity (c), synaptophysin (d), chromogranin (e), and CD56 (f), confirming the diagnosis of small cell lung carcinoma.

other malignancies such as lymphoma, thymic carcinoma, neuroblastoma, synovial carcinoma, nonseminomatous testicular germ cell tumours, and carcinoma of the gallbladder [6, 10–14]. Anti-Hu antibodies have also been identified in pediatric patients with autoimmune nonparaneoplastic limbic encephalitis [15].

3.3. Clinical Manifestations, Diagnostic Criteria, and Management of Anti-Hu Syndrome. In addition to the more common manifestations listed above, the most common cranial nerve manifestation in patients with anti-Hu syndrome is subacute sensorineural hearing loss [16, 17]. In anti-Hu syndrome, neurological symptoms typically precede tumour detection by a median of 7.5 months (range: 3–31 months) [18]. The neurological deficits associated with anti-Hu syndrome are typically progressive.

The presence of serum anti-Hu antibodies has been associated with improved prognosis in patients with underlying malignancies. In a series of 196 patients with SCLC, patients positive for anti-Hu antibodies (n = 32) demonstrated improved response to chemotherapy (55.6% versus 19.6%) and improved survival (14.9 versus 10.2 months), compared to those who were negative for anti-Hu antibodies [19]. It is hypothesized that the patients who produce anti-Hu antibodies are able to mount an immune response against the tumour, thus conferring them with a better prognosis. This was further alluded to in a case of spontaneous tumour regression seen in the setting of anti-Hu syndrome and SCLC [20].

Diagnostic criteria for paraneoplastic neuropathies were previously described and are divided into "definite" and "possible" based on the presence or absence of classical paraneoplastic phenomena and/or onconeural antibodies [21]. While our patient did not present with a classical paraneoplastic syndrome, she was found to have onconeural antibodies in her serum and would therefore meet criteria for definite paraneoplastic syndrome, as defined by Graus and Dalmau. The diagnosis of anti-Hu paraneoplastic syndrome requires 3 criteria: (1) clinical signs of central or peripheral neuropathy, (2) no direct tumour infiltration, compression, or metastasis to the nervous system, and (3) presence of serum anti-Hu antibodies [4]. Other systemic autoantibodies (such as anti-DNA, anti-centromere, anti-Ro, and anti-La) are present in up to 33% of patients with anti-Hu syndrome, and this may potentially confound the diagnosis. The diagnosis of anti-Hu syndrome should be followed by investigations to rule out an underlying malignancy, specifically SCLC.

The management of anti-Hu syndrome should be directed at identifying and treating the underlying malignancy, as well as rehabilitation of the neurological deficits. Immunosuppressants and immunomodulators previously described for use in anti-Hu syndrome include corticosteroids, rituximab, plasmapheresis, and intravenous immunoglobulins [4]. The outcomes of these therapies have not been studied extensively in large sample sizes, as documented by a recent Cochrane review [22]. The current body of literature consists only of small case series, case reports, and expert opinion. A recent example, an open-label study of sirolimus, did not find a significant improvement compared to other immunotherapies, with only 2 out of 17 patients demonstrating a response [23]. Currently, there is a lack of evidence endorsing the use of immunosuppressants and immunomodulators in anti-Hu syndrome.

4. Conclusion

We describe the second reported case of bilateral vocal cord immobility associated with anti-Hu paraneoplastic syndrome and small cell lung carcinoma. After ruling out more common etiologies, it may be helpful for the clinician to consider this diagnosis when investigating patients with bilateral vocal cord paralysis.

Competing Interests

None of the authors have conflict of interests to disclose.

Authors' Contributions

Jeffrey C. Yeung was involved in the patient's care, performed the literature review, and prepared the manuscript. C. Elizabeth Pringle was involved in the patient's care and contributed to manuscript preparation. Harmanjatinder S. Sekhon prepared and interpreted histopathologic slides and contributed to manuscript preparation. Shaun J. Kilty reviewed the manuscript and revised it critically for intellectual content. Kristian Macdonald was involved in the patient's care, reviewed the manuscript, and revised it critically for intellectual content. All authors read and approved the final manuscript.

References

[1] L. D. Holinger, P. C. Holinger, and P. H. Holinger, "Etiology of bilateral abductor vocal cord paralysis: a review of 389 cases," *Annals of Otology, Rhinology and Laryngology*, vol. 85, no. 4 I, pp. 428–436, 1976.

[2] C. Y. Chang, T. Martinu, and D. L. Witsell, "Bilateral vocal cord paresis as a presenting sign of paraneoplastic syndrome: case report," *Otolaryngology-Head and Neck Surgery*, vol. 130, no. 6, pp. 788–790, 2004.

[3] T. Martinu and A. S. Clay, "A 50-year-old woman with bilateral vocal cord paralysis and hilar mass," *Chest*, vol. 128, no. 2, pp. 1028–1031, 2005.

[4] F. Graus and J. Dalmau, "Paraneoplastic neuropathies," *Current Opinion in Neurology*, vol. 26, no. 5, pp. 489–495, 2013.

[5] F. Graus, F. Keime-Guibert, R. Reñe et al., "Anti-Hu-associated paraneoplastic encephalomyelitis: analysis of 200 patients," *Brain*, vol. 124, no. 6, pp. 1138–1148, 2001.

[6] H. Senties-Madrid and F. Vega-Boada, "Paraneoplastic syndromes associated with anti-Hu antibodies," *The Israel Medical Association Journal*, vol. 3, no. 2, pp. 94–103, 2001.

[7] F. Graus, C. Cordon-Cardo, and J. B. Posner, "Neuronal antinuclear antibody in sensory neuronopathy from lung cancer," *Neurology*, vol. 35, no. 4, pp. 538–543, 1985.

[8] W. Grisold and M. Drlicek, "Paraneoplastic neuropathy," *Current Opinion in Neurology*, vol. 12, no. 5, pp. 617–625, 1999.

[9] J. A. Tsou, M. Kazarian, A. Patel et al., "Low level anti-Hu reactivity: a risk marker for small cell lung cancer?" *Cancer Detection and Prevention*, vol. 32, no. 4, pp. 292–299, 2009.

[10] M. Hoosien, J. Vredenburgh, J. Lanfranco et al., "A myxoid chondrosarcoma associated with an anti-Hu-positive paraneoplastic encephalomyelitis," *Journal of Neuro-Oncology*, vol. 101, no. 1, pp. 135–139, 2011.

[11] S. Lukacs, N. Szabo, and S. Woodhams, "Rare association of anti-hu antibody positive paraneoplastic neurological syndrome and transitional cell bladder carcinoma," *Case Reports in Urology*, vol. 2012, Article ID 724940, 3 pages, 2012.

[12] J. K. Jakobsen, E. R. Zakharia, A. K. Boysen, H. Andersen, F. E. Schlesinger, and L. Lund, "Prostate cancer may trigger paraneoplastic limbic encephalitis: a case report and a review of the literature," *International Journal of Urology*, vol. 20, no. 7, pp. 734–737, 2013.

[13] H. Kalanie, A. A. Harandi, M. Mardani et al., "Trigeminal neuralgia as the first clinical manifestation of anti-Hu paraneoplastic syndrome induced by a borderline ovarian mucinous tumor," *Case Reports in Neurology*, vol. 6, no. 1, pp. 7–13, 2014.

[14] I. Pohley, K. Roesler, M. Wittstock, A. Bitsch, R. Benecke, and A. Wolters, "NMDA-receptor antibody and anti-Hu antibody positive paraneoplastic syndrome associated with a primary mediastinal seminoma," *Acta Neurologica Belgica*, vol. 115, no. 1, pp. 81–83, 2015.

[15] J. Honnorat, A. Didelot, E. Karantoni et al., "Autoimmune limbic encephalopathy and anti-Hu antibodies in children without cancer," *Neurology*, vol. 80, no. 24, pp. 2226–2232, 2013.

[16] C. F. Lucchinetti, D. W. Kimmel, and V. A. Lennon, "Paraneoplastic and oncologic profiles of patients seropositive for type 1 antineuronal nuclear autoantibodies," *Neurology*, vol. 50, no. 3, pp. 652–657, 1998.

[17] R. Renna, D. Plantone, and A. P. Batocchi, "Teaching NeuroImages: a case of hearing loss in a paraneoplastic syndrome associated with anti-Hu antibody," *Neurology*, vol. 79, no. 15, article e134, 2012.

[18] F. Keime-Guibert, F. Graus, A. Fleury et al., "Treatment of paraneoplastic neurological syndromes with antineuronal antibodies (Anti-Hu, Anti-Yo) with a combination of immunoglobulins, cyclophosphamide, and methylprednisolone," *Journal of Neurology Neurosurgery and Psychiatry*, vol. 68, no. 4, pp. 479–482, 2000.

[19] F. Graus, J. Dalmau, R. Reñé et al., "Anti-Hu antibodies in patients with small-cell lung cancer: association with complete response to therapy and improved survival," *Journal of Clinical Oncology*, vol. 15, no. 8, pp. 2866–2872, 1997.

[20] E. Mawhinney, O. M. Gray, F. McVerry, and G. V. McDonnell, "Paraneoplastic sensorimotor neuropathy associated with regression of small cell lung carcinoma," *BMJ Case Reports*, vol. 2010, 2010.

[21] F. Graus, J. Y. Delattre, J. C. Antoine et al., "Recommended diagnostic criteria for paraneoplastic neurological syndromes," *Journal of Neurology, Neurosurgery and Psychiatry*, vol. 75, no. 8, pp. 1135–1140, 2004.

[22] B. Giometto, R. Vitaliani, E. Lindeck-Pozza, W. Grisold, and C. Vedeler, "Treatment for paraneoplastic neuropathies," *Cochrane Database of Systematic Reviews*, vol. 12, Article ID CD007625, 2012.

[23] A. H. de Jongste, T. van Gelder, J. E. Bromberg et al., "A prospective open-label study of sirolimus for the treatment of anti-Hu associated paraneoplastic neurological syndromes," *Neuro-Oncology*, vol. 17, no. 1, pp. 145–150, 2015.

31

A Case of Reactive Cervical Lymphadenopathy with Fat Necrosis Impinging on Adjacent Vascular Structures

Albert Y. Han,[1,2] **Jacob F. Lentz,**[3] **Edward C. Kuan,**[4]
Hiwot H. Araya,[1] **and Mohammad Kamgar**[1]

[1]*Department of Medicine, David Geffen School of Medicine at UCLA, Los Angeles, CA 90095, USA*
[2]*Medical Scientist Training Program, David Geffen School of Medicine at UCLA, Los Angeles, CA 90095, USA*
[3]*Department of Emergency Medicine, David Geffen School of Medicine at UCLA, Los Angeles, CA 90095, USA*
[4]*Department of Head and Neck Surgery, David Geffen School of Medicine at UCLA, Los Angeles, CA 90095, USA*

Correspondence should be addressed to Albert Y. Han; alberthan@mednet.ucla.edu

Academic Editor: Yorihisa Orita

A tender neck mass in adults can be a diagnostic challenge due to a wide differential diagnosis, which ranges from reactive lymphadenopathy to malignancy. In this report, we describe a case of a young female with an unusually large and tender reactive lymph node with fat necrosis. The diagnostic imaging findings alone mimicked that of scrofula and malignancy, which prompted a complete workup. Additionally, the enlarged lymph node was compressing the internal jugular vein in the setting of oral contraceptive use by the patient, raising concern for Lemierre's syndrome or internal jugular vein thrombosis. This report shows how, in the appropriate clinical context, and especially with the involvement of adjacent respiratory or neurovascular structures, aggressive diagnostic testing can be indicated.

1. Case

A 19-year-old college student presented to a university emergency department with painful swelling on the left side of her neck. The swelling began two weeks earlier. It progressed slowly but had acutely worsened over the previous four days. She did not have a sore throat, but she endorsed worsening odynophagia since four days earlier. She denied any shortness of breath, stridor, or difficulty clearing secretions. She denied fever, skin rash, or axillary/inguinal lymphadenopathy. She recalled no inciting trauma or antecedent symptoms of sickness. She did, however, endorse night chills over the previous week.

The patient's medical history was limited to a diagnosis of streptococcal pharyngitis a month earlier, which had been treated with amoxicillin. Her surgical history included a bilateral tonsillectomy at the age of eight. She had no allergies, and her sole daily medication was an estrogen oral contraceptive pill (OCP). She recalled no family history of hematologic or head and neck malignancy.

The patient was born and raised in California, and she had never traveled outside of the United States or Europe. She had neither risk factors for tuberculosis (TB) nor TB contacts. She had no exposure to pets or animals. She denied drug and tobacco use, although she admitted to regular binge drinking episodes. Notably, the patient's recent strep pharyngitis diagnosis had occurred after a trip to a music festival in the California desert. Several of the friends with whom she had traveled developed similar symptoms, and in each of their cases the final diagnosis was strep pharyngitis.

1.1. Physical Exam Findings. The patient's vital signs upon arrival showed a blood pressure of 122/75, a pulse of 84, a temperature of 37.1 degrees Celsius, and respiratory rate of 12. Physical examination revealed a well-developed female in no acute distress. Oropharynx was clear, with no erythema or exudates. She had a nonerythematous, exquisitely tender mass on her left lateral neck over the sternocleidomastoid muscle, measuring approximately four centimeters (cm) in

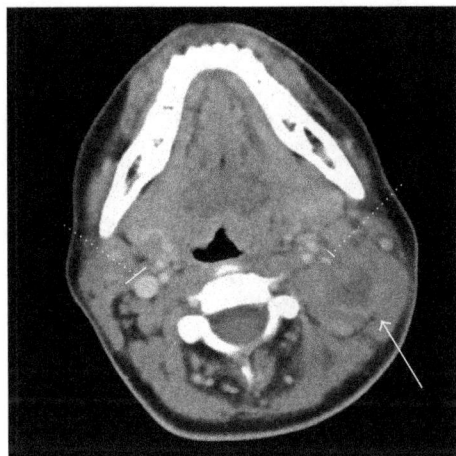

FIGURE 1: Computed tomography scan of the neck without contrast showing enlarged bilateral lymph nodes. On the patient's left, the largest lymph node (4.1 × 2.7 cm; white arrow) has a central hypodensity (1.9 × 1.2 cm) consistent with fatty necrosis. Additionally, the right internal jugular (IJ) vein measured 0.95 cm in the greatest diameter whereas the left IJ vein was 0.24.

diameter and three cm in height. The skin overlying the neck was intact. The remainder of the exam was unremarkable.

1.2. Laboratory Findings. The patient's electrolytes and liver function tests were within normal limits. The complete blood count (CBC) showed an elevated white blood cell count of 12.85, with a neutrophil predominance at 75 percent. The absolute neutrophil count was 9.6, and the absolute lymphocyte count was 2.1. The absolute monocyte count was slightly elevated at 1.1. Her CBC was otherwise unremarkable.

Human immunodeficiency virus (HIV), cytomegalovirus (CMV) IgM, human simplex virus 1/2 IgM, Epstein-Barr virus, *Bartonella henselae*, *Coccidioides*, and *Toxoplasma gondii* serologies were negative. QuantiFERON-TB Gold (Quant-Gold) test was also negative. The lactate dehydrogenase (LDH) level was normal.

1.3. Diagnostic Imaging. The patient's chest X-ray was unremarkable. A bedside ultrasound of the neck showed findings that were consistent with lymphadenopathy, with the location of the largest lymph node in Level IIB. A contrast-enhanced computed tomography (CT) of the neck revealed multilevel cervical lymphadenopathy bilaterally, with the largest mass measured at 4.1 × 2.7 cm in the left neck. A central hypodense area of this node measured 1.9 × 1.2 cm. The left internal jugular (IJ) vein remained patent but was decreased in caliber secondary to mass effect from the largest node (Figure 1). The diameter of the IJ vein was 0.95 cm on the right and 0.27 cm on the left. Radiology read this as a likely necrotic lymph node. (Figure 1).

Due to the impressive presentation, hypercoagulability (OCP use), venostasis (changes in IJ caliber), and concern for airway compromise, the patient was admitted for expedited evaluation and treatment. Furthermore, as a delayed diagnosis of head and neck cancer is associated with lower survival, otolaryngology was consulted immediately [1].

1.4. Hospital Course. The patient's airway remained patent and required no immediate intervention. Given the high suspicion for infection, the patient was started on empiric ampicillin-sulbactam. The swelling began to decrease over the course of treatment, and the patient's leukocyte count downtrended and normalized three days into treatment.

On hospital day 2, the patient underwent ultrasound-guided core needle biopsy. Tissue pathology showed fibroadipose tissue with acute inflammation and fat necrosis. A gram stain and acid-fast bacilli (AFB) stain of the specimen were negative, as was the gomori methenamine silver stain. The bacterial and fungal cultures of the aspirate were subsequently negative. Cytology revealed abundant neutrophils in a background of histiocytes and occasional scattered lymphocytes. Flow cytometry was negative for monoclonal proliferation (Figure 2).

The patient continued to improve. However, due to the diagnostic uncertainty from the core needle specimen, an excisional biopsy was performed on hospital day 4. The final pathology showed a mixture of T and B cells and irregular fragments of lymphoid cortex without light chain restriction, granulomas, or other focal lesions. These findings were consistent with reactive lymphoid tissue. The size and tenderness of the lymph node continued to decrease, and the patient was discharged with return precautions and outpatient follow-up on hospital day 6.

1.5. Diagnosis. The diagnosis was a reactive lymph node.

2. Discussion

A tender neck mass is a common presenting symptom in the adult population [2, 3]. The evaluation of a neck mass begins with a careful history related to the lesion (i.e., location, migration, temporal course, and associated symptoms). Patient-specific risk factors such as previous trauma, relevant travel, animal contact, and past medical history should be reviewed [2, 3]. Physical exam should not only include a characterization of the lesion but also an assessment of cranial nerve integrity and function. The security of the airway is crucial and must be checked during the initial assessment. Any sign of possible impending respiratory compromise warrants admission [4]. Possible odontogenic etiology, such as dental caries, must be considered, as complications from infection can negatively impact the course of treatment [3].

As a general rule, swollen nodes other than supraclavicular/Level V nodes usually result from reactive lymphadenopathy or infectious/viral lymphadenitis [5–7]. In the present case, a moderate leukocytosis and normal LDH lowered the suspicion of malignancy. However, a possible lymphatic spread of occult primary cancer remained on the differential, especially as the Level IIB nodes drain the oropharynx and the nasopharynx [8]. In this patient, the largest lymph node was in Level IIB, with a maximum

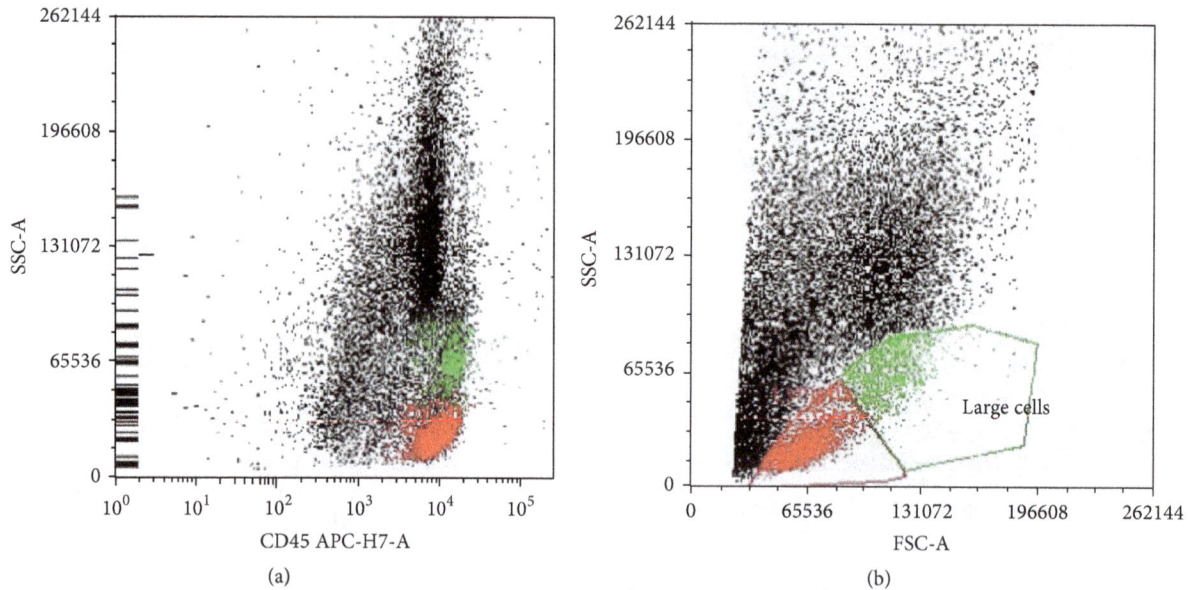

FIGURE 2: Multiparametric flow cytometry results. CD45+ lymphocyte gate (low SSC-A) was 14% of the total population (a). The lymphocytes were predominantly T cells (12% of total cells; (b)). (a) CD45 versus SSC and (b) FSC versus SSC.

diameter of 4.1 cm. The commonly accepted radiological criteria for lymph node malignancy is a ratio between the dimension of the long and short axes less than 2 [6, 9]. In the present case, the ratio was 1.52 with evidence of a necrotic core, and this prompted further investigation. Of note, CT of the neck is sensitive but not specific in differentiating an inflamed lymph node or abscess from metastatic cancer, as they often appear identical on imaging [2].

Tuberculosis cervical lymphadenitis (i.e., scrofula or King's evil) is perhaps the most famous etiology of a neck mass. Scrofula most commonly presents in young patients as large painless lymph nodes [10, 11]. Interestingly, only one-third of scrofula patients have a documented history of TB [12, 13]. The salient features of scrofula on a CT scan include central necrosis, nodal matting, and minimal peri-adenitis [14]. The gold standard test for diagnosing scrofula is tissue sampling and AFB stain and culture. However, the newer Quant-Gold test detects the release of interferon-γ by leukocytes, which are sensitized after incubation with synthetic peptides similar to *Mycobacterium tuberculosis* proteins. The Quant-Gold test can also detect nontuberculous mycobacteria, as identical proteins are also found in the species *Mycobacterium kansasii*, *Mycobacterium szulgai*, and *Mycobacterium marinum* [15, 16]. Although the patient in this case had a painful neck mass and a negative AFB stain and culture, it would have been critical to rule out pulmonary involvement if a diagnosis of scrofula had been made, as the public health implications for this are significant [11].

Other rare causes of neck masses include Kikuchi disease, Castleman disease, Kimura disease, and Rosai-Dorfman disease. Among these, Kikuchi disease was placed on the differential because it typically presents as cervical lymphadenopathy in a young woman associated with fever and constitutional symptoms [17]. Diagnosis is made by a tissue lymph node histology demonstrating paracortical areas of necrosis with the proliferation of histiocytes in the absence of neutrophils [18]. The natural history is benign and ultimately self-limiting [18]. The tissue analysis of the excisional biopsy in this case showed abundant neutrophils; this eliminated Kikuchi disease from the differential.

Bacterial infection can cause lymphadenopathy via an activated inflammatory response or direct hematogenous spread of bacteria into nodes. Reactive lymphadenopathy also emerges with the stimulation of the immune system by regional infectious processes, such as upper respiratory infections, stomatitis, or dental caries [14, 19]. Many viral infections, including HIV, infectious mononucleosis, and CMV, can result in significant cervical lymph node swelling via this mechanism. Bacteria from an odontogenic or salivary infection can directly travel to the cervical nodes, leading to frank abscess formation [2]. Patients with bacterial abscesses have pain, swelling, and erythema and possibly present with a fever. The bacterial abscess considered in this case was cat scratch disease, which is caused by the bacteria *Bartonella henselae* and is often found in patients younger than 21 years old with exquisitely tender lymph nodes [19, 20]. IgM/IgG serology is the diagnostic test of choice for *B. henselae* infection. In the present case, the serology was negative.

Poorly controlled odontogenic or pharyngeal infections can result in vascular complications. The patient in this case had at least two elements of Virchow's triad: hypercoagulation (OCP use) and stasis of blood flow (reduced caliber of IJ by 25%). Vascular complications are uncommon, but they include IJ venous thrombosis (IJVT) and thrombophlebitis of the IJ vein (Lemierre's syndrome). IJVT most commonly occurs in the setting of central line infection or tumor invasion into the vasculature [21, 22]. Lemierre's syndrome is characterized by a triad of recent oropharyngeal infection,

IJVT identified on CT, and confirmed anaerobic bacterial infection (most commonly *Fusobacterium necrophorum*) [23]. Approximately 30% of the patients experience a preceding upper respiratory infection. Upon first presentation, 23% of patients display a neck mass and approximately 20% complain of neck pain [24]. Although rare, the patient in this case had a recent history of pharyngitis and was at an increased risk for thrombosis due to her OCP use; she was therefore monitored closely during hospitalization.

It was ultimately concluded that an occult chronic bacterial infection was the cause of the patient's lymphadenopathy. It was hypothesized that her history of tonsillectomy left her oropharynx more prone to infection. Due to the degree of swelling and the significant compression of the left IJ in the setting of a hypercoagulable state, admission and extensive investigation were clinically warranted. Although neither this complication nor respiratory compromise developed, and while all stains, cultures, and serologies were negative, this case serves as a reminder that reactive lymph nodes can mimic many features of classic infectious and neoplastic processes, can grow to a formidable size, and can compress critically important adjacent structures.

Competing Interests

The authors declare that they have no competing interests.

Acknowledgments

The authors appreciate the insightful comments of Dr. Inderpreet Saini, Dr. Erin Dowling, Daria Gaut, Dr. Oz Simel, and Dr. Ashley Kita.

References

[1] E. Crozier and B. D. Sumer, "Head and neck cancer," *Medical Clinics of North America*, vol. 94, no. 5, pp. 1031–1046, 2010.

[2] T. L. Rosenberg, J. J. Brown, and G. D. Jefferson, "Evaluating the adult patient with a neck mass," *Medical Clinics of North America*, vol. 94, no. 5, pp. 1017–1029, 2010.

[3] J. Haynes, K. R. Arnold, C. Aguirre-Oskins, and S. Chandra, "Evaluation of neck masses in adults," *American Family Physician*, vol. 91, no. 10, pp. 698–706, 2015.

[4] M. Gleeson, A. Herbert, and A. Richards, "Management of lateral neck masses in adults," *British Medical Journal*, vol. 320, no. 7248, pp. 1521–1524, 2000.

[5] L. M. Weiss and D. O'Malley, "Benign lymphadenopathies," *Modern Pathology*, vol. 26, no. 1, pp. S88–S96, 2013.

[6] O. Sakai, H. D. Curtin, L. V. Romo, and P. M. Som, "Lymph node pathology: benign proliferative, lymphoma, and metastatic disease," *Radiologic Clinics of North America*, vol. 38, no. 5, pp. 979–998, 2000.

[7] K. T. Robbins, J. E. Medina, G. T. Wolfe, P. A. Levine, R. B. Sessions, and C. W. Pruet, "Standardizing neck dissection terminology. Official report of the Academy's Committee for Head and Neck Surgery and Oncology," *Archives of Otolaryngology—Head and Neck Surgery*, vol. 117, no. 6, pp. 601–605, 1991.

[8] V. Grégoire, K. Ang, W. Budach et al., "Delineation of the neck node levels for head and neck tumors: a 2013 update. DAHANCA, EORTC, HKNPCSG, NCIC CTG, NCRI, RTOG, TROG consensus guidelines," *Radiotherapy and Oncology*, vol. 110, no. 1, pp. 172–181, 2014.

[9] D. M. Gor, J. E. Langer, and L. A. Loevner, "Imaging of cervical lymph nodes in head and neck cancer: the basics," *Radiologic Clinics of North America*, vol. 44, no. 1, pp. 101–110, 2006.

[10] W. N. Gibbs, D. A. Bridges, and M. J. Opatowsky, "Bilateral lymphadenopathy in a young woman," *Proceedings (Baylor University. Medical Center)*, vol. 21, no. 4, pp. 430–432, 2008.

[11] J.-M. Fontanilla, A. Barnes, and C. F. von Reyn, "Current diagnosis and management of peripheral tuberculous lymphadenitis," *Clinical Infectious Diseases*, vol. 53, no. 6, pp. 555–562, 2011.

[12] Y.-F. Wei, Y.-S. Liaw, S.-C. Ku, Y.-L. Chang, and P.-C. Yang, "Clinical features and predictors of a complicated treatment course in peripheral tuberculous lymphadenitis," *Journal of the Formosan Medical Association*, vol. 107, no. 3, pp. 225–231, 2008.

[13] A. W. Artenstein, J. H. Kim, W. J. Williams, and R. C. Y. Chung, "Isolated peripheral tuberculous lymphadenitis in adults: current clinical and diagnostic issues," *Clinical Infectious Diseases*, vol. 20, no. 4, pp. 876–882, 1995.

[14] R. Restrepo, J. Oneto, K. Lopez, and K. Kukreja, "Head and neck lymph nodes in children: the spectrum from normal to abnormal," *Pediatric Radiology*, vol. 39, no. 8, pp. 836–846, 2009.

[15] G. H. Mazurek, J. Jereb, P. LoBue et al., "Guidelines for using the QuantiFERON-TB Gold test for detecting *Mycobacterium tuberculosis* infection, United States," *MMWR Recommendations and Reports*, vol. 54, no. 15, pp. 49–55, 2005.

[16] J. R. Starke, "Interferon-gamma release assays for diagnosis of tuberculosis infection and disease in children," *Pediatrics*, vol. 134, no. 6, pp. e1763–e1773, 2014.

[17] M. J. Bennie, K. M. Bowles, and S. C. Rankin, "Necrotizing cervical lymphadenopathy caused by Kikuchi-Fujimoto disease," *The British Journal of Radiology*, vol. 76, no. 909, pp. 656–658, 2003.

[18] C. B. Hutchinson and E. Wang, "Kikuchi-Fujimoto disease," *Archives of Pathology & Laboratory Medicine*, vol. 134, no. 2, pp. 289–293, 2010.

[19] J. D. Meier and J. F. Grimmer, "Evaluation and management of neck masses in children," *American Family Physician*, vol. 89, no. 5, pp. 353–358, 2014.

[20] S. Lang and B. Kansy, "Cervical lymph node diseases in children," *GMS Current Topics in Otorhinolaryngology, Head and Neck Surgery*, vol. 13, article Doc08, 2014.

[21] K. Chowdhurry, J. Bloom, M. J. Black, and K. Al-Noury, "Spontaneous and nonspontaneous internal jugular vein thrombosis," *Head & Neck*, vol. 12, no. 2, pp. 168–173, 1990.

[22] J. P. Cohen, M. S. Persky, and D. L. Reede, "Internal jugular vein thrombosis," *Laryngoscope*, vol. 95, no. 12, pp. 1478–1482, 1985.

[23] R. M. Centor, "Expand the pharyngitis paradigm for adolescents and young adults," *Annals of Internal Medicine*, vol. 151, no. 11, pp. 812–815, 2009.

[24] P. D. Karkos, S. Asrani, C. D. Karkos et al., "Lemierre's syndrome: a systematic review," *Laryngoscope*, vol. 119, no. 8, pp. 1552–1559, 2009.

32

Angiofibroma Originating outside the Nasopharynx: A Management Dilemma

Ashraf Nabeel Mahmood,[1] Rashid Sheikh,[2] Hamad Al Saey,[1,3] Sarah Ashkanani,[1] and Shanmugam Ganesan[2,3]

[1]Rhinology Section, Otorhinolaryngology, Head & Neck Surgery (ORL-HNS) Department, Rumailah Hospital, Hamad Medical Corporation, Doha, Qatar

[2]Otorhinolaryngology, Head & Neck Surgery (ORL-HNS) Department, Rumailah Hospital, Hamad Medical Corporation, Doha, Qatar

[3]Weill Cornell Medical College, Ar-Rayyan, Qatar

Correspondence should be addressed to Rashid Sheikh; rsheikh@hamad.qa

Academic Editor: Holger Sudhoff

Background. Angiofibroma is a benign tumor, consisting of fibrous tissue with varying degrees of vascularity, characterized by proliferation of stellate and spindle cells around the blood vessels. It most commonly arises from the nasopharynx, although it may rarely arise in extranasopharyngeal sites. *Case Report.* A 46-year-old male presented with left side nasal obstruction and epistaxis for one month. Clinical nasal examination revealed left sided polypoidal mass arising from the vestibular region of the lateral nasal wall. *Results.* CT scan and MRI showed highly vascular soft tissue mass occupying the anterior part of the left nostril. Preoperative selective embolization followed by transnasal excision was performed. Histopathological examination confirmed the diagnoses of nasal vestibular angiofibroma. *Conclusion.* Extranasopharyngeal angiofibroma is a very rare pathology. It should be kept in mind as a differential diagnosis with any unilateral nasal vestibular mass causing nasal obstruction and epistaxis. A biopsy without further investigation can cause life threatening bleeding in the patient.

1. Introduction

Angiofibroma is a benign tumor, consisting of fibrous tissue with varying degrees of vascularity, characterized by a proliferation of stellate and spindle cells around the blood vessels. It is originating from the pterygoid plate and the region of the sphenopalatine foramen. There are many theories trying to explain the pathology underlying this tumor, like genetic, hormonal, and developmental ones, but none of them had general acceptance. It has been hypothesized that angiofibroma is a testosterone-dependent tumor that arises from a fibrovascular nidus in the nasopharynx that lies dormant until the onset of puberty; hence the incidence is more in males with peak incidence between the ages of 14 and 18 years [1]. Histologically, angiofibroma is made up of fibrous and vascular components, with varying ratio between both of

them. Mostly, the vessels are just endothelium-lined spaces without muscle coat, and that accounts for the severe bleeding as the vessels lose the ability to contract [2]. It is the most common vascular neoplasm of the nasal cavity, representing 0.5% of all head and neck tumors [1, 3, 4]. Although it is a benign tumor, it is locally invasive. Progressive nasal obstruction is the most common presenting symptom [5]. Despite the fact that it most commonly arises from the nasopharynx, it may rarely arise in extranasopharyngeal sites, like maxillary sinus which is the most common site (24.6%–32%) [4–7]. Other rare reported sites include ethmoid and sphenoid sinuses, nasal septum, middle turbinate, inferior turbinate, conjunctiva, molar and retromolar region, and tonsil and larynx [1]. Here, we report a very rare case of extranasopharyngeal angiofibroma originating from the lateral wall of the left nasal vestibular area.

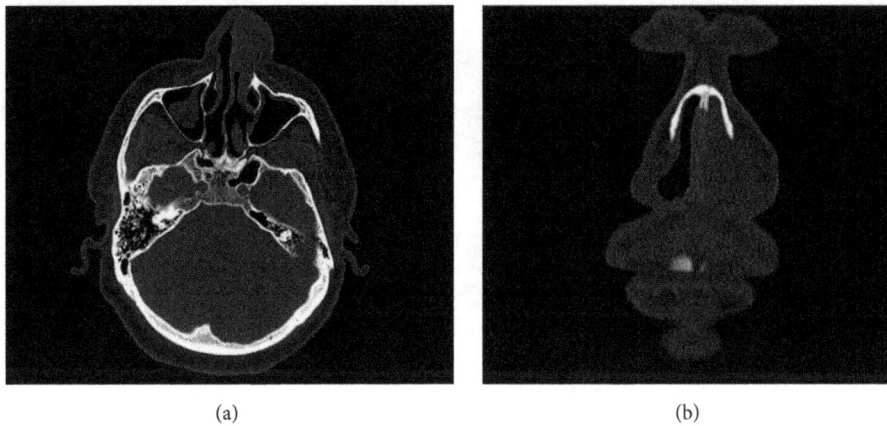

(a)   (b)

FIGURE 1: (a) shows axial and (b) shows coronal CT images. Both show a soft tissue mass occupying the left nasal vestibular area.

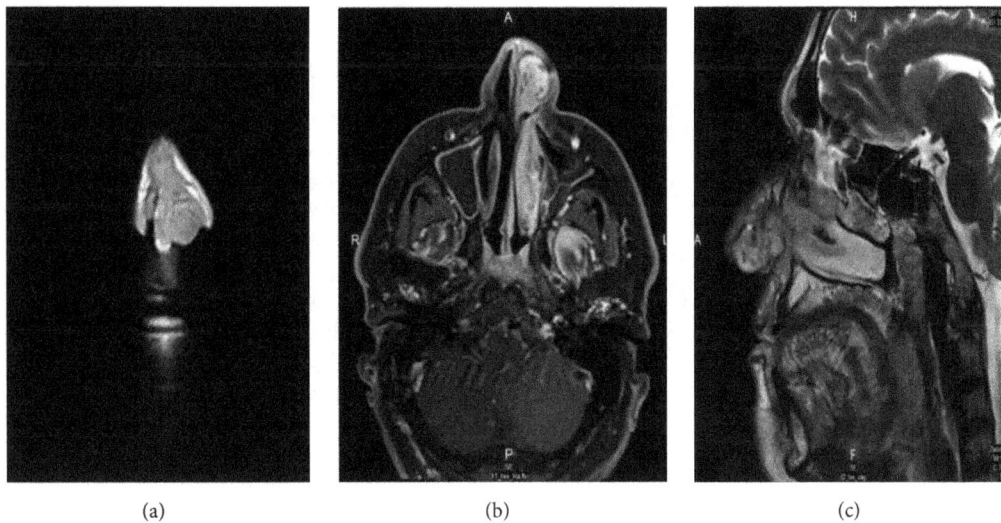

(a)   (b)   (c)

FIGURE 2: MRI of nose and paranasal sinuses showing a highly vascular mass occupying the left nasal vestibular area. (a) shows T1 coronal view, (b) shows T1 postcontrast axial view, and (c) shows a T2 sagittal view.

2. Case Report

A 46-year-old male, not known to have any chronic illness, presented to the emergency department in Hamad Medical Corporation due to one-month history of left side intermittent anterior nasal bleeding increasing in severity and associated with nasal blockage. He had a history of decreased sense of smell and headache for one month. There was no history of trauma, infection, nasal allergies, or bleeding disorders. ENT examination showed mildly deviated nasal septum to the right side with a left sided pinkish colored polypoidal mass originating from the vestibular region of the left lateral nasal wall, easily bleeding upon manipulation. Ears and throat examination was normal. Silver nitrate cauterization was done and bleeding was controlled. So the patient was discharged and he was referred to ORL-HNS clinic for follow-up. The white blood cells count (WBC) was $8.8 \times 10^3/mm^3$, hemoglobin (Hb) level 12.5 g/100 mL, and platelets count (Plt) $278 \times 10^3/mm^3$. Liver and kidney

function tests were normal. CT scan of paranasal sinuses showed $3.4 \times 2.5 \times 1.9$ cm mass localized to the anterior part of the left side of the nasal cavity with no extension to the choana or to the paranasal sinuses (Figures 1(a) and 1(b)). MRI (done to rule out hypervascularity of the mass before surgical intervention) showed a hypervascular mass in the same previously described position (Figures 2(a), 2(b), and 2(c)). 24 hours before the surgery, angiography was done which showed hypervascular left side nasal mass supplied by the distal branches of the left internal maxillary artery and distal branches of the left facial artery. Selective embolization was done, to decrease the intraoperative bleeding, with polyvinyl alcohol temporary occlusive particles (PVA), which reduced 85% of the blood flow to the area (Figures 3(a) and 3(b)).

The removal of the tumor was performed under general anesthesia. The pedicle had been completely transected with bipolar diathermy, with insignificant bleeding which was controlled with electrocautery. Nasal pack was inserted in the left nostril only. The postoperative period was uneventful, and

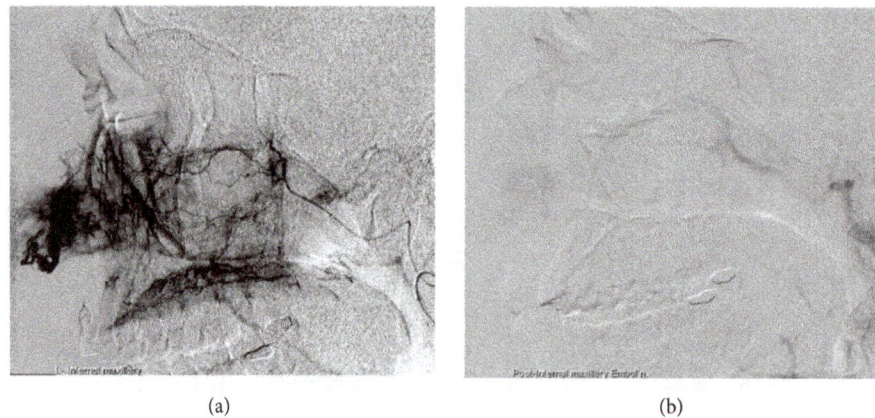

(a)   (b)

FIGURE 3: (a) Angiography showing hypervascular nasal mass supplied by the distal branches of the left internal maxillary artery and distal branches of the left facial artery. (b) The mass after embolization of the internal maxillary artery.

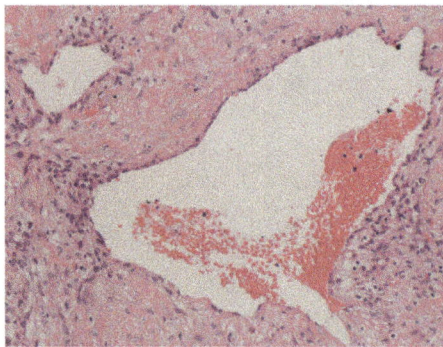

FIGURE 4: Richly vascular lesion which has variable-sized thin-walled vessels surrounded by a fibroblastic stroma. The vessels have a single endothelial cell lining without a muscularis layer (H&E 20x).

the pack was removed on the third postoperative day with no bleeding, and the patient was discharged on the same day. The mass was sent for histopathology. Immunohistochemical staining was performed for AE1/3, vimentin, SMA, desmin, S-100, CD34, CD31, CD117, CD99 BCL-2, and ki-67. The histomorphology and immunohistochemical staining profile supported the diagnosis of angiofibroma (Figure 4). The patient was followed up in the clinic and clinical examination during his last visit (6 months after surgery) showed no recurrence and clear site of operation.

3. Discussion

The nasal vestibule is lined with keratinizing squamous epithelium and contains different components such as sebaceous glands and sweat glands. So the pathologic lesions in the nasal vestibule are different from those in the nasal cavity proper; they can be infectious, inflammatory, benign, or malignant tumors. Differential diagnoses can include nasal vestibule cyst, fibroma, squamous papilloma, trichofolliculoma, pseudoepitheliomatous hyperplasia, sebaceous cyst carcinoma, hidradenoma, rhinoscleroma, and malignant

melanoma [8, 9]. Here we report a case of nasal vestibule angiofibroma, which is the only hypervascular tumor among all the other mentioned diagnoses.

The presenting symptoms of the nasal vestibular angiofibroma are nasal obstruction and epistaxis [2, 3, 5]. The main differences in clinical presentation of extranasopharyngeal angiofibroma (ENA) versus nasopharyngeal angiofibroma (NA) are the sex predilection, age of presentation, and vascularity. With regards to gender predilection, NA is predominantly a disease of males. However, ENA is of a greater incidence relative to NA in females. Also ENA presents in older age group more than NA, with mean age of 22 years and 17 years, respectively [3, 7], while for nasal vestibule angiofibroma the mean age is 43 years. The administration of contrast agent in NA leads to a strong and usually homogeneous enhancement on CT and MRI, while EN varies from strong to minimal or even no enhancement, due to the frequent poor vascularity of the tumor [10].

The management of any vestibular mass should include preoperative radiological examination. CT scan and MRI (with contrast) are essential for evaluating the extension and vascularity of the lesion. However, signs of suspected hypervascularity, upon CT scan or MRI, indicate the need for angiography with selective embolization prior to any surgical intervention, to reduce the risk of bleeding during the surgery. The use of angiography and selective embolization should have a high threshold, that is, only if there is radiological evidence of diffuse, large, and hypervascular lesion, as these procedures come with their own complications. There are three cases of nasal vestibule angiofibroma previously reported in the literature with no preoperative embolization; all had different amount of intraoperative bleeding varying from minimal to profuse (Table 1). Perhaps smaller lesions can be excised without the need for such elaborate perioperative measures like angiography and embolization. However, the diagnosis should be confirmed by sending the excised lesion for histopathology. The NA have a recurrence rate ranging from 6 to 27.5% [7], while no recurrence was reported in the literature for ENA.

TABLE 1: Reported cases of vestibular extranasopharyngeal angiofibroma.

Authors	Year	Age	Sex	Location	Symptoms	Onset	Therapy	Pre-op embolization
Kim et al. [8]	2013	56 years	Female	Right nasal vestibule	Progressive swelling	3 years	Endonasal resection (bleeding)	No
Pillenahalli Maheshwarappa et al. [1]	2013	10 years	Male	Left nasal vestibule	Nasal obstruction and epistaxis	4 months	Endoscopic excision (profuse bleeding)	No
Sharanabasappa [11]	2013	60 years	Male	Left nasal vestibule	Nasal mass	1 year	Transnasal resection (minimal bleeding)	No
Present case	2014	46 years	Male	Left nasal vestibule	Recurrent epistaxis and nasal obstruction	1 month	Transnasal resection (insignificant bleeding)	Yes

4. Conclusion

(1) Although extranasopharyngeal angiofibroma is very rare diagnosis, it should be kept in mind as a differential diagnosis with any unilateral nasal vestibular mass causing nasal obstruction and epistaxis.

(2) CT scan and MRI are essential in the preoperative evaluation of a vestibular mass to assess for hypervascularity.

(3) The use of angiography and selective embolization should have a high threshold, that is, only if there is radiological evidence of diffuse, large, and hypervascular lesions which are predictive factors of intraoperative profuse bleeding.

Ethical Approval

The case at hand has already been approved by the authors' institution's medical research and ethics committee at the research center.

Consent

The patient's consent was taken for the publication of the case report and the figures.

Competing Interests

Authors have no conflict of interests or financial interest, real or perceived, to disclose.

References

[1] R. Pillenahalli Maheshwarappa, A. Gupta, J. Bansal, M. V. Kattimani, S. S. Shabadi, and S. C. Baser, "An unusual location of juvenile angiofibroma: a case report and review of the literature," *Case Reports in Otolaryngology*, vol. 2013, Article ID 175326, 3 pages, 2013.

[2] P. L. Dhingra and S. Dhingra, *Diseases of Ear, Nose & Throat*, Elsevier, 5th edition, 2010.

[3] M. Uyar, M. Turanli, I. Pak, S. Bakir, and U. Osma, "Extranasopharyngeal angiofibroma originating from the nasal septum: a case report," *Kulak Burun Boğaz İhtisas Dergisi*, vol. 19, no. 1, pp. 41–44, 2009.

[4] S. K. Bhargava and S. Phatak, "Angiofibroma arising from nasal septum in adult male—a rare occurence," *Indian Journal of Otolaryngology and Head and Neck Surgery*, vol. 47, no. 1, pp. 39–41, 1995.

[5] J. A. S. Makhasana, M. A. Kulkarni, S. Vaze, and A. S. Shroff, "Juvenile nasopharyngeal angiofibroma," *Journal of Oral and Maxillofacial Pathology*, vol. 20, no. 2, article 330, 2016.

[6] L. Garcia-Rodriguez, K. Rudman, C. H. Cogbill, T. Loehrl, and D. M. Poetker, "Nasal septal angiofibroma, a subclass of extranasopharyngeal angiofibroma," *American Journal of Otolaryngology—Head and Neck Medicine and Surgery*, vol. 33, no. 4, pp. 473–476, 2012.

[7] A. Szymańska, M. Szymański, K. Morshed, E. Czekajska-Chehab, and M. Szczerbo-Trojanowska, "Extranasopharyngeal angiofibroma: clinical and radiological presentation," *European Archives of Oto-Rhino-Laryngology*, vol. 270, no. 2, pp. 655–660, 2013.

[8] S. J. Kim, S. W. Byun, and S.-S. Lee, "Various tumors in the nasal vestibule," *International Journal of Clinical and Experimental Pathology*, vol. 6, no. 12, pp. 2713–2718, 2013.

[9] S.-H. Zhou, Y.-Y. Xu, S.-Q. Wang, L. Ling, H.-T. Yao, and G.-P. Ren, "Analysis of 60 masses in the nasal vestibule," *Zhonghua Er Bi Yan Hou Ke Za Zhi*, vol. 39, no. 6, pp. 337–339, 2004.

[10] I. Tasca and G. C. Compadretti, "Extranasopharyngeal angiofibroma of nasal septum. A controversial entity," *Acta Otorhinolaryngologica Italica*, vol. 28, no. 6, pp. 312–314, 2008.

[11] R. M. Sharanabasappa, "Extranasopharyngeal angiofibroma from nasal vestibule: a rare presentation," *JP Journals*, vol. 5, no. 3, pp. 169–172, 2013.

33

Chronic Invasive Nongranulomatous Fungal Rhinosinusitis in Immunocompetent Individuals

Ozge Turhan,[1] **Asli Bostanci,**[2] **Irem Hicran Ozbudak,**[3] **and Murat Turhan**[2]

[1]*Department of Infectious Diseases, Akdeniz University School of Medicine, Antalya, Turkey*
[2]*Department of Otolaryngology, Head and Neck Surgery, Akdeniz University School of Medicine, Antalya, Turkey*
[3]*Department of Pathology, Akdeniz University School of Medicine, Antalya, Turkey*

Correspondence should be addressed to Asli Bostanci; draslibostanci@gmail.com

Academic Editor: Rong-San Jiang

Chronic invasive nongranulomatous fungal rhinosinusitis is a well-described but uncommon type of fungal rhinosinusitis (FRS). While the prevalence of chronic FRS is 0.11% in healthy individuals, only 1.3% of them are in nongranulomatous invasive nature. The majority of the cases in the literature have been reported from developing countries mostly located in the tropical regions, as typically occurring in the background of diabetes mellitus or corticosteroid treatment. The current paper reports four consecutive cases, who were diagnosed within a short period of six months at a single center of a country located outside the tropical climate zone. None of the patients had a comorbid disease that may cause immune suppression or a history of drug use. The only risk factor that may have a role in development of chronic invasive nongranulomatous FRS was that all of our patients were people working in greenhouse farming. Three cases underwent endoscopic sinus surgery, and one case underwent surgery with both endoscopic and external approaches. Systemic antifungal therapy was initiated in all cases in the postoperative period with voriconazole 200 mg orally twice a day. All patients achieved a complete clinical remission. Chronic invasive nongranulomatous FRS should be kept in mind in the presence of long-standing nonspecific sinonasal symptoms in immunocompetent individuals, particularly with a history of working in greenhouse farming.

1. Introduction

Fungal rhinosinusitis (FRS) encompasses a spectrum of sinonasal diseases with distinct clinical courses, histopathologies, and disease outcomes. FRS is classified into two groups as invasive and noninvasive depending on invasion of the mucosal layer by fungi. Noninvasive FRS includes saprophytic fungal infestation, fungal ball, and allergic FRS. Invasive FRS is subdivided into acute invasive, chronic nongranulomatous invasive, and chronic granulomatous types [1].

Chronic nongranulomatous invasive FRS is a well-described but uncommon type of FRS. While the prevalence of chronic FRS is 0.11% in healthy individuals, only 1.3% of them are in nongranulomatous invasive nature [2]. In this paper, four consecutive immunocompetent patients with chronic invasive nongranulomatous FRS, who were diagnosed over a period of 6 months at a single center (June 2015–October 2015), were presented along with the literature.

2. Case Presentation

The current study was conducted in accordance with the Declaration of Helsinki and with approval from the Institutional Ethics Committee. Written informed consent was obtained from the patients.

All patients were farmers from rural areas. A comprehensive head and neck examination was performed in all cases. Complete blood cell counts and serum chemistry panel, including hepatic and renal function tests, were evaluated. Radiological evaluation was carried out by computed tomography (CT) scan. None of the patients had a comorbid disease that may cause immune suppression or a history of drug use. Three cases underwent endoscopic sinus surgery, and one case underwent sinus surgery with both endoscopic and external approaches. A Gomori methenamine-silver stain was used in the histopathological diagnosis. The diagnosis of chronic invasive FRS was made by the demonstration of silver

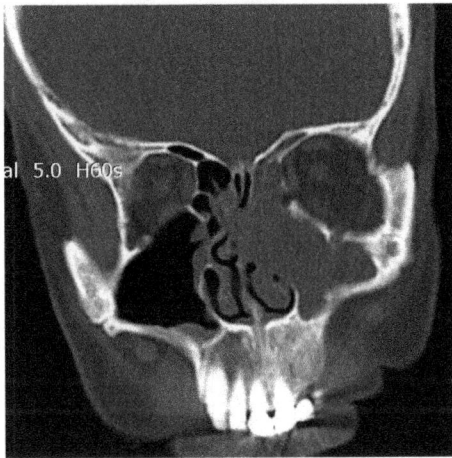

FIGURE 1: Paranasal sinus computed tomography showing a soft tissue lesion eroding the left maxillary sinus medial wall, filling the ethmoidal cells and frontal sinus and destructing the lamina papyracea.

accumulation in the fungal cell wall, the presence of hyphal forms within the submucosa, and the demonstration of tissue necrosis accompanied by minimal host inflammatory cell infiltration [3]. It was distinguished from granulomatous FRS by dense accumulation of hyphae, occasional angioinvasion, sparse inflammatory infiltrate, and lack of submucosal granulomatous inflammation containing giant cells [4]. Histopathological diagnosis was confirmed by fungal culture, although it was not an absolute requirement [5].

Systemic antifungal therapy was initiated in all cases in the postoperative period with voriconazole 200 mg orally twice a day. The duration of treatment was decided at the discretion of the institutional local committee on infectious diseases. Although the treatment was maintained for six weeks in three cases, it was terminated in the third week in one case due to the adverse effects. Patients were followed up for recurrence once every three months by physical and endoscopic examinations. Demographic, clinical, and radiological data were recorded for all patients (Table 1).

2.1. Case 1. A 58-year-old male patient was admitted with a 6-month history of nasal obstruction, swelling on the left side of the face, and left orbital pain. Endoscopic examination revealed a polypoid mass and intense purulent secretion in the left nasal cavity and middle meatus. On paranasal sinus CT, an expansive soft tissue lesion that erodes the left maxillary sinus medial wall, fills the ethmoidal cells and frontal sinus, and leads to the destruction of lamina papyracea was observed (Figure 1). A gray-white, cheesy material was completely removed from all sinuses by endoscopic sinus surgery. Tissue culture identified the fungus as *Aspergillus fumigatus*. No recurrence was detected during a follow-up period of 10 months after systemic antifungal therapy was discontinued.

2.2. Case 2. A 43-year-old male patient was referred to our clinic with the complaints of nasal obstruction, headache, and

facial pain which existed for about two years. It was learned that he had received multiple medications for rhinosinusitis without improvement of his symptoms. Endoscopic examination showed intense purulent discharge in the left nasal cavity and middle meatus. Paranasal sinus CT scan revealed a soft tissue mass that fills the left nasal cavity and ethmoid, frontal, and sphenoid sinuses and indents the medial rectus muscle by destructing the lamina papyracea (Figure 2(a)). Ophthalmologic examination was unremarkable. Left maxillary, ethmoid, frontal, and sphenoid sinuses were opened endoscopically, and a yellow-green gelatinous material was drained (Figure 2(b)). The left orbital medial wall was observed to be eroded, and the orbital adipose tissue was found to be exposed. An external surgical approach was performed to clear the tissues located at the most lateral part of the left frontal sinus. Histopathological examination was consistent with chronic nongranulomatous invasive FRS (Figures 2(c)-2(d)), while *Aspergillus flavus* was isolated in the culture. No recurrence occurred during a follow-up period of eight months, although the antifungal therapy was stopped on postoperative day 21 due to the adverse effects including blurred vision, vision color changes, and skin rashes.

2.3. Case 3. A 60-year-old female patient presented with a history of dizziness, headache, and postnasal drainage for nine months. Endoscopic examination of the nasal cavity and osteomeatal complex was unremarkable. A tattletale gray cheesy material was observed in the sphenoethmoidal recess. Paranasal sinus CT scan showed a soft tissue mass that fills the right posterior ethmoidal cells and sphenoid sinus and erodes the posterior wall of the sphenoid sinus and floor of the sella (Figures 3(a)-3(b)). She underwent total sphenoethmoidectomy through transnasal and transethmoidal approaches. Sphenoid sinus was fully filled by a yellow-green caseous material (Figure 3(c)). Fungal debris and underlying hypertrophic mucosa were excised. The floor of the sella was eroded, but the dura was intact (Figure 3(d)). Fungal culture was positive for *Aspergillus fumigatus*. The patient is disease-free at seven months after antifungal therapy.

2.4. Case 4. A 68-year-old male patient presented with a history of nasal obstruction, headache, and left retroorbital pain for six months. Nasal endoscopy revealed drainage of purulent secretion from the right sphenoid sinus ostium. Paranasal sinus CT showed a hypodense mass filling the right sphenoid sinus (Figures 4(a)–4(c)). The patient underwent total sphenoethmoidectomy, and the caseous material within the sphenoid sinus was completely removed (Figure 4(d)). While the histopathological examination was consistent with chronic nongranulomatous invasive FRS, no growth was evident in the fungal culture. Six months postoperatively, he is free of symptoms and is doing well.

3. Discussion

Rhinosinusitis is a common public health problem that affects approximately 20% of the population [2]. While viruses and bacteria are the infectious agents detected in the majority of

TABLE 1: Characteristics and outcome of the patients.

	Case 1	Case 2	Case 3	Case 4
Age/gender	58 yrs/male	43 yrs/male	60 yrs/female	68 yrs/male
Immune suppression	–	–	–	–
Symptom onset to diagnosis	6 months	24 months	9 months	6 months
Symptoms at presentation	Left orbital pain Swelling on the face Nasal obstruction	Nasal obstruction Headache Facial pain	Dizziness Headache Postnasal drip	Headache Left retroorbital pain
Anatomic subsite involvement				
Nasal cavity	+	+	–	–
Osteomeatal complex	+	+	–	–
Maxillary sinus	+	–	–	–
Ethmoidal sinuses	+	+	+ (right posterior)	+ (right posterior)
Sphenoid sinus	+ (left side)	+ (left side)	+ (right side)	+ (right side)
Frontal sinus	+	+	–	–
Bilateral involvement	–	–	–	–
Orbital involvement	LP destruction	LP destruction	–	–
Intracranial extension	–	–	+	–
Surgical treatment	ESS	ESS combined with external frontal sinus surgery	ESS	ESS
Organism				
Microbiology	A. fumigatus	A. flavus	A. fumigatus	–
Histopathology	Nongranulomatous CIFRS	Nongranulomatous CIFRS	Nongranulomatous CIFRS	Nongranulomatous CIFRS
Medical treatment				
Voriconazole	+	+	+	+
Follow-up time	10 months	8 months	7 months	5 months
Disease recurrence	–	–	–	–

LP: lamina papyracea, ESS: endoscopic sinus surgery, and CIFRS: chronic invasive fungal rhinosinusitis.

(a)

(b)

(c)

(d)

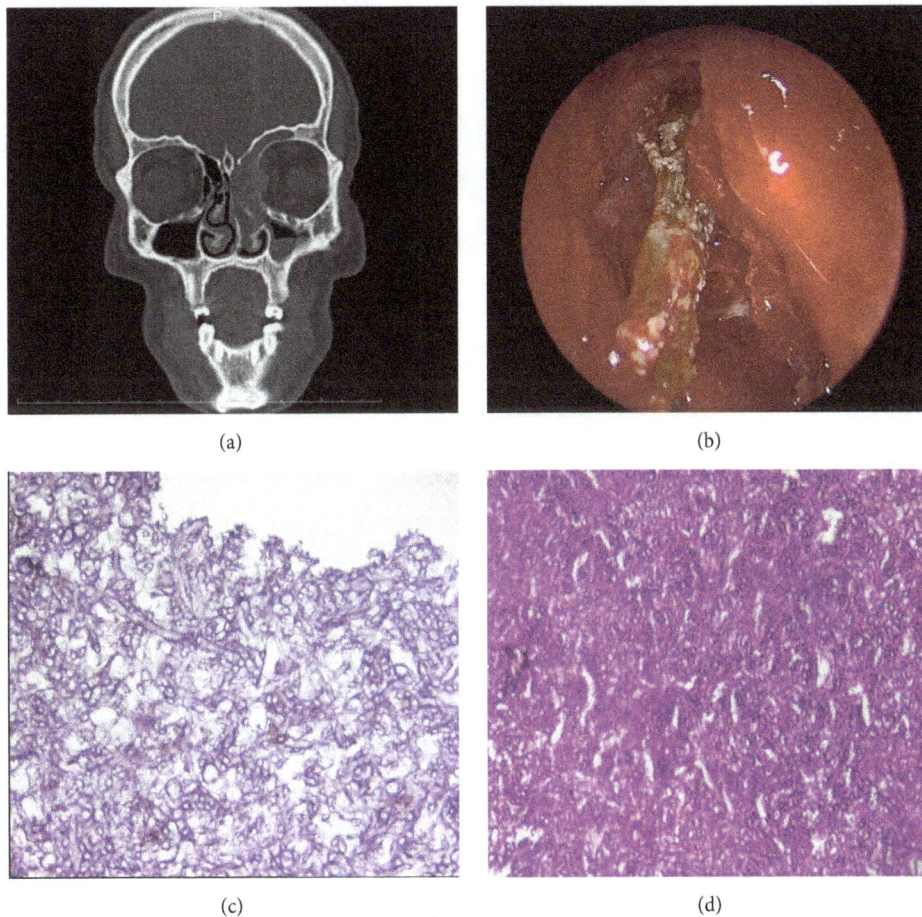

FIGURE 2: (a) Paranasal sinus computed tomography showing a soft tissue mass filling the left nasal cavity and ethmoid, frontal, and sphenoid sinuses and indenting the medial rectus muscle by destructing the lamina papyracea. (b) Endoscopic view of the yellow-green colored fungal debris. (c) Hematoxylin and eosin stain of the tissue revealing a group of narrow branching septate hyphae (×400). (d) Periodic acid-Schiff stain of the tissue showing branching septate hyphae.

cases, fungi are responsible for certain particular subtypes [6].

Acute invasive FRS is an opportunistic fungal infection almost exclusively affecting immunocompromised individuals. Classical hosts include those receiving multiagent chemotherapy for a hematologic malignancy and those who are neutropenic or those with aplastic anemia [7]. The disease manifests with an acute onset and has a fulminant course. In a case series of 29 patients, Monroe et al. reported a six-month overall survival of only 18% [8].

In contrast to acute invasive disease, chronic forms of invasive FRS including granulomatous and nongranulomatous types are mostly seen in apparently healthy individuals [2]. Although these two forms of chronic invasive FRS are considered separate entities, they share many clinical and pathologic features. *Aspergillus* species are the most common fungi isolated in both forms. Tissue invasion by fungi occurs over a prolonged period (several weeks or months), rather than hours as in acute invasive FRS [7]. Patients often present with nonspecific symptoms and have an indolent clinical course. Therefore, they are usually associated with delayed

diagnosis, which may increase the morbidity as well as mortality [7]. Despite the lack of comparative data, no significant differences in disease outcomes have been documented [1]. Both forms are treated in a similar fashion [5].

The distinction between granulomatous and nongranulomatous types of chronic invasive FRS is primarily based on pathological findings [1]. Granulomatous type is characterized by the presence of submucosal noncaseating granuloma consisting of foreign body or Langhans-type giant cells. Fungal hyphae are usually sparse, and there is extensive fibrosis. In contrast, there is a dense accumulation of hyphae in nongranulomatous type but the inflammatory infiltrate is sparse [4].

The majority of chronic invasive FRS cases in the literature have been reported from developing countries mostly located in the tropical regions of South Asia, Middle East, Africa, and South America [9]. The hot and humid climate in these regions creates a suitable environment for fungal growth and proliferation of spores. In addition, the high number of people working in agricultural activities increases the risk of intense exposure to fungal spores and development

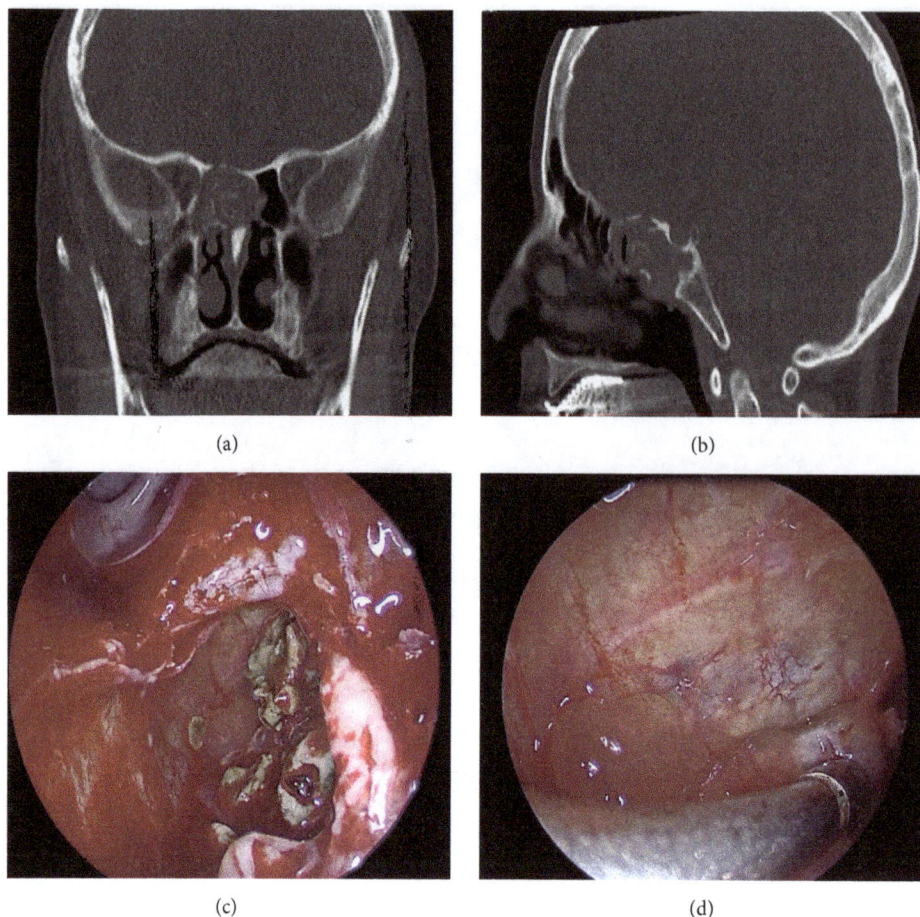

(a)

(b)

(c)

(d)

FIGURE 3: (a, b) Paranasal sinus computed tomography of a soft tissue mass filling the right posterior ethmoidal cells and sphenoid sinus. (c) Endoscopic view of the yellow-green colored caseous material in the right sphenoid sinus. (d) Endoscopic view of the intact dura mater in the right sphenoid sinus.

of fungal infection in a healthy individual. However, most of these reported cases include examples of granulomatous type.

Available data regarding chronic nongranulomatous invasive FRS are relatively sparse as compared to acute invasive and chronic granulomatous FRS. In most instances, the disease occurs in the background of diabetes mellitus or prolonged corticosteroid treatment [1]. In a multi-institutional analysis including 18 patients with invasive FRS (of them 8 were chronically nongranulomatous and 10 were acutely invasive), Pagella et al. reported a disease-related mortality rate of 25% for chronic invasive nongranulomatous FRS compared with 40% for acute invasive disease [10]. The majority of patients with chronic invasive disease had diabetes mellitus (87.5%) as comorbidity. On the other hand, in a small case series of 6 patients with chronic nongranulomatous invasive FRS, D'Anza et al. reported that all patients were free of disease at last follow-up, with a range of 1 to 27 months [11]. In this series, also all patients had systemic comorbidities, with diabetes mellitus being the most common.

In contrast to previous reports, none of the patients in our series had any comorbidities or history of corticosteroid use that may alter immune functions. In addition, our country remains outside the tropical climate zone. Apparently,

the only risk factors in our patients were that they were rural and were working in greenhouse farming and the fact that four cases are being reported from a single center within a short period of six months is clinically important.

The treatment of invasive FRS, including both acute and chronic subtypes, requires an effective surgical debridement and systemic antifungal therapy [5]. The aim of the surgery is to provide adequate sinus ventilation by the removal of devitalized tissues and to facilitate the penetration of antifungal agents. Amphotericin B, voriconazole, itraconazole, posaconazole, and caspofungin are antifungal agents that are effective against *Aspergillus* species [12]. In the single randomized controlled trial comparing voriconazole with amphotericin B, voriconazole was associated with better response and survival rates and fewer side effects than amphotericin B [13]. The duration of antifungal therapy has not been optimally defined in clinical practice guidelines. On the other hand, immune status of the patient, extent of the disease, and stabilization of all clinical and radiographic manifestations have been proposed to be the main factors in decision making for duration of treatment [12]. An important issue that should be considered in the use of voriconazole is that it may lead to transient visual disturbances (44%) [13].

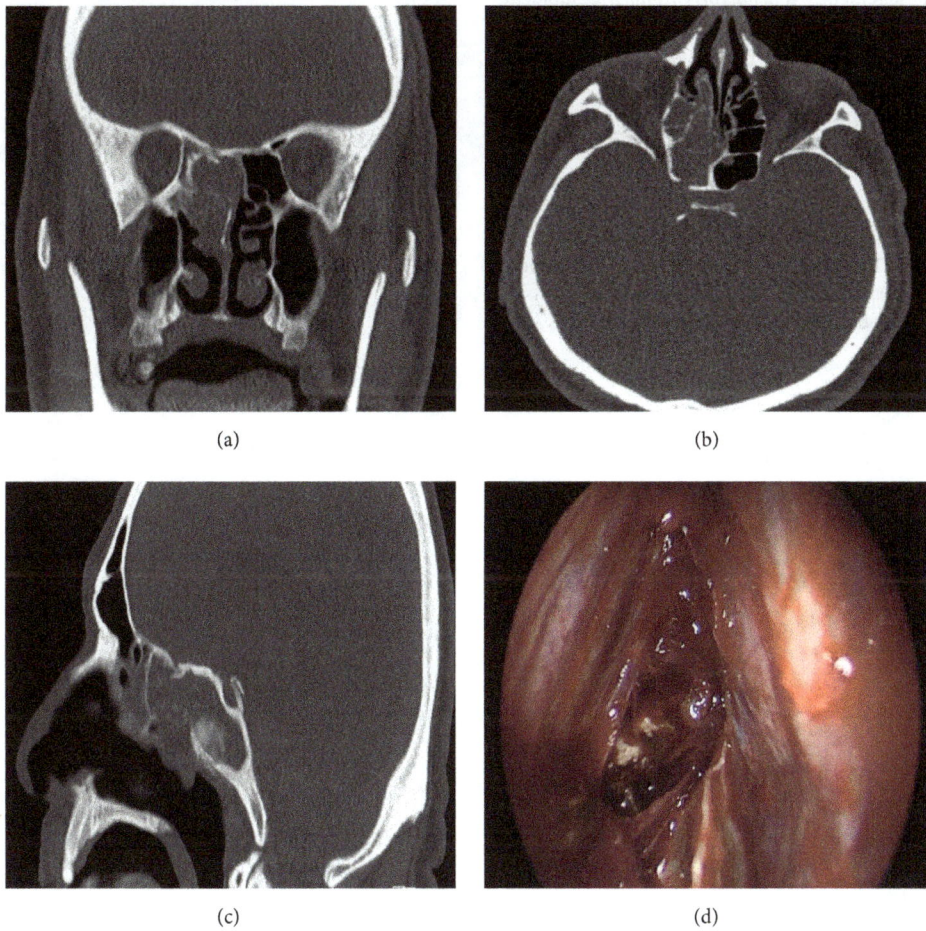

(a)

(b)

(c)

(d)

FIGURE 4: (a, b, and c) Paranasal sinus computed tomography of a hypodense mass filling the right sphenoid sinus (a-coronal, b-axial c-sagittal planes). (d) Endoscopic view of the caseous material filling the right sphenoid sinus.

In one of the cases in our series, a partial visual impairment occurred in the third week of the treatment; however it resolved spontaneously within 72 hours after stopping voriconazole.

In conclusion, chronic invasive nongranulomatous FRS should be kept in mind in the presence of long-standing nonspecific sinonasal symptoms in immunocompetent individuals with a history of working in greenhouse farming.

Competing Interests

The authors declare that they have no conflict of interests.

References

[1] A. Chakrabarti, D. W. Denning, B. J. Ferguson et al., "Fungal rhinosinusitis: a categorization and definitional schema addressing current controversies," *Laryngoscope*, vol. 119, no. 9, pp. 1809–1818, 2009.

[2] A. Chakrabarti, S. M. Rudramurthy, N. Panda, A. Das, and A. Singh, "Epidemiology of chronic fungal rhinosinusitis in rural India," *Mycoses*, vol. 58, no. 5, pp. 294–302, 2015.

[3] V. A. Epstein and R. C. Kern, "Invasive fungal sinusitis and complications of rhinosinusitis," *Otolaryngologic Clinics of North America*, vol. 41, no. 3, pp. 497–524, 2008.

[4] K. T. Montone, "Pathology of fungal rhinosinusitis: a review," *Head and Neck Pathology*, vol. 10, no. 1, pp. 40–46, 2016.

[5] T. J. Walsh, E. J. Anaissie, D. W. Denning et al., "Treatment of aspergillosis: clinical practice guidelines of the Infectious Diseases Society of America," *Clinical Infectious Diseases*, vol. 46, no. 3, pp. 327–360, 2008.

[6] B. F. Marple, J. A. Stankiewicz, F. M. Baroody et al., "Diagnosis and management of chronic rhinosinusitis in adults," *Postgraduate Medicine*, vol. 121, no. 6, pp. 121–139, 2009.

[7] C. Chang, M. E. Gershwin, and G. R. Thompson III, "Fungal disease of the nose and sinuses: an updated overview," *Current Allergy and Asthma Reports*, vol. 13, no. 2, pp. 152–161, 2013.

[8] M. M. Monroe, M. McLean, N. Sautter et al., "Invasive fungal rhinosinusitis: a 15-year experience with 29 patients," *Laryngoscope*, vol. 123, no. 7, pp. 1583–1587, 2013.

[9] A. Chakrabarti, S. S. Chatterjee, A. Das, and M. R. Shivaprakash, "Invasive aspergillosis in developing countries," *Medical Mycology*, vol. 49, supplement 1, pp. S35–S47, 2011.

[10] F. Pagella, F. De Bernardi, D. Dalla Gasperina et al., "Invasive fungal rhinosinusitis in adult patients: our experience in

diagnosis and management," *Journal of Cranio-Maxillofacial Surgery*, vol. 44, no. 4, pp. 512–520, 2016.

[11] B. D'Anza, J. Stokken, J. S. Greene, T. Kennedy, T. D. Woodard, and R. Sindwani, "Chronic invasive fungal sinusitis: characterization and shift in management of a rare disease," *International Forum of Allergy & Rhinology*, 2016.

[12] H. W. Boucher, A. H. Groll, C. C. Chiou, and T. J. Walsh, "Newer systemic antifungal agents: pharmacokinetics, safety and efficacy," *Drugs*, vol. 64, no. 18, pp. 1997–2020, 2004.

[13] R. Herbrecht, D. W. Denning, T. F. Patterson et al., "Voriconazole versus amphotericin B for primary therapy of invasive aspergillosis," *The New England Journal of Medicine*, vol. 347, no. 6, pp. 408–415, 2002.

34

Metastatic Renal Cell Carcinoma Presenting as a Paranasal Sinus Mass: The Importance of Differential Diagnosis

Massimo Ralli,[1] **Giancarlo Altissimi,**[2] **Rosaria Turchetta,**[2] **and Mario Rigante**[3]

[1]*Department of Oral and Maxillofacial Sciences, Sapienza University of Rome, Rome, Italy*
[2]*Department of Sense Organs, Audiology Section, Policlinico Umberto I, Sapienza University of Rome, Rome, Italy*
[3]*Department of Otorhinolaryngology, Catholic University of Sacred Heart, Rome, Italy*

Correspondence should be addressed to Massimo Ralli; massimo.ralli@uniroma1.it

Academic Editor: Marco Berlucchi

Metastases in the paranasal sinuses are rare; renal cell carcinoma is the most common cancer that metastasizes to this region. We present the case of a patient with a 4-month history of a rapidly growing mass of the nasal pyramid following a nasal trauma, associated with spontaneous epistaxis and multiple episodes of hematuria. Cranial CT scan and MRI showed an ethmoid mass extending to the choanal region, the right orbit, and the right frontal sinus with an initial intracranial extension. Patient underwent surgery with a trans-sinusal frontal approach using a bicoronal incision combined with an anterior midfacial degloving; histological exam was compatible with a metastasis of clear cell renal cell carcinoma. Following histological findings, a total body CT scan showed a solitary 6 cm mass in the upper posterior pole of the left kidney identified as the primary tumor. Although rare, metastatic renal cell carcinoma should always be suspected in patients with nasal or paranasal masses, especially if associated with symptoms suggestive of a systemic involvement such as hematuria. A correct early-stage diagnosis of metastatic RCC can considerably improve survival rate in these patients; preoperative differential diagnosis with contrast-enhanced imaging is fundamental for the correct treatment and follow-up strategy.

1. Introduction

Renal cell carcinoma (RCC) is the most common kidney cancer, with approximately 35,000 new cases in the US each year [1]; RCC mainly affects male patients between 40 and 60 years old [2]. Common presentation symptoms include hematuria (40%), flank pain (40%), and a palpable abdominal mass (25%) [3]. Approximately 30% of patients with renal cell carcinoma present with metastatic disease [4]; target organs are lung (75%), soft tissues (36%), bone (20%), liver (18%), cutaneous sites (8%), and central nervous system (8%) [5, 6]. Metastases in the paranasal sinuses are rare [7]; however, RCC is the most common cancer that metastasizes to this region. Prognosis of metastatic RCC is poor [8]; the survival rate ranges between 15 and 30% at 5 years [9] in case of a single metastasis and between 0 and 7% in patients with multiple metastases [10]. Metastatic RCC is often resistant to chemotherapy and radiotherapy [11]; numerous agents targeting VEGF and non-VEGFR pathways have been proposed during the last decade for the treatment of advanced RCC [12–18].

We present the case of a patient with a single, rapidly growing mass in the upper portion of the nasal pyramid, with late, postnasal surgery histological diagnosis of renal cell carcinoma that allowed primary tumor identification.

2. Case Presentation

A 72-year-old man was referred to our institution with a 4-month history of a voluminous mass in the upper portion of the nasal pyramid following a nasal trauma. He had been treated a few weeks earlier at a different ENT service for a massive spontaneous epistaxis. The patient also reported a long history of hematuria, previously attributed to renal tuberculosis occurring over 40 years before. At admission, a cranial CT scan showed a large soft tissue ethmoid mass extending to the right and left choanal region, the right orbit, the right frontal sinus, and an initial intracranial extension

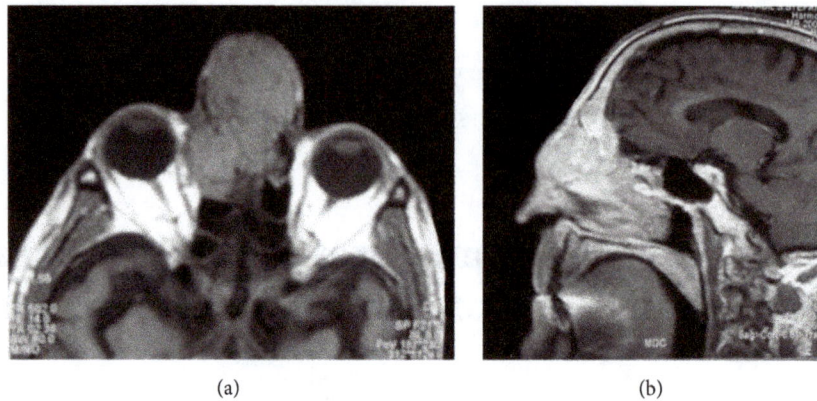

(a)   (b)

FIGURE 1: MRI in the axial (a) and sagittal (b) planes showing a soft tissue ethmoid mass extending to the right and left choanal region, the right orbit, the right frontal sinus, and an initial intracranial extension with partial erosion of the crista galli.

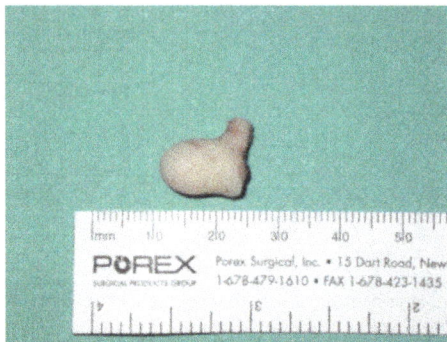

FIGURE 2: The excised mass; histological exam was consistent with a clear cell renal cell carcinoma.

with partial erosion of the crista galli. MRI confirmed the evidence found at computed tomography (Figure 1). Fine needle aspiration showed typical epithelial tissue and clear-cytoplasm cells interpreted as pericytes. Preoperative local biopsy was not performed due to the history of severe epistaxis and the high risk of massive bleeding during the procedure.

The patient underwent surgery with a trans-sinusal frontal approach using a bicoronal incision combined with an anterior midfacial degloving to excise the mass; however, the right orbital and especially the initial intracranial extension did not allow a complete removal of the neoplasm. Considerable bleeding occurred during surgery. The histological exam revealed a clear cell renal cell carcinoma (Figure 2). Based on these findings, the patient underwent a total body CT scan that showed a solitary 6 cm mass in the upper posterior pole of the left kidney. Bone scintigraphy also revealed increased uptake in the ethmoid and orbital region. Due to the poor general conditions, no surgery was performed to remove the primary tumor; the patient died 4 months later.

3. Discussion

Nasal cavity and paranasal sinus cancers are usually primary tumors. Metastases to the paranasal sinuses are rarely found;

among them, renal cell carcinoma is the most common cancer to metastasize to this region (49%) followed, respectively, by bronchus, urogenital ridge, breast, and gastrointestinal tract [19, 20]. RCC can metastasize to any region of the body, with a prevalence for lungs (75% of cases), regional lymph nodes (65%), bone (40%), and liver (40%) [21]. Metastasis to the head and neck regions account for about 15% of the cases, targeting in order of frequency the paranasal sinuses, the larynx, jaws, temporal bones, thyroid, and parotid glands [22].

RCC tumor cells can reach the sinonasal region via two routes: the first includes inferior vena cava, lungs, heart, and the maxillary artery; the second involves the communication of the avalvular vertebral venous plexus and the intracranial venous plexus [23]. Maxillary sinuses are the most commonly involved sinuses by metastatic tumors (36%), followed by the ethmoid (25%), frontal and sphenoid sinuses (17%), and nasal cavity (11%) [24, 25]. One of the first reports available in recent literature to describe a renal clear cell carcinoma metastatic to the paranasal sinuses has been published by Matsumoto and Yanagihara in 1982 [26]; afterwards several authors described case reports of RCC presenting as metastatic diseases in the paranasal sinuses. Available literature describes presentation of RCC metastasis as a solitary periorbital [27] and orbital mass [28], as a frontal sinus mass [29], as an ethmoid sinus mass [30, 31], in the nasal cavity [32, 33], in the maxillary [34, 35], and sphenoid sinus [36–38]. In some cases, the extension of the metastasis to the skull base has been described [39].

Metastatic RCC to the sinonasal district has been reported as the presenting sign of this disease in a few cases [29, 34], while in others it followed or occurred simultaneously to primary cancer diagnosis. Presentation symptoms are often limited to recurrent epistaxis [40–43] and the presence of a primary renal cell carcinoma is recognized only after surgical removal of the metastatic tumor via histologic examination supported by immunohistochemical staining of the specimen [5]. Rarely, metastasis in the sinonasal cavities followed RCC diagnosis and treatment [44–46]; cases of postsurgery metastasis in the head and neck district have been described up to 12 years after surgery [47].

The key point in RCC presenting with a sinonasal metastasis is differential diagnosis with primary tumors such as adenocarcinomas, angiofibromas, hemangiopericytomas, melanomas, hemangiomas, metastatic tumors from the breast and lungs, and, more rarely, systemic diseases such as Wegener's and midline granulomas [48]. In fact, in such cases diagnostic delays, misdiagnosis, undertreatment, and mismanagement could occur due to (1) the attribution of the mass to a primary sinonasal cancer given the rare nature of sinonasal metastasis or (2) to the overlook of presenting symptoms such as recurrent epistaxis, swelling, pain, and nasal obstruction. Hematuria can be considered as an indicator of RCC; it has been reported that about 10% of patients with RCC with distant metastasis exhibit massive hematuria. However, intermittent hematuria may be present in 90% of cases [3]. For this reason, patients presenting with nasosinusal tumors also reporting hematuria should always undergo systemic evaluation. Radiological examination with CT scan and, secondly, MRI and angiography are necessary in assessing the extent of the metastatic lesion. However, it should be considered that RCC metastases have similar radiological appearances to primary malignant lesions of sinonasal cavities; some indicators of renal origin at CT scan are enhancement, destruction, and lack of tumoral calcification [6].

In this case, CT scan allowed the identification of a neoformed paranasal sinus mass; however, only histological exam identified the mass as a metastasis of RCC and led to the execution of total body CT scan to identify primary tumor. Although difficult, differential preoperative diagnosis is fundamental for the correct treatment and follow-up strategy; contrast-enhanced imaging plays a central role since a preoperative biopsy of the nasal mass may be difficult in these patients due to massive recurring bleeding and, in some cases, may result in only necrotic tissue inconclusive on histopathology [42]. The ENT specialist, therefore, should always suspect metastatic disease from primary sites external to the head and neck region in patients with hypervascular mass in the nasal cavity or paranasal sinuses and a history of massive nasal bleeding and should complete preoperative workup with total body CT scan. Furthermore, it is important to remark that metastatic tumors originating from primary kidney masses are highly vascularized and surgeons should expect significant haemorrhage during surgical removal. One of the main advantages of a preoperative diagnosis of RCC when approaching a patient with sinonasal mass is the preparation for management of severe perioperative bleeding, thus implementing strategies to optimise the patient's tolerance to bleeding and to reduce the amount of bleeding morbidity and mortality.

Prognosis of metastatic RCC is poor; however, a correct early-stage diagnosis of metastatic disease can considerably improve survival rate: literature reports that excision of solitary metastatic lesion of renal cell carcinoma following nephrectomy results in a 41% survival at 2 years and 13% survival at 5 years [48]. The sole excision of the metastatic lesion, instead, significantly lowers survival rate [49]; patients with multiple metastases have a 5-year survival rate between 0 and 7% [10].

Although metastatic RCC is often resistant to chemotherapy and radiotherapy, numerous agents targeting VEGF and non-VEGFR pathways should be taken into account for the treatment of advanced RCC. Multitargeted VEGF tyrosine kinase inhibitors (TKIs) include sorafenib [12], sunitinib [13], pazopanib [14], axitinib [15], and bevacizumab [16]; mTOR inhibitors include temsirolimus [17] and everolimus [18]. Unfortunately, especially in cases of advanced neoplasms, benefits are still time-limited and treatment decisions should be based not only on guidelines but also on clinical considerations, such as patient comorbidities, treatment toxicity, prognostic factors, and molecular aspects of disease. In this case, the poor general conditions of the patient prevented additional treatment except for palliative pain management.

In conclusion, metastatic renal cell carcinoma should always be suspected in patients with nasal or paranasal masses, especially if associated with symptoms suggestive of a systemic involvement such as hematuria; early-stage diagnosis of metastatic disease can considerably limit perioperative complications and improve survival rate.

Competing Interests

The authors declare that they have no competing interests.

References

[1] A. Jemal, R. C. Tiwari, T. Murray et al., "Cancer Statistics, 2004," *CA: A Cancer Journal for Clinicians*, vol. 54, no. 1, pp. 8–29, 2004.

[2] R. Y. Lim, D. F. Bastug, and B. L. Caldwell, "Metastatic renal cell carcinoma of the nasal septum," *The West Virginia Medical Journal*, vol. 85, no. 4, pp. 143–145, 1989.

[3] D. G. Skinner, C. D. Vermillion, R. C. Pfister, and W. F. Leadbetter, "Renal cell carcinoma," *American Family Physician*, vol. 4, no. 4, pp. 89–94, 1971.

[4] R. C. Flanigan, S. C. Campbell, J. I. Clark, and M. M. Picken, "Metastatic renal cell carcinoma," *Current Treatment Options in Oncology*, vol. 4, no. 5, pp. 385–390, 2003.

[5] J. Singh, V. Baheti, S. S. Yadav, and R. Mathur, "Occult renal cell carcinoma manifesting as nasal mass and epistaxis," *Reviews in Urology*, vol. 16, no. 3, pp. 145–148, 2014.

[6] P. M. Som, K. I. Norton, J. M. Shugar et al., "Metastatic hypernephroma to the head and neck," *American Journal of Neuroradiology*, vol. 8, no. 6, pp. 1103–1106, 1987.

[7] M. Ziari, S. Shen, R. J. Amato, and B. S. Teh, "Metastatic renal cell carcinoma to the nose and ethmoid sinus," *Urology*, vol. 67, no. 1, pp. 199.e21–199.e23, 2006.

[8] M. H. Ather, N. Masood, and T. Siddiqui, "Current management of advanced and metastatic renal cell carcinoma," *Urology Journal*, vol. 7, no. 1, pp. 1–9, 2010.

[9] B. Torres Muros, R. Bonilla Parrilla, J. R. Solano Romero, J. G. Rodríguez Baró, and J. Verge González, "Metastasis in maxilar sinus as only manifestation of disseminate renal adenocarcinoma," *Anales Otorrinolaringológicos Ibero-Americanos*, vol. 34, no. 3, pp. 231–236, 2007.

[10] E. T. Cheng, D. Greene, and R. J. Koch, "Metastatic renal cell carcinoma to the nose," *Otolaryngology—Head and Neck Surgery*, vol. 122, no. 3, p. 464, 2000.

[11] R. J. Motzer, P. Russo, D. M. Nanus, and W. J. Berg, "Renal cell carcinoma," *Current Problems in Cancer*, vol. 21, no. 4, pp. 185–232, 1997.

[12] B. Escudier, N. Lassau, E. Angevin et al., "Phase I trial of sorafenib in combination with IFN α-2a in patients with unresectable and/or metastatic renal cell carcinoma or malignant melanoma," *Clinical Cancer Research*, vol. 13, no. 6, pp. 1801–1809, 2007.

[13] R. J. Motzer, M. D. Michaelson, J. Rosenberg et al., "Sunitinib efficacy against advanced renal cell carcinoma," *Journal of Urology*, vol. 178, no. 5, pp. 1883–1887, 2007.

[14] C. N. Sternberg, I. D. Davis, J. Mardiak et al., "Pazopanib in locally advanced or metastatic renal cell carcinoma: results of a randomized phase III trial," *Journal of Clinical Oncology*, vol. 28, no. 6, pp. 1061–1068, 2010.

[15] B. I. Rini, B. Melichar, T. Ueda et al., "Axitinib with or without dose titration for first-line metastatic renal-cell carcinoma: a randomised double-blind phase 2 trial," *The Lancet Oncology*, vol. 14, no. 12, pp. 1233–1242, 2013.

[16] B. Escudier, A. Pluzanska, P. Koralewski et al., "Bevacizumab plus interferon alfa-2a for treatment of metastatic renal cell carcinoma: a randomised, double-blind phase III trial," *The Lancet*, vol. 370, no. 9605, pp. 2103–2111, 2007.

[17] G. Hudes, M. Carducci, P. Tomczak et al., "Temsirolimus, interferon alfa, or both for advanced renal-cell carcinoma," *New England Journal of Medicine*, vol. 356, no. 22, pp. 2271–2281, 2007.

[18] R. J. Motzer, B. Escudier, S. Oudard et al., "Efficacy of everolimus in advanced renal cell carcinoma: a double-blind, randomised, placebo-controlled phase III trial," *The Lancet*, vol. 372, no. 9637, pp. 449–456, 2008.

[19] P. Sountoulides, L. Metaxa, and L. Cindolo, "Atypical presentations and rare metastatic sites of renal cell carcinoma: a review of case reports," *Journal of Medical Case Reports*, vol. 5, article no. 429, 2011.

[20] E. Evgeniou, K. R. Menon, G. L. Jones, H. Whittet, and W. Williams, "Renal cell carcinoma metastasis to the paranasal sinuses and orbit," *BMJ Case Reports*, vol. 2012, 2012.

[21] E. E. Lang, N. Patil, R. M. Walsh, M. Leader, and M. A. Walsh, "A case of renal cell carcinoma metastatic to the nose and tongyue," *Ear, Nose and Throat Journal*, vol. 82, no. 5, pp. 382–383, 2003.

[22] F. Ö. Dinçbas, B. Atalar, D. Ç. Öksüz, F. V. Aker, and S. Koca, "Unusual metastasis of renal cell carcinoma to the nasal cavity," *Journal of B.U.ON.*, vol. 9, no. 2, pp. 201–204, 2004.

[23] M. D. Gottlieb and J. T. Roland Jr., "Paradoxical spread of renal cell carcinoma to the head and neck," *Laryngoscope*, vol. 108, no. 9, pp. 1301–1305, 1998.

[24] M. Kovačić, A. Krvavica, and M. Rudić, "Renal cell carcinoma metastasis to the sinonasal cavity: case report," *Acta Clinica Croatica*, vol. 54, no. 2, pp. 223–226, 2015.

[25] J. M. Bernstein, W. W. Montgomery, and K. Balogh, "Metastatic tumors to the maxilla, nose, and paranasal sinuses," *Laryngoscope*, vol. 76, no. 4, pp. 621–650, 1966.

[26] Y. Matsumoto and N. Yanagihara, "Renal clear cell carcinoma metastatic to the nose and paranasal sinuses," *Laryngoscope*, vol. 92, no. 10, part 1, pp. 1190–1193, 1982.

[27] J. J. Homer and N. S. Jones, "Renal cell carcinoma presenting as a solitary paranasal sinus metastasis," *Journal of Laryngology and Otology*, vol. 109, no. 10, pp. 986–989, 1995.

[28] J. W. Jung, S. C. Yoon, D. H. Han, and M. Chi, "Metastatic renal cell carcinoma to the orbit and the ethmoid sinus," *Journal of Craniofacial Surgery*, vol. 23, no. 2, pp. e136–e138, 2012.

[29] T. Ikeuchi, N. Asai, T. Hori et al., "Renal cell carcinoma detected by metastasis to the frontal sinus: a case report," *Acta Urologica Japonica*, vol. 44, no. 2, pp. 89–92, 1998.

[30] G. K. Maheshwari, H. A. Baboo, M. H. Patel, and G. Usha, "Metastatic renal cell carcinoma involving ethmoid sinus at presentation," *Journal of Postgraduate Medicine*, vol. 49, no. 1, pp. 96–97, 2003.

[31] N. Terada, K. Hiruma, M. Suzuki, T. Numata, and A. Konno, "Metastasis of renal cell cancer to the ethmoid sinus," *Acta Oto-Laryngologica, Supplement*, no. 537, pp. 82–86, 1998.

[32] S. Vreugde, R. Duttmann, A. Halama, and P. Deron, "Metastasis of a renal cell carcinoma to the nose and paranasal sinuses," *Acta Oto-Rhino-Laryngologica Belgica*, vol. 53, no. 2, pp. 129–131, 1999.

[33] R. Nason and R. L. Carrau, "Metastatic renal cell carcinoma to the nasal cavity," *American Journal of Otolaryngology—Head and Neck Medicine and Surgery*, vol. 25, no. 1, pp. 54–57, 2004.

[34] B. Torres Muros, J. R. Solano Romero, J. G. Rodríguez Baró, and R. Bonilla Parrilla, "Maxillary sinus metastasis of renal cell carcinoma," *Actas Urologicas Espanolas*, vol. 30, no. 9, pp. 954–957, 2006.

[35] Y. He, J. Chen, W. Xu et al., "Case report metastatic renal cell carcinoma to the left maxillary sinus," *Genetics and Molecular Research*, vol. 13, no. 3, pp. 7465–7469, 2014.

[36] S. Koscielny, "The paranasal sinuses as metastatic site of renal cell carcinoma," *Laryngorhinootologie*, vol. 78, no. 8, pp. 441–444, 1999.

[37] R. Simo, A. J. Sykes, S. P. Hargreaves et al., "Metastatic renal cell carcinoma to the nose and paranasal sinuses," *Head and Neck*, vol. 22, no. 7, pp. 722–727, 2000.

[38] J. G. Pereira Arias, V. Ullate Jaime, F. Valcárcel Martín et al., "Epistaxis as initial manifestation of disseminated renal adenocarcinoma," *Actas Urologicas Espanolas*, vol. 26, no. 5, pp. 361–365, 2002.

[39] P. K. Parida, "Renal cell carcinoma metastatic to the sinonasal region: three case reports with a review of the literature," *Ear, Nose and Throat Journal*, vol. 91, no. 11, pp. E11–E16, 2012.

[40] M. Szymański, A. Szymańska, K. Morshed, and H. Siwiec, "Renal cell carcinoma metastases to nose and paranasal sinuses presenting as recurrent epistaxis," *Wiadomosci Lekarskie*, vol. 57, no. 1-2, pp. 94–96, 2004.

[41] H. Lee, H. J. Kang, and S. H. Lee, "Metastatic renal cell carcinoma presenting as epistaxis," *European Archives of Oto-Rhino-Laryngology*, vol. 262, no. 1, pp. 69–71, 2005.

[42] D. R. Nayak, K. Pujary, S. Ramnani, C. Shetty, and P. Parul, "Metastatic renal cell carcinoma presenting with epistaxis," *Indian Journal of Otolaryngology and Head and Neck Surgery*, vol. 58, no. 4, pp. 406–408, 2006.

[43] R. Kumar, K. Sikka, R. Kumar, and P. Chatterjee, "Nephrogenic epistaxis," *Singapore Medical Journal*, vol. 55, no. 7, pp. e112–e113, 2014.

[44] V. Montoro Martínez, M. López Vilas, M. Gurri Freixa, E. De Dios Orán, J. R. Montserrat Gili, and J. M. Fabra Llopis, "Nasal sinus metastasis of renal carcinoma. A case report," *Acta Otorrinolaringológica Española*, vol. 50, no. 8, pp. 653–656, 1999.

[45] H. Sawazaki, T. Segawa, K. Yoshida et al., "Bilateral maxillary sinus metastasis of renal cell carcinoma: a case report," *Acta Urologica Japonica*, vol. 53, no. 4, pp. 231–234, 2007.

[46] S.-L. Hong, D.-W. Jung, H.-J. Roh, and K.-S. Cho, "Metastatic renal cell carcinoma of the posterior nasal septum as the first presentation 10 years after nephrectomy," *Journal of Oral and Maxillofacial Surgery*, vol. 71, no. 10, pp. 1813.e1–1813.e7, 2013.

[47] G. Fyrmpas, A. Adeniyi, and S. Baer, "Occult renal cell carcinoma manifesting with epistaxis in a woman: a case report," *Journal of Medical Case Reports*, vol. 5, article 79, 2011.

[48] M. K. Dineen, R. D. Pastore, L. J. Emrich, and R. P. Huben, "Results of surgical treatment of renal cell carcinoma with solitary metastasis," *Journal of Urology*, vol. 140, no. 2, pp. 277–279, 1988.

[49] D. G. Skinner, R. B. Colvin, C. D. Vermillion, R. C. Pfister, and W. F. Leadbetter, "Diagnosis and management of renal cell carcinoma. A clinical and pathologic study of 309 cases," *Cancer*, vol. 28, no. 5, pp. 1165–1177, 1971.

35

Case of Chronic Otitis Media with Intracranial Complication and Contralateral Extracranial Presentation

X. Y. Yeoh, P. S. Lim, and K. C. Pua

Department of Otorhinolaryngology, Penang General Hospital, Jalan Residensi, 10990 Penang, Malaysia

Correspondence should be addressed to X. Y. Yeoh; xy.yeoh@gmail.com

Academic Editor: Rong-San Jiang

Intracranial complications of chronic otitis media have been on the decline with advent of antibiotics. Septic thrombosis of the sigmoid sinus is rarer compared to commoner complications such as otogenic brain abscesses and meningitis. This patient presented with recurrent infection after left mastoidectomy secondary to cholesteatoma and a contralateral internal jugular vein thrombosis with parapharyngeal abscess, which was drained. He recovered well postoperatively with antibiotics.

1. Introduction

Otitis media is potentially serious due to its life-threatening complications. The complications arising from this condition can be further divided into intracranial and extracranial. These complications, from being common with high morbidity and mortality rates, have become rare now with arrival of the antibiotic era. A retrospective study by Lund talks of the mortality rate due to intracranial complications being at 36% between 1939 and 1949, 6% from 1950 to 1960, and 0% from 1961 to 1971, demonstrating the drastic change in the incidence [1].

2. Case Report

A 23-year-old Nepali, with history of left modified radical mastoidectomy 2 months prior for cholesteatoma, presented with one-week history of fever, right otalgia, neck pain, and right neck swelling, with reduced neck movement. On examination, he appeared ill with high spiking fever; there was a presence of House Brackmann grade II facial nerve palsy on the left (present only postoperatively) and the left postauricular wound dehiscence was discharging pus. He also had torticollis to the right, associated with fullness over the right upper neck (Figure 1). Otoscopy on the left revealed copious amounts of mucopus in the middle ear and mastoid cavity and, on the right, an inflamed but dull

tympanic membrane (Figure 2). Due to financial constraints, a myringotomy was performed on the right ear, yielding only mucoid material, and a failed aspiration over the fullness of the right neck was done. An exploration of the left wound was performed under local anaesthesia; draining pus and packing was done. His fever persisted, and an urgent brain and neck Contrast Enhanced Computed Tomography (CECT) was done, showing soft tissue within the left mastoid cavity, right parapharyngeal abscess, and bilateral internal jugular vein (IJV) thrombosis (Figure 3). Patient was subjected to drainage of the right parapharyngeal abscess under general anaesthesia. He became afebrile immediately postoperatively, and the torticollis resolved. Pus culture of the left postauricular wound grew *Pseudomonas aeruginosa* and of the right neck grew *Bacteroides* spp. He completed 10 days of IV Rocephine, Amikacin, and metronidazole and was discharged with oral antibiotics after secondary suturing was done over his right neck wound. He decided to continue his treatment in Nepal.

3. Discussion

Chronic suppurative otitis media (CSOM) affects 65–330 million individuals with draining ears, and accounts for 28000 deaths in 1990. The Western Pacific and Southeast Asian regions contribute 85–90% of this global burden from CSOM, with India and China accounting for most cases [2]. The majority of intracranial complications were

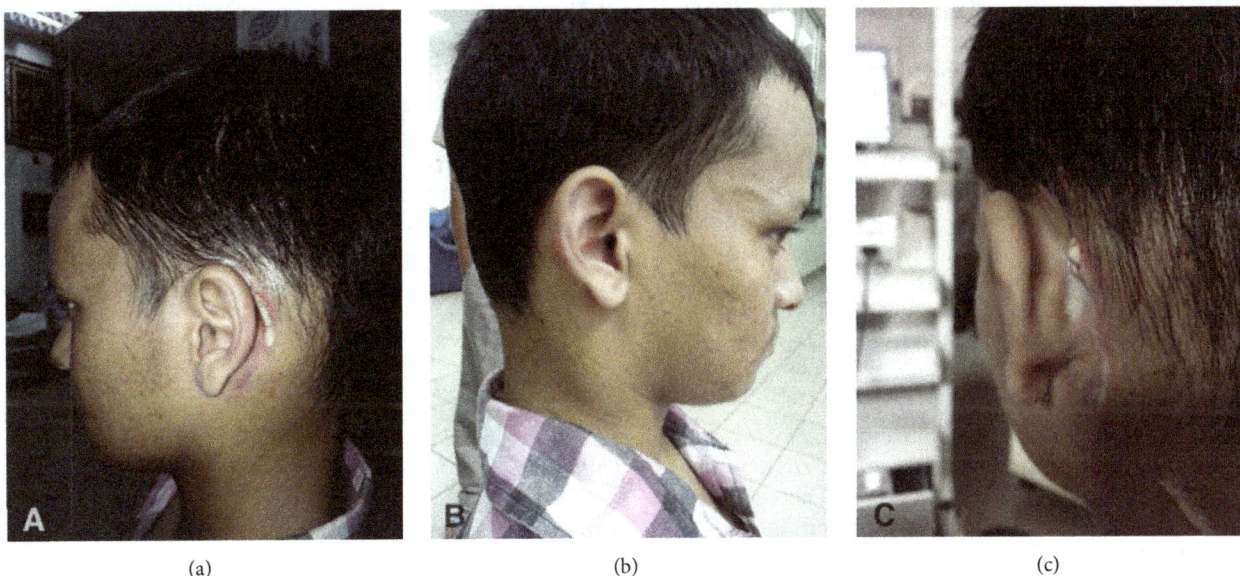

FIGURE 1: (a and c) Wound dehiscence of the left mastoidectomy site discharging pus. (b) Right neck fullness.

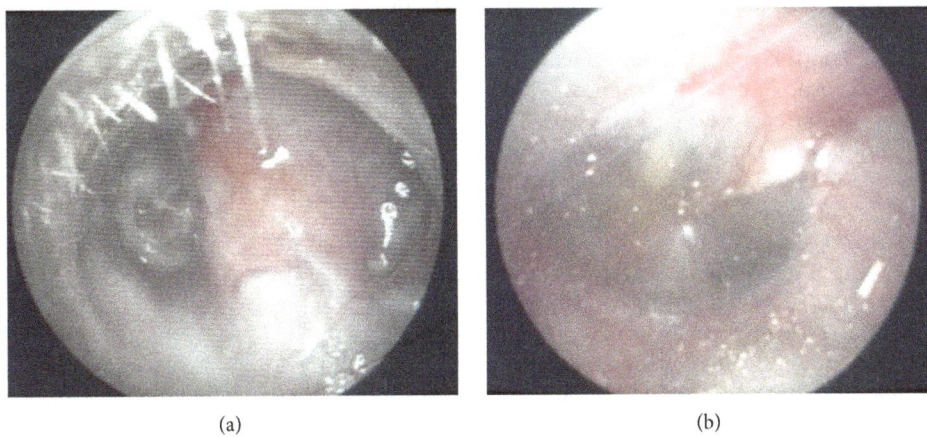

FIGURE 2: (a) Left otoscopy showing mucopus at the mastoid cavity and external auditory canal. (b) Right inflamed and dull tympanic membrane.

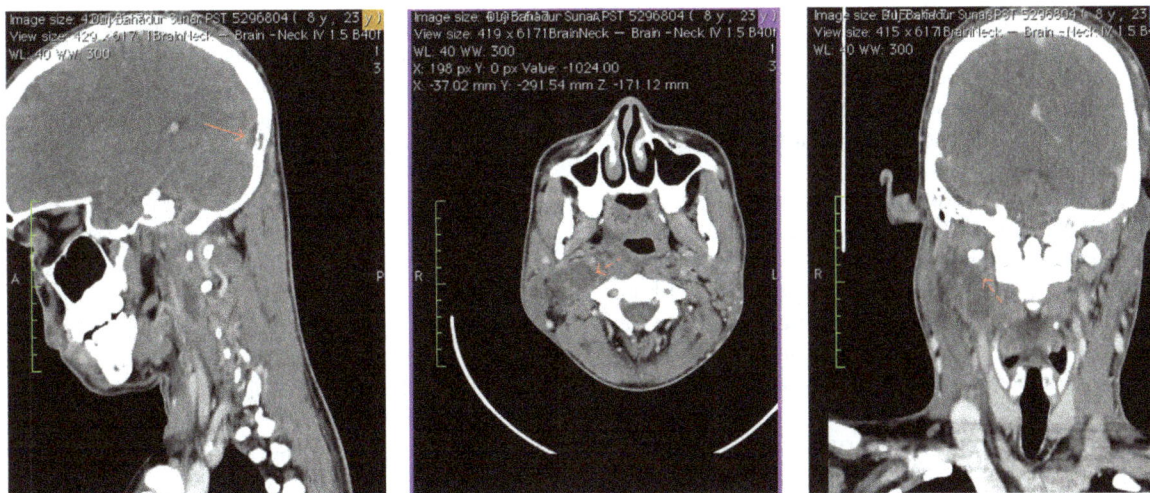

FIGURE 3: CECT showing right IJV thrombosis with right parapharyngeal abscess and delta sign at the transverse sinus.

caused by chronic otitis media and cholesteatoma (95.8%), and these complications occur more frequently in the first three decades of life with a higher incidence in males [3]. The commonest to occur are meningitis and brain abscess (temporal or cerebellar) and one or more complications may present in a single patient [4, 5]. They may present with headache, neck stiffness, vomiting, and fits associated with otorrhea and decreased hearing. However, these may be difficult to recognize and present atypically and more subtly as the symptoms can be masked by use of antibiotics. The commonest presentation of patients with lateral sinus thrombosis is sustained or spiking fever, associated with otorrhea, postauricular oedema, and otalgia [6], which were evident in this patient.

Sinus thrombosis occurs by bone erosion of the mastoid over the sinus, due to either cholesteatoma or granulomatous processes, forming a perisinus abscess. This abscess creates pressure on the bone, causing necrosis on the anterior portion of the sinus and the intima, with adherence of fibrin, red blood cells, and platelets, forming a mural thrombus. This thrombus might propagate towards the jugular vein bulb, and to other sites, or subcutaneous tissue, or it might throw emboli [7]. This patient had a left cholesteatoma with sigmoid sinus thrombosis, with retrograde propagation to the transverse sinus and contralateral sigmoid sinus, and IJV, resulting in parapharyngeal abscess formation over the right side. Lemierre's syndrome, according to a systematic review, is rarely due to middle ear or mastoid infections (2%), commoner causes being the tonsil, pharynx, or the chest. However, this patient's presentation of neck pain and swelling is the commonest for patients with IJV thrombosis [8].

Organisms involved in septic IJV are determined by the etiology. In intravenous catheter related IJV, the most likely organism is *Staphylococcus aureus*, and, in oropharyngeal infections, anaerobes are common. In otologic infections, *Proteus* and *Pseudomonas* are the most common organisms isolated [9]. This patient grew *Pseudomonas* from cultures of the left mastoidectomy site. CECT aids in the diagnosis of intracranial complications of otitis media, be it an abscess or a sinus thrombosis, which will demonstrate the "delta sign" (central nonenhancing clot surrounded by enhancing dural sinus wall) [10]. It is therefore imperative that CECT or an MRI be performed if sinus thrombosis is suspected as a plain HRCT of the temporal region, which is normally performed for patients with cholesteatoma undergoing surgery and would miss this fairly rare intracranial complication nowadays.

This patient's presentation was interesting as he presented with a unilateral discharging ear, he was diagnosed to have cholesteatoma, and mastoidectomy was performed after a HRCT temporal. He has currently presented with an extracranial extension of an intracranial complication on the contralateral side, and this septic thrombosis has caused the formation of a parapharyngeal abscess, which was adequately addressed with drainage.

In infected IJV thrombosis, the primary site of infection should be treated first; for example, neck abscesses should be drained and mastoidectomy should be done for mastoiditis [9], as in this patient. Most patients with infected

IJV thrombosis do well on antibiotics alone, and the choice depends on the most likely organism. Migirov et al. have demonstrated that combination antibiotics are effective in treating intracranial complications in his series as many of his patients have been prescribed antibiotics prior to presentation [11]. In the case of a primary ear infection, the patient should be treated with Amikacin to cover Gram-negative organisms [9]. This patient was started on appropriate antibiotics, namely, Rocephin, Amikacin, and Metronidazole, and he responded to combined medical and surgical treatment that was rendered.

4. Conclusion

A contralateral presentation of the right parapharyngeal abscess due to septic IJV thrombosis resulting from chronic otitis media is rare. A high index of suspicion is required for diagnosis for proper treatment to be initiated.

Consent

Written consent has been obtained from the subject and full confidentiality will be maintained.

Competing Interests

There are no competing interests regarding this paper.

Authors' Contributions

The authors have participated in managing this patient and production of the paper.

References

[1] W. S. Lund, "A review of 50 cases of intracranial complications from otogenic infection between 1961 and 1977," *Clinical Otolaryngology and Allied Sciences*, vol. 3, no. 4, pp. 495–501, 1978.

[2] WHO, *Chronic Suppurative Otitis Media: Burden of Illness and Management Options*, WHO, Geneva, Switzerland, 2004.

[3] N. D. O. Penido, A. Borin, L. C. N. Iha et al., "Intracranial complications of otitis media: 15 years of experience in 33 patients," *Otolaryngology—Head and Neck Surgery*, vol. 132, no. 1, pp. 37–42, 2005.

[4] J.-F. Wu, Z. Jin, J.-M. Yang, Y.-H. Liu, and M.-L. Duan, "Extracranial and intracranial complications of otitis media: 22-year clinical experience and analysis," *Acta Oto-Laryngologica*, vol. 132, no. 3, pp. 261–265, 2012.

[5] S. P. Dubey and V. Larawin, "Complications of chronic suppurative otitis media and their management," *Laryngoscope*, vol. 117, no. 2, pp. 264–267, 2007.

[6] D. M. Kaplan, M. Kraus, M. Puterman, A. Niv, A. Leiberman, and D. M. Fliss, "Otogenic lateral sinus thrombosis in children," *International Journal of Pediatric Otorhinolaryngology*, vol. 49, no. 3, pp. 177–183, 1999.

[7] M. S. Miura, R. C. Krumennauer, and J. F. Lubianca Neto, "Intracranial complications of chronic suppurative otitis media in children," *Revista Brasileira de Otorrinolaringologia*, vol. 71, no. 5, pp. 639–643, 2005.

[8] P. D. Karkos, S. Asrani, C. D. Karkos et al., "Lemierre's syndrome: a systematic review," *Laryngoscope*, vol. 119, no. 8, pp. 1552–1559, 2009.

[9] N. E. Jonas and J. J. Fagan, "Internal jugular vein thrombosis: a case study and review of literature," *The Internet Journal of Otorhinolaryngology*, vol. 6, no. 2, pp. 1–4, 2007.

[10] H. Seven, A. E. Ozbal, and S. Turgut, "Management of otogenic lateral sinus thrombosis," *American Journal of Otolaryngology—Head and Neck Medicine and Surgery*, vol. 25, no. 5, pp. 329–333, 2004.

[11] L. Migirov, S. Duvdevani, and J. Kronenberg, "Otogenic intracranial complications: a review of 28 cases," *Acta Oto-Laryngologica*, vol. 125, no. 8, pp. 819–822, 2005.

36

A Case of Ameloblastic Fibroodontoma Extending Maxillary Sinus with Erupted Tooth: Is Transcanine Approach with Alveolectomy Feasible?

Mustafa Aslıer,[1] **Mustafa Cenk Ecevit,**[1] **Sülen Sarıoğlu,**[2] **and Semih Sütay**[1]

[1]*Department of Otorhinolaryngology, Dokuz Eylul University School of Medicine, Izmir, Turkey*
[2]*Department of Pathology, Dokuz Eylul University School of Medicine, Izmir, Turkey*

Correspondence should be addressed to Mustafa Aslıer; mustafa.aslier@gmail.com

Academic Editor: Emilio Mevio

Ameloblastic fibroodontoma (AFO) is a rare entity of mixed odontogenic tumors and frequently arises from posterior portion of the maxilla or mandible in first two decades of life. Herein, a 35-year-old woman with a noncontributory medical history who presented with a progressive left maxillary toothache, left maxillary first molar tooth mobility, and swelling in the left maxillary molar area for the last 2 months was reported. Radiologically, a tumor that originated from periapical area of the second mature molar teeth of maxilla was seen and additively unerupted tooth was not detected. The histopathologic examination revealed AFO. The patient is disease-free for five years after treated with limited segmental alveolectomy combining with Caldwell-Luc procedure.

1. Introduction

Ameloblastic fibroodontoma (AFO) is an uncommon mixed odontogenic tumor of odontogenic epithelium and mesenchyme origin [1, 2]. According to the latest World Health Organization (WHO) classification, AFO is a lesion resembling ameloblastic fibroma which also shows inductive alterations composed of both enamel and dentin [3]. Typical features of AFO show a slow growth swelling from posterior portion of the maxilla or mandible generally in the first and rarely in the second decades of life. It is generally associated with unerupted teeth of the affected area. Radiological appearance shows a well-defined radiolucent border with radiopaque foci containing density similar to that of dental hard tissues [4, 5]. Conservative enucleation or curettage is enough for adequate treatment of AFO and radical surgical procedures such as segmental resection or hemimandibulectomy are infrequently needed [5, 6]. Here in, a case of AFO arising from the posterior portion of the maxilla of a middle-aged female was presented.

2. Case Report

A 35-year-old female presented with a 2-month history of progressive left maxillary toothache, left maxillary first molar tooth mobility, and swelling in the left maxillary molar area. There was no history of chronic nasal problems or odontogenic surgery. Swelling on the left side of the maxillary alveolar arch was revealed by intraoral inspection. The rest of the ENT examination was unremarkable. Preoperative oral panoramic radiograph (OPR) and computer tomography imaging (CTI) of the paranasal sinus revealed a radiolucent expansive lesion containing multiple radiopaque foci on the left side maxillary sinus (Figure 1). An incisional biopsy was performed through canine fossae approach. The histopathological examination revealed fibroblastic connective tissue matrix containing ameloblastic and odontogenic epithelial component was shown on the histopathological examination. After completion of diagnostic investigation, curative resection was approved. Under general anaesthesia with transnasal intubation, five-centimetre mucosal incision was made in the

(a)

(b)

(c)

(d)

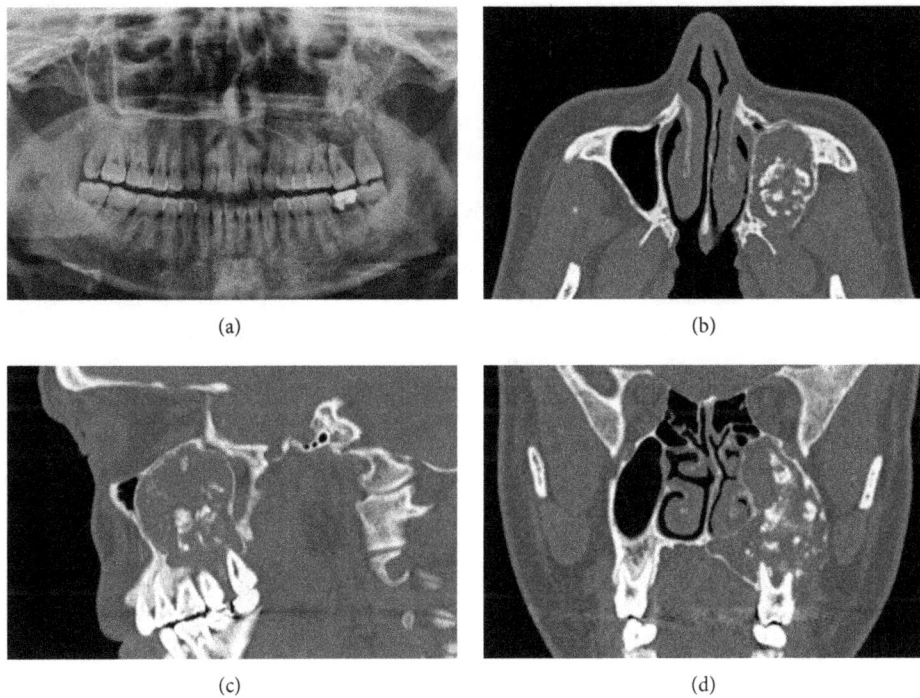

FIGURE 1: (a) Preoperative OPR showing a radiopaque mass with a radiolucent border in the left upper jaw. (b, c, d) Preoperative CTI showing a radiolucent expansive lesion containing multiple radiopaque foci on the left side maxillary sinus.

gingivolabial sulcus, extending from the canine tooth to the first molar tooth. Soft tissue and periosteum were elevated and four-centimetre diameter fenestration was made on the anterior wall of the maxillary sinus. Thereafter, tumor was dissected quite easily from the anterior, medial, and superior walls of the sinus. Posterior dissection was hardly performed because of bleeding. Next, all of the three molar teeth of maxilla were extracted and tumor resection was completed combining with limited segmental alveolectomy. Tumor originated from the second molar teeth of maxilla and progressed into maxillary sinus was detected when the specimen was examined. At the final stage, mucosal incisions were then closed using absorbable sutures. Postoperative healing was uneventful. Definitive pathology report was similar to the previously examined and tumor was diagnosed as AFO (Figure 2). The patient remains clinical and radiological disease-free up till a five-year follow-up period. Postoperative magnetic resonance imaging (MRI) revealed mucosal thickening in the maxillary without any evidence of tumor recurrence (Figure 3).

3. Discussion

Ameloblastic fibroodontoma is a rare entity of mixed odontogenic tumors and frequently arises from posterior portion of the maxilla or mandible in first two decades of life [1, 7, 8]. But as it is seen in our case, it may be presented at middle age period. Histologically, the WHO classification defines AFO as "a lesion similar to ameloblastic fibroma (AF), but also showing inductive changes that lead to formation of both dentin

and enamel" [3]. Most investigators suggested that the age of the patient was the essential distinction between AF and AFO [1]. However, pathological examination combining immunohistochemical staining shows important evidences of AFO [2, 7]. In the present study, histopathologically ameloblastic and odontoid ectomesenchymal tissues including dentin-like calcified structures in fibroid stroma were seen and according to these findings the final diagnosis was AFO in a 35-year-old female.

Asymptomatic slow growth swelling and delayed tooth eruptions are the most common symptoms of AFO especially at early ages [2, 8, 9]. The tumor is predominantly related unerupted tooth but at times it may arise from a supernumerary or deciduous tooth [10]. The patient presented in this report had no unerupted tooth. According to this feature AFO may occur after the tooth eruption process completed. Therefore, tooth problems like toothache and tooth mobility may also be included to the signs and symptoms of AFO at advanced ages.

Radiological findings of the AFO were described in the previous studies. Dental like radiopaque foci surrounding well-defined radiolucent borders are the most detectable feature of AFO in radiological examinations [4, 5]. Radiological findings of the AFO were similar in the present patient. Preoperative oral panoramic radiograph and CTI showed radiopaque foci containing multiple dental like densities surrounding radiolucent area and sclerotic border which were suggesting AFO (Figure 1).

The curative treatment of AFO involves enucleation or curettage. These approaches are frequently sufficient if the

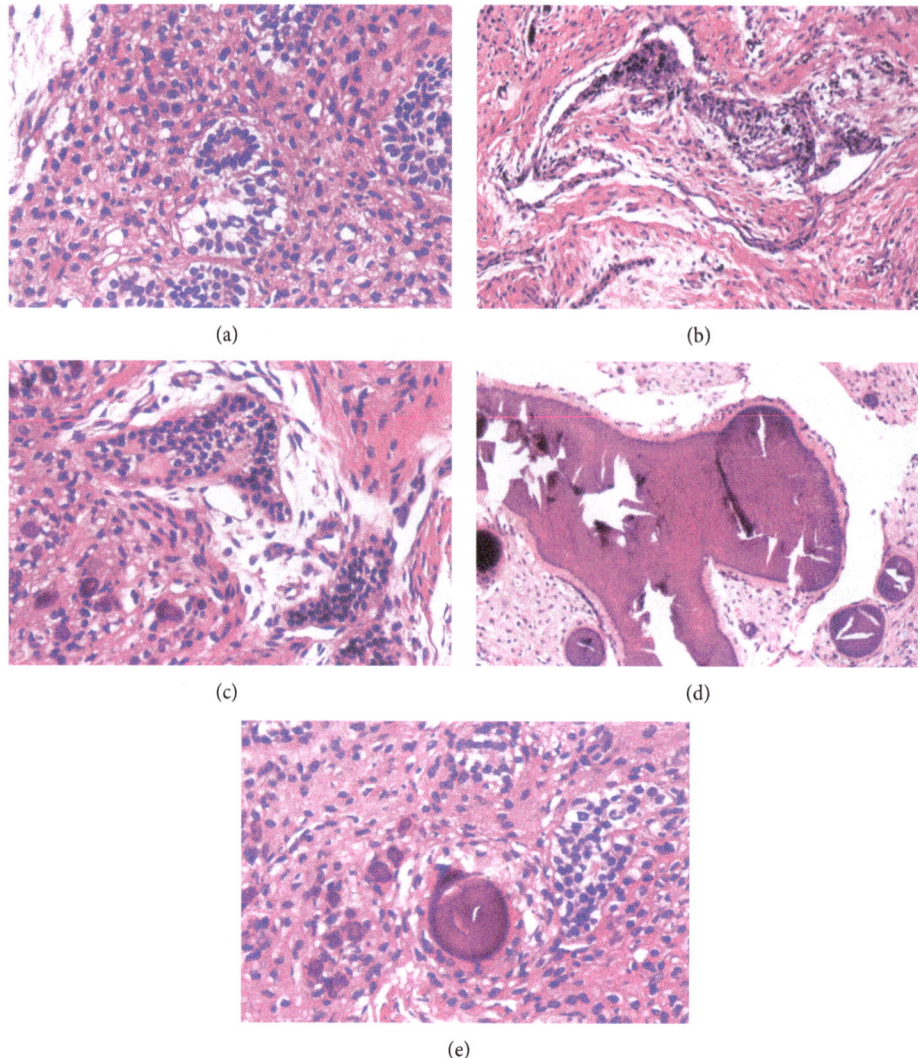

FIGURE 2: (a) Ameloblastic epithelium in the fibroblastic stroma (H&E ×20). (b) Odontogenic epithelium forming premature tooth like pattern (H&E ×10). (c) Odontogenic epithelium forming material consistent with dentine (H&E ×10). (d) Calcific zones surrounded with dentine (H&E ×10). (e) Focal zones consistent with cementifying changes (H&E ×20).

lesion is associated with unerupted teeth and the affected area is limited. In a small group of patients who have giant, extensive, and destructive disease, partial maxillectomy or segmental mandibulectomy may be needed [1, 2]. But even AFO is believed to have low potential for recurrence; according to Boxberger, almost all cases of recurrences were related to incomplete removal of the lesion at the initial surgery [11]. In this report, lesion was originated from the periapical area of the left maxillary second molar tooth and grown into the maxillary sinus. Anterior, superior, and medial walls of the sinus were preserved. By the reasons of these features, partial maxillectomy was found super abound and unnecessary. Limited segmental alveolectomy combining with Caldwell-Luc procedure was done and the patient was disease-free for five years. We suggest combination of trans-canine-fossa approach with segmental alveolectomy as an uncomplicated, safe, and feasible approach for AFO extending to the maxillary sinus.

In conclusion, AFO may also occur at advanced ages with odontogenic symptoms and the extension of lesion manages the curative treatment alternatives.

Consent

Patient consent had been obtained as a written document.

Disclosure

The current address of Mustafa Aslıer, due to mandatory state work, is Silopi Devlet Hastanesi, Yenişehir Mah. 8 Cadde., No. 73, Silopi, Şırnak, Turkey.

Competing Interests

None of the authors have any conflict of interests that could inappropriately influence (bias) the work.

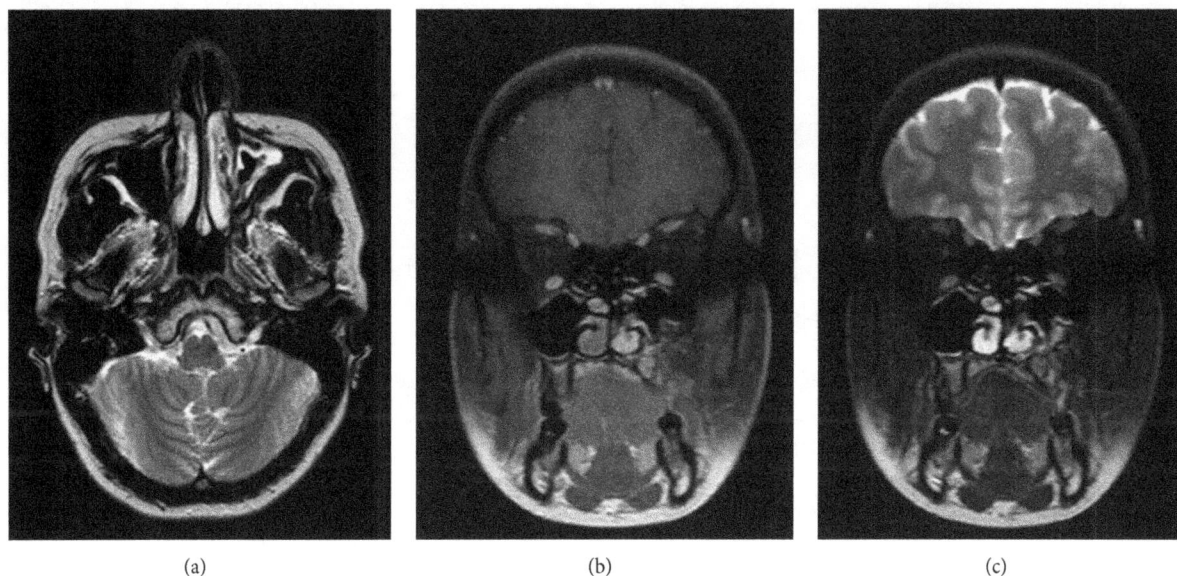

(a)　　　　　　　　(b)　　　　　　　　(c)

FIGURE 3: (a, b, c) Respectively, axial T2, coronal T1, and coronal T2 postoperative MRI showing mucosal thickening in the maxillary without any evidence of tumor recurrence.

Authors' Contributions

The authors confirmed that they all have viewed and agreed to the submission.

References

[1] G. De Riu, S. M. Meloni, M. Contini, and A. Tullio, "Ameloblastic fibro-odontoma. Case report and review of the literature," *Journal of Cranio-Maxillofacial Surgery*, vol. 38, no. 2, pp. 141–144, 2010.

[2] H. A. R. Pontes, F. S. C. Pontes, A. G. Lameira et al., "Report of four cases of Ameloblastic fibro-odontoma in mandible and discussion of the literature about the treatment," *Journal of Cranio-Maxillo-Facial Surgery*, vol. 40, no. 2, pp. e59–e63, 2012.

[3] Y. Takeda and C. E. Tomich, "Ameloblastic fibro-odontoma," in *World Health Organization Classification of Tumours Pathology and Genetics. Head and Neck Tumors*, L. Barnes, J. W. Eveson, P. Reichart, and D. Sidransky, Eds., p. 309, IARC Press, Lyon, France, 2005.

[4] D. Dolanmaz, A. A. Pampu, A. Kalayci, O. A. Etöz, and S. Atici, "An unusual size of ameloblastic fibro-odontoma," *Dentomaxillofacial Radiology*, vol. 37, no. 3, pp. 179–182, 2008.

[5] E. M. G. Piette, H. Tideman, and P. C. Wu, "Massive maxillary ameloblastic fibro-odontoma: case report with surgical management," *Journal of Oral and Maxillofacial Surgery*, vol. 48, no. 5, pp. 526–530, 1990.

[6] Y.-P. Hu, B. Liu, T. Su, W.-F. Zhang, and Y.-F. Zhao, "A huge ameloblastic fibro-odontoma of the maxilla," *Oral Oncology Extra*, vol. 42, no. 4, pp. 160–162, 2006.

[7] H. P. Philipsen, P. A. Reichart, and F. Praetorius, "Mixed odontogenic tumours and odontomas. Considerations on interrelationship. Review of the literature and presentation of 134 new cases of odontomas," *European Journal of Cancer Part B: Oral Oncology*, vol. 33, no. 2, pp. 86–99, 1997.

[8] A. Buchner, P. W. Merrell, and W. M. Carpenter, "Relative frequency of central odontogenic tumors: a study of 1,088 cases from Northern California and comparison to studies from other parts of the world," *Journal of Oral and Maxillofacial Surgery*, vol. 64, no. 9, pp. 1343–1352, 2006.

[9] P. J. Slootweg, "An analysis of the interrelationship of the mixed odontogenic tumors—ameloblastic fibroma, ameloblastic fibroodontoma, and the odontomas," *Oral Surgery, Oral Medicine, Oral Pathology*, vol. 51, no. 3, pp. 266–276, 1981.

[10] M. Ghandehari-Motlagh, Z. Khosravi, G. Meighani, and Y. Baradaran-Nakhjavani, "Ameloblastic fibro-odontoma in a 4-year-old boy," *Iranian Journal of Pediatrics*, vol. 26, no. 2, p. 3124, 2016.

[11] N. R. Boxberger, R. B. Brannon, and C. B. Fowler, "Ameloblastic fibro-odontoma: a clinicopathologic study of 12 cases," *Journal of Clinical Pediatric Dentistry*, vol. 35, no. 4, pp. 397–404, 2011.

37

Sudden Sensorineural Hearing Loss in the Only Hearing Ear: Large Vestibular Aqueduct Syndrome

Kemal Koray Bal, Onur Ismi, Helen Bucioglu, Yusuf Vayısoğlu, and Kemal Gorur

Department of Otorhinolaryngology, Faculty of Medicine, University of Mersin, Mersin, Turkey

Correspondence should be addressed to Onur Ismi; dronurismi@gmail.com

Academic Editor: Guangwei Zhou

Sudden hearing loss in the only hearing ear cases are rarely published in the English literature; most of the cases are idiopathic. It is an otologic emergency needing urgent treatment. Delayed diagnosis can interfere with patient's social life with interrupting the verbal communication. In this case report we presented a 33-year-old female patient having sudden sensorineural hearing loss in the only hearing ear diagnosed as bilateral large vestibular aqueduct syndrome.

1. Introduction

Sudden sensorineural hearing loss (SSHL) can be described as at least 30 dB sensorineural hearing loss (SNHL) in at least three consecutive frequencies within a three-day period [1]. It is an important otolaryngological emergency needing thorough investigation and urgent treatment. SHL occurring in the only hearing ear is a more serious problem, since it increases patient's morbidity and the sequel in the only hearing ear can affect the patient's social life dramatically with interrupting the verbal communication. SSHL in the only hearing ear cases are rarely published in the English literature [2–6] and most of these cases are idiopathic. In this case report we presented a large vestibular aqueduct syndrome (LVAS) patient admitting with a sudden hearing loss in the only hearing ear.

2. Case Report

A 33-year-old woman was admitted with complaints of sudden hearing loss in the right ear for one day. She had no vertigo or dizziness complaint. On her medical history, she had total hearing loss in the left ear from the childhood. She had no additional illnesses. Otoscopic examination was normal. In the pure tone audiometry she had 52 dB sensorineural hearing loss in the right ear and a profound sensorineural hearing loss in the left ear (Figure 1). She had no history of triggering factors such as head trauma. Vestibular tests were in normal limits. Head impulse and head shaking tests revealed no pathological nystagmus. Romberg test was normal. The patient was hospitalized, and complete blood cell count, serum biochemistry, viral and immunological markers, and contrast enhanced temporal magnetic resonance imaging (MRI) were performed. The only positive sign was bilateral LVAS on MRI (Figure 2). 1 mg/kg/day of oral methylprednisolone was started. Pendred syndrome gene mutation analysis was planned, but price of the genetic assessment was much more than the patient could pay. Thyroid ultrasound imaging and thyroid function tests were in normal limits. Oral steroid treatment had no benefit on hearing on the second day of the follow-up. 8 mg intratympanic dexamethasone application with hyperbaric oxygen treatment for two weeks with a 10 kPa/minute pressure was added to treatment protocol. At the end of the second week hearing loss decreased to 40 dB. Hearing aid was recommended to patient with a successful fitting. On the sixth-month follow-up she had still 40 dB hearing loss. She is under follow-up in our institution.

3. Discussion

The vestibular aqueduct (VA) is a bony canal extending from medial wall of the vestibule to the posterior fossa dura at the level of anterior part of the sigmoid sinus. Ductus

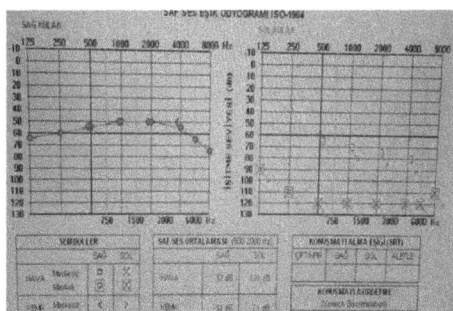

FIGURE 1: Pure tone audiogram of the patient at first admission was presented.

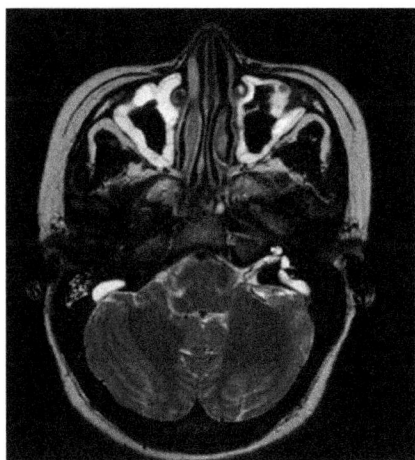

FIGURE 2: Magnetic resonance imaging of the inner ear showing the bilateral large vestibular aqueduct was demonstrated.

endolymphaticus is the main structure that courses in the VA. Normal VA diameter is reported to be between 0.4 and 1 mm, and large VA is mostly accepted to be a VA greater than 1.5 mm at its anteroposterior diameter or greater than 2.0 mm as measured at the midway the common crus and external aperture [7]. LVAS is a clinical entity in which large VA accompanies audiovestibular symptoms such as hearing loss and vestibulopathy [7]. It is a congenital disorder and affects mostly children [8]. The hearing loss is mild at the few years of life, but it worsens with an average of 4 dB/year causing a profound hearing loss in the adulthood [9]. The characteristic hearing loss is a progressive or fluctuating type sensorineural hearing loss; acute deteriorations can be seen especially with mild head trauma [6, 9]. The higher pressure of cerebrospinal fluid transmission to the inner ear by enlarged VA may be the main reason of the sensorineural hearing loss [6]. Repeated increase in intracochlear pressure causes irreversible injury to hair cells and at the end profound hearing loss occurs [8]. Endolymphatic sac obliteration has been advised to decrease the pressure load in case of progressive sensorineural hearing loss [6] but shown to have no benefit for hearing preservation [9]. Cochlear implantation is the main surgical option for

cases with profound hearing loss [9]. Spontaneous perilymphatic fistula can be seen; exploratory tympanotomy may also be considered [8]. For acute deterioration of hearing, steroids should be thought in treatment protocol [6]; hyperbaric oxygen therapy has promising results for sudden exhaustion of hearing thresholds [6, 9]. Hearing aids are also another nonsurgical treatment option [9]. Our case showed that combination of intratympanic steroid with hyperbaric oxygen may be a suitable treatment option for LVAS cases that are refractory to oral steroid treatment.

Sudden hearing loss in the only hearing ear is an audiological emergency interrupting the patient's verbal communication as well as psychological and social health status [2]. Due to scarcity of case reports and series, underlying pathogenesis is not fully understood; most of the patients are idiopathic [2–5, 10]. Berrettini et al. [2] proposed four different hypotheses including genetic and microscopic labyrinthine malformations and viral and autoimmune causes regarding the pathogenesis. In the series of Lee et al. [5] with 25 patients, Pyykkö et al. [4] with 10 patients, and Stahl and Cohen [3] with 9 patients, none of the patients had LVAS in the sudden hearing loss ear. Berrettini et al. [2] presented one case of bilateral LVAS in their 34 patients with sensorineural hearing loss in the only hearing ear. The hearing loss was a fluctuating type rather than a sudden hearing loss. Nakashima et al. [6] presented a bilateral LVAS causing SSHL in the only hearing ear similar to our case treated with hyperbaric oxygen. Different from our patient, the patient presented by Nakashima et al. [6] was a child. As seen, our case is unique showing an adult LVAS causing SSHL in the only hearing ear. There is no universally accepted treatment algorithm for SSHL in the only hearing ear. Stahl and Cohen [3] and and Lee et al. [5] argue that SSHL in the only hearing ear can be treated as the same way with SSHL with normal hearing contralateral ear. Pyykkö et al. [4] advised immunosuppressive treatment with azathioprine and corticosteroid combination for these cases. Berrettini et al. [2] recommended osmotic diuretics when delayed endolymphatic hydrops in the contralateral ear was suspected. Since our patient had no vestibular complaints, delayed endolymphatic hydrops in the contralateral ear was not thought and diuretic treatment was not applied. For the treatment of SSHL, steroids, whether systemic or intratympanic, remain the most widely used treatment options [11], although the meta-analysis of randomized controlled trials does not support the beneficial effect over placebo [12]. Antivirals are no sooner advised due to lack of supporting evidence [1]. Intratympanic steroids have beneficial effect when used as a salvage treatment of oral steroids [11]. Hyperbaric oxygen treatment is favorable when used early in the treatment protocol [1]. Our case showed that combination of intratympanic steroids with hyperbaric oxygen can be used as a salvage treatment for oral steroid treatment regimen in the SSHL.

In conclusion, for cases with sudden hearing loss in the only hearing ear, LVAS must also be considered in differential diagnosis. Early addition of intratympanic steroid and hyperbaric oxygen treatment modalities to oral steroids may have supportive effect on hearing, rescuing the patient from cochlear implantation surgery.

Competing Interests

The authors declare that they have no competing interests.

References

[1] A. M. Metrailer and S. C. Babu, "Management of sudden sensorineural hearing loss," *Current Opinion in Otolaryngology & Head and Neck Surgery*, vol. 24, no. 5, pp. 403–406, 2016.

[2] S. Berrettini, A. De Vito, L. Bruschini et al., "Idioptahic sensorineural hearing loss in the only hearing ear," *Acta Otorhinolaryngologica Italica*, vol. 36, pp. 119–126, 2016.

[3] N. Stahl and D. Cohen, "Idiopathic sudden sensorineural hearing loss in the only hearing ear: patient characteristics and hearing outcome," *Archives of Otolaryngology—Head and Neck Surgery*, vol. 132, no. 2, pp. 193–195, 2006.

[4] I. Pyykkö, H. Ishizaki, and M. Peltomaa, "Azathioprine with cortisone in treatment of hearing loss in only hearing ear," *Acta Oto-Laryngologica. Supplementum*, vol. 529, pp. 83–85, 1997.

[5] S. S. Lee, H. H. Cho, C. H. Jang, and Y. B. Cho, "Fate of sudden deafness occurring in the only hearing ear: outcomes and timing to consider cochlear implantation," *Journal of Korean Medical Science*, vol. 25, no. 2, pp. 283–286, 2010.

[6] T. Nakashima, H. Ueda, A. Furuhashi et al., "Large vestibular aqueduct syndrome treated by hyperbaric oxygen," *International Journal of Pediatric Otorhinolaryngology*, vol. 51, no. 3, pp. 207–210, 1999.

[7] G. M. Pyle, "Embryological development and large vestibular aqueduct syndrome," *The Laryngoscope*, vol. 110, no. 11, pp. 1837–1842, 2000.

[8] I. H. Can, H. Göçmen, A. Kurt, and E. Samim, "Sudden hearing loss due to large vestibular aqueduct syndrome in a child: should exploratory tympanotomy be performed?" *International Journal of Pediatric Otorhinolaryngology*, vol. 68, no. 6, pp. 841–844, 2004.

[9] H. Shilton, M. Hodgson, and G. Burgess, "Hyperbaric oxygen therapy for sudden sensorineural hearing loss in large vestibular aqueduct syndrome," *The Journal of Laryngology & Otology*, vol. 128, supplement 1, pp. S50–S54, 2014.

[10] D. B. Hawkins, "Hearing rehabilitation in a patient with sudden sensorineural hearing loss in the only hearing ear," *Journal of the American Academy of Audiology*, vol. 19, no. 3, pp. 267–274, 2008.

[11] B. P. O'Connell, J. B. Hunter, and D. S. Haynes, "Current concepts in the management of idiopathic sudden sensorineural hearing loss," *Current Opinion in Otolaryngology & Head and Neck Surgery*, vol. 24, no. 5, pp. 413–419, 2016.

[12] R. A. Crane, M. Camilon, S. Nguyen, and T. A. Meyer, "Steroids for treatment of sudden sensorineural hearing loss: a meta-analysis of randomized controlled trials," *The Laryngoscope*, vol. 125, no. 1, pp. 209–217, 2015.

38

Myoepithelioma of the Nasal Septum: A Rare Case of Extrasalivary Gland Involvement

Gustavo Barreto da Cunha, Tatiane Costa Camurugy,
Thiago Cavalcante Ribeiro, Nara Nunes Barbosa Costa, Amanda Canário Andrade Azevedo,
Eriko Soares de Azevedo Vinhaes, and Nilvano Alves de Andrade

Santa Casa de Misericórdia da Bahia, Hospital Santa Izabel, Salvador, BA, Brazil

Correspondence should be addressed to Gustavo Barreto da Cunha; gbarretocunha@hotmail.com

Academic Editor: Emilio Mevio

Introduction. The myoepithelioma is a rare benign tumor, most frequently found in the salivary glands. The extrasalivary gland involvement is even rarer and few cases involving the nasal cavity have been reported in the literature. *Case Report.* MES, a 54-year-old woman, complaining of progressive nasal obstruction and mild epistaxis through the right nostril which had developed 1 year previously. Computed tomography scan showed tumor with heterogeneous contrast enhancement occupying the right nasal cavity, moving contralaterally in the nasal septum. Excisional biopsy was performed through endoscopic surgery of the mass that was inserted at the nasal septum. Pathological and immunohistochemical exams concluded myoepithelioma. *Discussion.* The main symptoms of nasal myoepitheliomas are nasal obstruction and epistaxis. Immunohistochemistry is necessary to confirm the diagnosis, typically positive for cytokeratin and S-100, calponin, smooth muscle actin, myosin, vimentin, glial fibrillary acidic protein (GFAP), and carcinoembryonic antigen. The main marker for myoepithelioma is the S-100 protein. In our case, it was positive for cytokeratin, S-100, calponin, actin smooth muscle, and GFAP. In all cases reported in the literature surgical treatment was performed and the recurrence was associated with incomplete tumor resection. *Final Comments.* The myoepithelioma is a rare differential diagnosis of nasal tumors and its treatment is the total lesion excision.

1. Introduction

Myoepithelioma is a rare benign tumor, most frequently found in the salivary glands, representing, however, only 1% of all tumors of these glands. In the major salivary glands there is a predilection for the parotid and in the minor salivary glands for the palate and oral cavity [1, 2]. The extrasalivary involvement is even rarer and just few cases involving the nasal cavity have been reported in the literature. This is a case of myoepithelioma of the nasal septum and the discussion about its diagnosis and treatment.

2. Case Report

MES, a 54-year-old woman, presented at our hospital complaining of progressive nasal obstruction and mild epistaxis through the right nostril which had developed 1 year previously. She denied smoking and had no known toxic exposure or family history of neoplasms. Nasofibroscopy revealed irregular vascular lesion which occupied the right nasal cavity almost completely. Computed tomography (CT) scan showed heterogeneous contrast enhancement by the tumor, which displaced contralaterally the nasal septum (Figure 1). Complete endoscopic resection of the lesion that had originated from the nasal septum was performed. Ipsilateral septal mucosa and septal cartilage as surgical margin were removed, opting for the preservation of the contralateral mucosa, which was found apparently free of disease (Figure 2).

The material that consisted of several brown tissue fragments measuring together $6,0 \times 3,0 \times 1,0$ cm was sent for pathological examination, which showed morphological features compatible with myoepithelioma, despite the

(a)

(b)

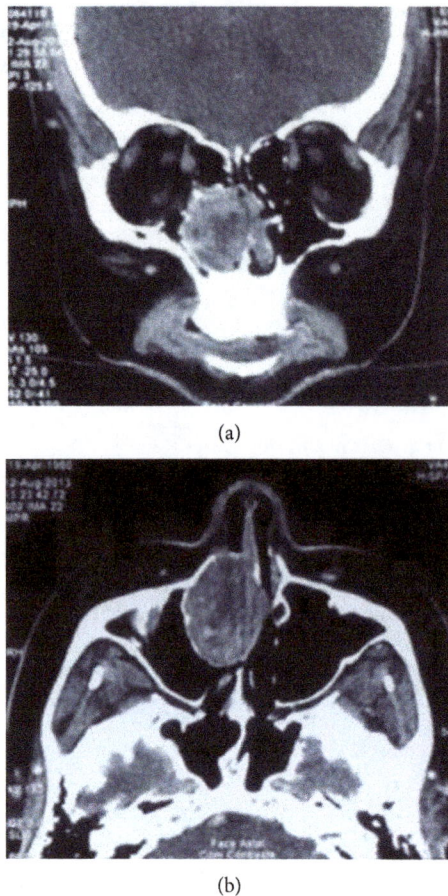

FIGURE 1: Computed tomography. Coronal (a) and axial (b) planes demonstrate heterogeneous contrast enhancement by the tumor.

(a)

(b)

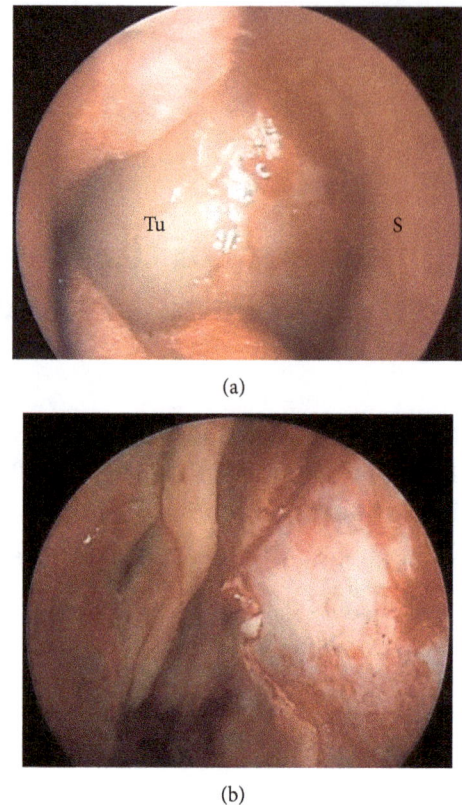

FIGURE 2: Endoscopic appearance. Preoperative (a) and immediately after resection (b). Tu = tumor. S = nasal septum.

focal presence of chondroid matrix and occasional ductal structures. Immunohistochemistry presented positivity for glial fibrillary acidic protein (GFAP), smooth muscle actin, cytokeratin (AE1AE3 and MNF116), calponin, P63, S100, and CD99. The septal margin was found to be affected by the tumor but was chosen for follow-up, and after two years of follow-up there was no evidence of tumor recurrence or metastasis.

3. Discussion

Nasal cavity and paranasal sinus tumors are very infrequent, accounting for less than 1% of all head and neck tumors [3]. Nasal mucosa contains mucous glands, minor salivary glands, melanocytes, and olfactory neuroepithelial cells [4]. Myoepithelioma is a benign slow-growing tumor of the salivary glands described by Sheldom in 1943 [5]. The main symptoms of nasal myoepitheliomas are nasal obstruction, due to tumor growth, and epistaxis [6–8], symptoms presented by the patient reported in this paper. The CT does not have a well-defined standard, but it is an important test for therapeutic planning. No relationship was found between sex, age, and injury presented.

Myoepithelioma is composed of myoepithelial cells and may have pattern of solid growth, myxoid or reticular. The cell types found are fusiform, plasmacytoid, epithelioid, and clear cells. The pattern of growth and cell type does not change the prognosis of the disease [9–12]. This is a tumor classically defined as not having a ductal differentiation, but several authors have adopted a less rigid definition, including the presence of a small number of ducts (presence in less than 5% of the examined field) as well as in the present case (Figure 3) and also in other reported cases of myoepitheliomas of the nasal cavity [6–8, 13]. The main differential diagnosis is the pleomorphic adenoma, but it presents myoepithelial cells in varied proportions and ductal formations are numerous [9, 10, 12].

Immunohistochemistry is necessary to confirm the diagnosis, typically positive for cytokeratin, S-100, calponin, smooth muscle actin, myosin, vimentin, glial fibrillary acidic protein (GFAP), and carcinoembryonic antigen [14, 15]. The main marker for myoepithelioma is the S-100 protein and the diagnosis will hardly be made if negative [12]. The leiomyomas and squamous cell cancers are negative for S-100 protein. The schwannomas are positive but have their own histological features [1]. In our case, it was positive for cytokeratin, S-100, calponin, smooth muscle actin, and GFAP.

In all cases reported the surgical treatment was performed and the recurrence has been associated with incomplete resection of tumor, which proves the aggressive biological behavior of this tumor [16, 17]. Histologically this tumor is well circumscribed, so complete excision is possible [18]. This

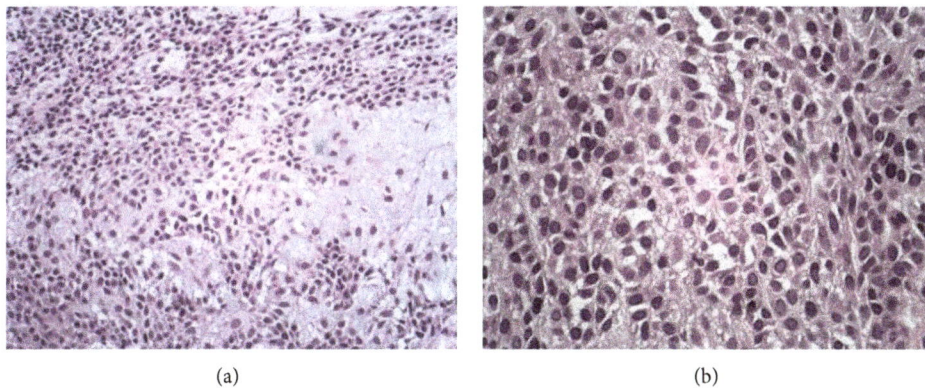

FIGURE 3: Microscopic view, H and E stain, 200x (a) and ×400 (b). Typical plasmacytoid myoepithelial cells among myxoid stroma.

neoplasm is not radio- or chemosensitive and it needs a long-term follow-up since recurrence varied from 35% to 50% and metastasis rates from 8.1% to 25% in different reports [19]. This case had neither recurrence nor metastasis two years after surgery.

There are very few cases of myoepithelioma involving the nasal cavity reported in the literature. However in the last few years the publications of its extrasalivary gland involvement increased substantially, which makes the authors question if it is an underdiagnosed disease. The advances in pathology and immunohistochemistry knowledge and techniques may help us to diagnose it more and more commonly in the future. Therefore, although it is rare, we have to consider it as a differential diagnosis of nasal tumors.

Competing Interests

The authors declared no conflict of interests with respect to the authorship and/or publication of this article.

References

[1] C. T-Ping, G. U. Pizarro, S. Pignatari, and L. L. Weckx, "Mioepitelioma de glândula salivar menor em base de língua: relato de caso," *Revista Brasileira de Otorrinolaringologia*, vol. 70, no. 5, pp. 701–704, 2004.

[2] A. Piattelli, M. Fioroni, and C. Rubini, "Myoepithelioma of the gingiva. Report of a case," *Journal of Periodontology*, vol. 70, no. 6, pp. 683–687, 1999.

[3] B. Schick and J. Dlugaiczyk, "Benign tumors of the nasal cavity and paranasal sinuses," in *Rhinology and Facial Plastic Surgery*, F. J. Stucker, C. Souza, G. S. Kenyon, T. S. Lian, W. Draf, and B. Schick, Eds., pp. 377–383, Springer, Berlin, Germany, 2009.

[4] R. J. Wong and D. H. Kraus, "Cancer of the nasal cavity and paranasal sinuses," in *Cancer of the Head and Neck*, J. P. Shah and B. C. Decker, Eds., pp. 204–224, 2001.

[5] F. P. García, M. J. Carcasés, S. Martínez, M. C. Beiva, R. Durán, and J. R. Malluguiza, "Mioepitelioma en glándulas salivares," *Acta Otorrinolaringológica Española*, vol. 52, no. 3, pp. 269–272, 2001.

[6] T. Fujikura and K. Okubo, "Nasal myoepithelioma removed through endonasal endoscopic surgery: a case report," *Journal of Nippon Medical School*, vol. 77, no. 5, pp. 273–276, 2010.

[7] L. R. Begin, L. Rochon, and S. Frenkiel, "Spindle cell myoepithelioma of the nasal cavity," *American Journal of Surgical Pathology*, vol. 15, no. 2, pp. 184–190, 1991.

[8] S. S. Lateef, M. Castillo, S. K. Mukherji, and L. L. Cooper, "Myoepithelioma of the nasal piriform aperture: CT findings," *American Journal of Roentgenology*, vol. 173, no. 5, pp. 1413–1414, 1999.

[9] L. Barnes, B. N. Appel, H. Perez, and A. Moneim El–Attar, "Myoepitheliomas of the head and neck: case report and review," *Journal of Surgical Oncology*, vol. 28, no. 1, pp. 21–28, 1985.

[10] M. Michal, A. Skálová, R. H. W. Simpson, V. Rychterová, and I. Leivo, "Clear cell malignant myoepithelioma of the salivary glands," *Histopathology*, vol. 28, no. 4, pp. 309–315, 1996.

[11] T. Nagao, I. Sugano, Y. Ishida et al., "Salivary gland malignant myoepithelioma: a clinicopathologic and immunohistochemical study of ten cases," *Cancer*, vol. 83, no. 7, pp. 1292–1299, 1998.

[12] J. J. Sciubba and R. B. Brannon, "Myoepithelioma of salivary glands: report of 23 cases," *Cancer*, vol. 49, no. 3, pp. 562–572, 1982.

[13] A. Cardesa and L. Alos, "Myoepithelioma," in *World Health Organization Classification of Tumours. Pathology and Genetics, Head and Neck Tumours*, L. Barnes, J. W. Eveson, P. Reichart, and D. Sidransky, Eds., pp. 259–260, IARC Press, Lyon, France, 2005.

[14] S. I. Sayed, R. A. Kazi, M. V. Jagade, R. S. Palav, V. V. Shinde, and P. V. Pawar, "A rare myoepithelioma of the sinonasal cavity: case report," *Cases Journal*, vol. 1, no. 1, article 29, 2008.

[15] F. C. Zelaya, D. Q. Rivera, J. L. TapiaVazquez, C. Paez Valencia, and L. A. GaitanCepeda, "Plasmacytoid myoepithelioma of the palate. Report of one case and review of the literature," *Medicina Oral, Patología Oral y Cirugía Bucal*, vol. 12, no. 8, pp. E552–E555, 2007.

[16] C. Gore, N. Panicker, S. Chandanwale, and B. Singh, "Myoepithelioma of minor salivary glands—a diagnostic challenge: report of three cases with varied histomorphology," *Journal of Oral and Maxillofacial Pathology*, vol. 17, no. 2, pp. 257–260, 2013.

[17] M. Policarpo, V. Longoni, P. Garofalo, P. Spina, and F. Pia, "Voluminous myoepithelioma of the minor salivary glands involving the base of the tongue," *Case Reports in Otolaryngology*, vol. 2016, Article ID 3785979, 5 pages, 2016.

[18] A. Ghosh, S. Saha, V. P. Saha, A. Sadhu, and S. Chattopadhyay, "Infratemporal fossa myoepithelial carcinoma—a rare case

report," *Oral and Maxillofacial Surgery*, vol. 13, no. 1, pp. 59–62, 2009.

[19] A. Ghosh, S. Saha, and S. Pal, "Myoepithelial neoplasm of nasal cavity: an uncommon tumor presenting with an unusual clinical presentation," *Journal of Ear, Nose, and Throat*, vol. 24, no. 1, pp. 42–45, 2014.

39

Leiomyosarcoma Ex Pleomorphic Adenoma of the Parotid Gland: A Case Report and Literature Review

Michael Coulter,[1] Jingxuan Liu,[2] and Mark Marzouk[3]

[1]*Health Science Center, Stony Brook University School of Medicine, Stony Brook, NY 11794, USA*
[2]*Department of Pathology, Stony Brook University Hospital, 101 Nicolls Road, Stony Brook, NY 11794, USA*
[3]*Department of Otolaryngology, Upstate University Hospital, 750 E. Adams, Syracuse, NY 13210, USA*

Correspondence should be addressed to Michael Coulter; michael.coulter@stonybrookmedicine.edu

Academic Editor: Abrão Rapoport

There is only one previously reported incident in the English literature of sarcoma ex pleomorphic adenoma of the parotid and there are only 8 cases of primary parotid leiomyosarcoma. In our case, a 79-year-old female patient presented to our care with left preauricular pain, swelling, and facial weakness. After CT imaging, she underwent left total parotidectomy. A spindle cell lesion was identified intraoperatively and the facial nerve was sacrificed. Subsequent analysis of the lesion yielded a diagnosis of leiomyosarcoma ex pleomorphic adenoma. After 30 fractions of radiation therapy, scans were negative for tumor. However, 18 months after first experiencing symptoms, she was found to have metastases to the brainstem and lung. When diagnosing sarcoma ex pleomorphic adenoma of the parotid gland, it is important to perform thorough immunohistochemical staining and exclude a previous history of sarcoma or other sources of metastases. Complete resection is critical due to the tumor's local aggressiveness and metastatic potential. Although these tumors are not very responsive to chemotherapy or radiation, adjuvant treatment is commonly used when margins are unclear.

1. Introduction

Of all major salivary gland neoplasms, only 0.3 to 1.5% are diagnosed as sarcomas [1, 2]. Of the salivary gland sarcomas, malignant schwannoma and fibrosarcoma are the most common [2]. A rare occurrence is a primary leiomyosarcoma of the parotid gland, as only 8 cases [2–9] have been reported in the English literature, as detailed in Table 1. From this data, there seems to be no sex or age predilection; 4 were female and 4 were male with an average age of 40 ± standard deviation of 20.8 years. Leiomyosarcomas of the head and neck reportedly uncommonly metastasize to cervical lymph nodes and have a low potential for distant metastasis [4, 6]. However, 4 of the 8 primary parotid lesions reported metastases: 2 to lymph nodes, 1 to the scalp and lymph nodes, and 1 to the lungs [4, 6, 7, 9]. In order to diagnose a primary leiomyosarcoma of the parotid gland, Luna et al. proposed four basic criteria: (a) negative history of sarcoma at other sites must be excluded; (b) metastasis from the upper aerodigestive tract must be ruled out; (c) the macroscopic and histologic appearance must be consistent with an origin within the gland, instead of invasion by nearby soft tissue; (d) carcinosarcoma must be excluded by histologic analysis of multiple sections [1].

Leiomyosarcoma can have a primary site of origin anywhere in the body with smooth muscle. Although sparse in the head and neck region, smooth muscle is found mainly in the walls of blood vessels and erector pili muscles of the skin. Presenting symptoms of this tumor in the head and neck region are usually nonspecific and occurring due to mass effect. Histology and immunohistochemical studies are required for diagnosis. Leiomyosarcomas appear grossly hemorrhagic and soft. Microscopically, they exhibit pleomorphism and may show abnormal mitotic figures and coagulative tumor cell necrosis. Staining must be positive for smooth muscle markers such as smooth muscle actin and/or H-caldesmon, which excludes a myofibroblastic tumor [3]. They are nonreactive to S-100 and cytokeratin [4].

TABLE 1: Literature review of eight primary parotid leiomyosarcomas.

Study	Age (years)	Gender	Presenting symptoms	Metastases	Treatment	Local recurrence	Followup
[2]	59	Female	Not reported	None	SX, RT	No	In remission 9 years postop.
[3]	78	Male	Painless mass	None	SX	No	In remission 5 years postop.
[4]	8	Male	Painless mass	Lungs	CRT	N/A	Lost to followup
[5]	45	Female	Painless mass	None reported (only local extension)	RT	N/A	Expired 5 years after presentation. Tumor directly extended into ipsilateral temporal lobe penetrating the orbit, maxillary sinus, zygomatic arch, ethmoid bone, sella turcica, and nares
[6]	33	Female	Painless mass	Lymph nodes & scalp	SX, RT	No	In remission 5 years postop.
[7]	17	Female	Painful mass	Lymph nodes	SX (three times, the last included excision of SCM and block dissection of cervical lymph nodes)	Thrice	Not reported
[8]	44	Male	Painless mass	None	SX, RT	No	In remission 3 years postop.
[9]	36	Male	Painful mass	Lymph nodes & facial nerve	SX, CRT	No	Not reported

SX: surgical excision; RT: radiation therapy; CRT: chemoradiation; N/A: not applicable.

The mitotic activity could be helpful for determining malignancy as well as metastatic potential [10]. Based on the limited data, leiomyosarcoma of the head and neck behaves more aggressively locally and has a relatively poor prognosis [9, 11, 12]. Early surgical removal with wide margins has resulted in the best outcomes while the tumor is still small and in situ. These tumors are generally not very responsive to chemotherapy or radiation, although adjunctive treatment is still commonly used when margins are unclear or tumor cells are left behind.

Most of the salivary sarcomas and carcinosarcomas arise as de novo neoplasms. Pleomorphic adenomas may undergo malignant change to carcinoma ex pleomorphic adenoma, true malignant mixed tumor (carcinosarcoma), or metastasizing pleomorphic adenoma. Only one other case has been reported in which pure sarcomatous change was observed with no epithelial carcinomatous component and thus was diagnosed as a sarcoma ex pleomorphic adenoma [13]. In that case, a 59-year-old man presented with a parotid mass and subsequent FNA suggested findings of benign mixed tumor and thus a parotidectomy was performed. The tumor showed a high-grade sarcoma exhibiting metaplastic bone with evidence of vascular and capsular invasion within a background of an otherwise typical mixed tumor. Examination of additional sections demonstrated the same. The patient received chemotherapy after further workup demonstrated a recurrent and progressive disease with lung metastasis. The patient expired with complications 2 years after first presentation. The extremely rare occurrence of a leiomyosarcoma ex pleomorphic adenoma of the parotid presents not only significant academic interest and diagnostic conundrum but also important clinical support for aggressive management of this tumor with poor prognosis, comparable to all leiomyosarcomas of the head and neck.

2. Case Report

A 79-year-old female presented to the emergency department with 2 weeks of left jaw pain and swelling as well as left facial weakness and droop. As seen in Figure 1, an MRI with IV contrast revealed a 1.5 × 1.5 × 1.8 cm heterogenous, low-intensity, peripherally enhancing lesion located in the deep lobe of the left parotid gland, abutting the posterior aspect of the left lateral pterygoid muscle. It demonstrated likely pathologic involvement of the facial nerve within the parotid gland and in the region of the stylomastoid foramen. She was subsequently referred to our office and was found to have weakness of the marginal branch of the facial nerve and diminished gag reflex.

Due to high malignancy suspicion, a left total parotidectomy with facial nerve resection was performed as well as facial nerve reconstruction. The tumor was noted to be very firm and was encountered deep in the parotid gland, extending to the deep muscles in the neck but not adherent to any surrounding structures. The margins were distorted during the excision. Surgical pathology included 2 tumor excisions exhibiting spindle cell morphologies and 5 lymph nodes labeled benign. The first parotid excision was 2.5 cm and

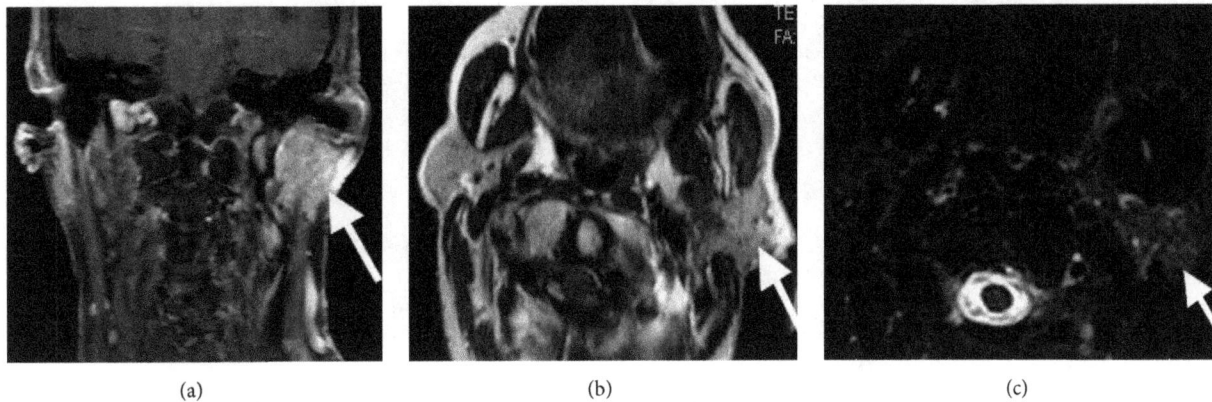

(a)   (b)   (c)

FIGURE 1: MRI revealing a mass in the deep lobe of the parotid gland abutting the posterior aspect of the lateral pterygoid muscle, likely extending towards the stylomastoid foramen exhibiting low T1 signal intensity in (a) coronal and (b) axial planes as well as low STIR signal intensity in (c) axial plane.

showed extensive calcification and hyalinization. The second was 1.9 cm, surrounded nerve bundles, and was noted to have focal necrosis. Diagnosis was a sarcoma ex pleomorphic adenoma with the sarcomatous component being consistent with a leiomyosarcoma.

The patient began external radiation 2 months postoperatively to the left total parotidectomy tumor bed using generous margins and tracing the path of the left facial nerve back to the stylomastoid foramen. Lymph nodes were not included since the surgical specimens were negative and spindle cell sarcomas do not generally metastasize to lymph nodes. Left facial droop improved over the course of 6 weeks of 30 radiation treatment fractions. Six months after surgery, PET scan of the head and neck showed no abnormal hypermetabolic foci within the head and neck region to suggest metastatic disease. Nonspecific bilateral hilar hypermetabolic densities were appreciated, so a repeat CAT scan 3 months later was recommended. At a one-year postoperative followup, the patient had no complaints and only marginal facial nerve palsy was noted on exam.

While vacationing in Florida, the patient presented to the local hospital with 2 days of symptoms including ataxia, diplopia in the right eye, and bilateral hand numbness. MRI revealed a homogenously enhancing mass in the left paramedian inferior pontine region of the brainstem measuring about 9×9 mm. Chest CT also revealed a lobulated 5.2×2 cm mass along the peripheral portions of the right upper lobe. The brainstem and lung masses were assumed to be metastatic sarcoma from the left parotid. She was not deemed a surgical candidate and was recommended to undergo palliative radiation therapy, but she preferred hospice care just 18 months after first experiencing symptoms.

2.1. Pathology Report. The parotid specimen was prepared on H&E and immunohistochemical stained slides, shown in Figure 2. Observations included the following: identifiable foci of pleomorphic adenoma with presence of benign glandular/tubular structures identified within a predominantly acellular hyalinized and focally calcified nodular area.

There was also variably differentiated spindle-shaped cellular proliferation extensively involving periparotid soft tissues including perineural and perivascular invasion, as well as invasion of the parotid parenchyma. The lesion showed fascicular to storiform growth comprised of elongated cigar-shaped nuclei. There was increased mitotic activity including atypical mitoses and focal necrosis. The IHC stains were variably reactive for smooth muscle actin, smooth muscle myosin heavy chain, desmin, and calponin but negative for pan-cytokeratin, S100 protein, CD34, and ALK1. This is consistent with leiomyosarcoma. While there was focal moderate nuclear pleomorphism, the nuclear morphology was relatively bland lacking features of a histologic high-grade neoplasm. Diagnosis is a sarcoma ex pleomorphic adenoma with the sarcomatous component being consistent with a leiomyosarcoma. The absence of epithelial malignancy precludes a diagnosis of carcinosarcoma. The specimen was defined as histologic grade 2, including perineural and perivascular invasion with tumor extension into periparotid soft tissue. 12 lymph nodes were examined and 0 were noted for malignancy. Thus, the stage of the tumor was $T_1N_0M_0$.

3. Discussion

Our case would be only the second reported sarcoma ex pleomorphic adenoma and is unique because of the sarcomatous component being consistent with leiomyosarcoma. A primary leiomyosarcoma of the parotid gland is also extremely rare. Thus, even after thorough H&E and immunohistochemical staining, this case is very difficult to diagnose. The differential is vast and the possibility of metastasis must be ruled out. Other possibilities include carcinosarcoma, sarcomatoid carcinoma, melanoma, and sarcoma of any origin. Also, it is important to suspect a metastasis from a primary site more commonly home to these neoplasms, such as the uterus in females. Saiz et al. presented the case of a uterine leiomyosarcoma that metastasized to the parotid gland 6 years before any clinical presentation in the uterus [14].

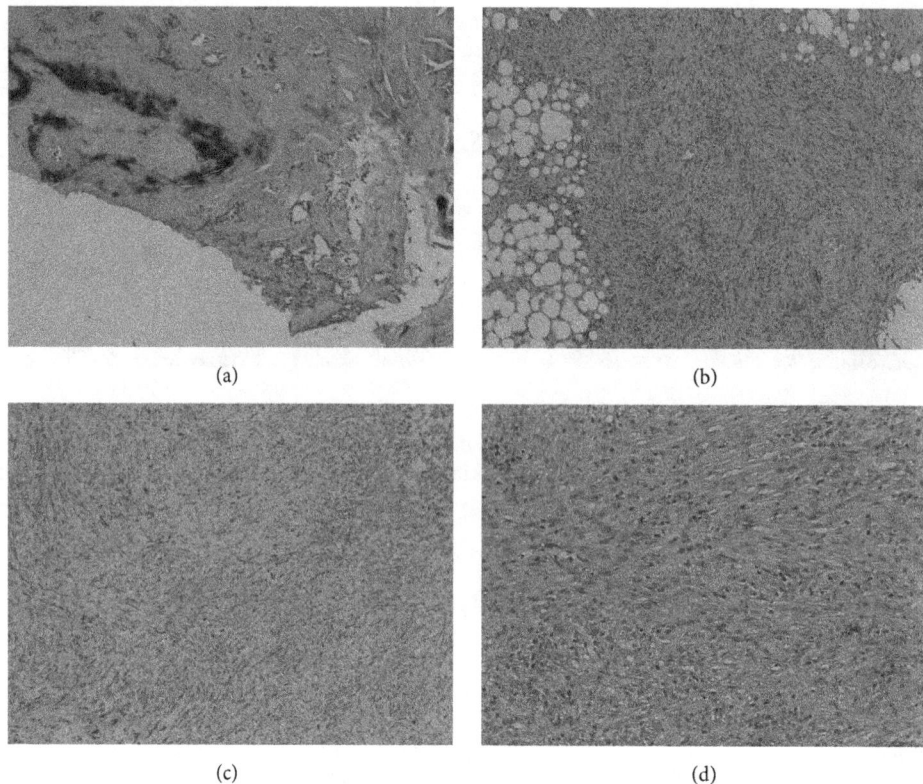

FIGURE 2: 100x magnification of (a) calcifications around benign glandular tissue, (b) spindle cells infiltrating periparotid adipose tissue, and (c) smooth muscle stain of parotid lesion being positive. 200x magnification of (d) spindle cell lesion.

Although smooth muscle cells have been thought to be the origin of leiomyosarcomas, some authors have claimed that they may derive from pluripotent mesenchymal cells. When leiomyosarcomas of any anatomic site metastasize, they usually do so hematogenously as observed in 20% of cases. Lung involvement is seen in about 75% of cases due to the pulmonary vascular bed's filtering function [6]. As observed in the limited number of cases of primary parotid lesions, they seem to disseminate hematogenously and lymphatically. Local recurrence was only seen in one case, where it recurred thrice.

4. Conclusion

Leiomyosarcoma ex pleomorphic adenoma and primary leiomyosarcoma of the parotid gland are extremely rare occurrences, and diagnosis is challenging. It is important to perform thorough immunohistochemical staining and exclude a previous history of sarcoma or other sources of metastases, such as the upper aerodigestive tract or uterus. As with other sarcomas of the head and neck, complete resection of the primary tumor with tumor-free margins is critical especially due to the local aggressiveness and metastatic potential.

Competing Interests

The authors declare that they have no competing interests.

Acknowledgments

The authors acknowledge Bruce Wenig, M.D., as consulting pathologist.

References

[1] M. A. Luna, M. E. Tortoledo, N. G. Ordonez, R. A. Frankenthaler, and J. G. Batsakis, "Primary sarcomas of the major salivary glands," *Archives of Otolaryngology—Head and Neck Surgery*, vol. 117, no. 3, pp. 302–306, 1991.

[2] P. L. Auclair, J. M. Langloss, S. W. Weiss, and R. L. Corio, "Sarcomas and sarcomatoid neoplasms of the major salivary gland regions: a clinicopathologic and immunohistochemical study of 67 cases and review of the literature," *Cancer*, vol. 58, no. 6, pp. 1305–1315, 1986.

[3] S. Krüger and K. Sommer, "Leiomyosarcoma of the parotid gland: a case report," *European Archives of Oto-Rhino-Laryngology*, vol. 263, no. 10, pp. 951–954, 2006.

[4] A. Sethi, S. Mrig, D. Sethi, A. K. Mandal, and A. K. Agarwal, "Parotid gland leiomyosarcoma in a child: an extremely unusual neoplasm," *Oral and Maxillofacial Pathology*, vol. 102, pp. 82–84, 2006.

[5] M. C. Wheelock and T. J. Madden, "Uncommon tumors of the salivary glands," *Surgery, Gynecology & Obstetrics*, vol. 88, no. 6, pp. 776–782, 1949.

[6] G. K. Maheshwari, H. A. Baboo, M. H. Patel, M. K. Wadhwa, and U. Gopal, "Leiomyosarcoma of the parotid gland metastatic to the scalp: a rare primary location with unusual metastatic

lesion," *Turkish Journal of Cancer*, vol. 33, no. 4, pp. 191–194, 2003.

[7] S. Sandhyamani, A. K. Mahapatra, and B. M. Kapur, "Leiomyosarcoma of the parotid gland," *Australian and New Zealand Journal of Surgery*, vol. 53, no. 2, pp. 179–181, 1983.

[8] J. Kang, J. A. Levinson, and I. F. Hitti, "Leiomyosarcoma of the parotid gland: a case report and review of the literature," *Head and Neck*, vol. 21, no. 2, pp. 168–171, 1999.

[9] S. Oncel, M. Doganay, A. Ozer, S. Arslanoglu, M. Ermetet, and N. Erdogan, "Leiomyosarcoma of the parotid gland," *The Journal of Laryngology and Otology*, vol. 110, pp. 401–403, 1996.

[10] A. Kuruvilla, B. M. Wenig, D. M. Humphrey, and D. K. Heffner, "Leiomyosarcoma of the sinonasal tract. A clinicopathologic study of nine cases," *Archives of Otolaryngology—Head and Neck Surgery*, vol. 116, no. 11, pp. 1278–1286, 1990.

[11] M. E. Schenberg, P. J. Slootweg, and R. Koole, "Leiomyosarcomas of the oral cavity. Report of four cases and review of the literature," *Journal of Cranio-Maxillofacial Surgery*, vol. 21, no. 8, pp. 342–347, 1993.

[12] R. L. Josephson, R. L. Blair, and Y. C. Bedard, "Leiomyosarcoma of the nose and paranasal sinuses," *Otolaryngology—Head and Neck Surgery*, vol. 93, no. 2, pp. 270–274, 1985.

[13] N. Said-Al-Naief, C. Moran, and M. Luna, "Sarcoma ex-pleomorphic adenoma: a case report of a unique entity," *Oral Surgery, Oral Medicine, Oral Pathology, Oral Radiology, and Endodontology*, vol. 103, no. 4, pp. e28–e29, 2007.

[14] A. D. Saiz, U. Sachdev, M. L. Brodman, and L. Deligdisch, "Metastatic uterine leiomyosarcoma presenting as a primary sarcoma of the parotid gland," *Obstetrics & Gynecology*, vol. 92, no. 4, pp. 667–668, 1998.

40

Oncocytoma of the Submandibular Gland: Diagnosis and Treatment Based on Clinicopathology

Betty Chen,[1] **Joshua I. Hentzelman,**[1] **Ronald J. Walker,**[1] **and Jin-Ping Lai**[2]

[1]*Department of Otolaryngology-Head and Neck Surgery, Saint Louis University School of Medicine, St. Louis, MO 63104, USA*
[2]*Department of Pathology, Saint Louis University School of Medicine, St. Louis, MO 63104, USA*

Correspondence should be addressed to Jin-Ping Lai; jinpinglai@slu.edu

Academic Editor: Rong-San Jiang

Background. Submandibular oncocytomas are rare benign salivary gland neoplasms. They are typically found in Caucasian patients aged 50–70 years with no gender preference. Due to the overlapping histological and clinical features of head and neck tumors, they are often misdiagnosed. *Methods.* We report a case of unilateral submandibular gland oncocytoma in a 63-year-old Caucasian man. *Results.* The patient underwent unilateral submandibular gland resection and histopathologic analysis of the tumor specimen. On follow-up at 2 weeks and 1 year, no recurrence was identified. *Conclusion.* Submandibular oncocytomas are best diagnosed with preoperative FNA and CT imaging and have distinctive findings on cytology and histology. CT followed by fine-needle aspiration cytology would be the preferred diagnostic modalities. Due to its low rate of malignant transformation and recurrence, the best treatment is local resection with follow-up as necessary.

1. Introduction

Oncocytomas are rare benign neoplasms composed of oncocytes or polyhedral cells with eosinophilic cytoplasm made up of abundant mitochondria and dark centrally located nuclei [1–3]. Hürthle first described oncocytes in a canine thyroid gland in 1894 [4, 5]. The term "oncocytoma" was first used by Schaefer to describe "granular swollen cells" in ducts and acini of salivary glands [1, 6]. In 1931, Hamperl reported oncocytomas in numerous glandular structures including major salivary glands, thyroid and parathyroid glands, pituitary glands, testicles, pancreas, liver, and stomach [1, 7].

Salivary gland oncocytomas are primarily found in the parotid gland and rarely found in the submandibular glands [3]. To the best of our knowledge, there have only been 33 cases of submandibular oncocytoma reported in previous literature, including our case. Despite its rarity, submandibular oncocytoma is an important area of study because it has a distinct clinical course compared to more common salivary neoplasms such as pleomorphic adenoma and Warthin's tumor. Pleomorphic adenomas have 1.5% and 9.5% malignant potential on follow-up at 5 and 15 years, respectively [8],

and can recur after resection [9]. In addition, 37 cases of carcinoma arising from previous Warthin's tumor have been reported [10]. In contrast, oncocytomas have extremely low malignant potential, and those in the submandibular gland have not been found to recur after surgery [11]. In other words, submandibular oncocytomas favor a better prognosis.

Submandibular oncocytomas can present asymptomatically or as tender, enlarging neck masses over weeks to years. Typical patients are Caucasians 50–70 years of age with no gender preference. There are no clear etiologies for the development of submandibular oncocytomas, although there have been cases associated with radiation exposure [11].

This report aims to evaluate the clinical and histopathological features of submandibular oncocytomas through a single case report at St. Louis University hospital and will include a review of previous literature with an emphasis on diagnostic criteria and future treatment of such cases.

2. Case Presentation

A 63-year-old Caucasian male presented with a 3-year history of tender right neck mass. He denied other symptoms and

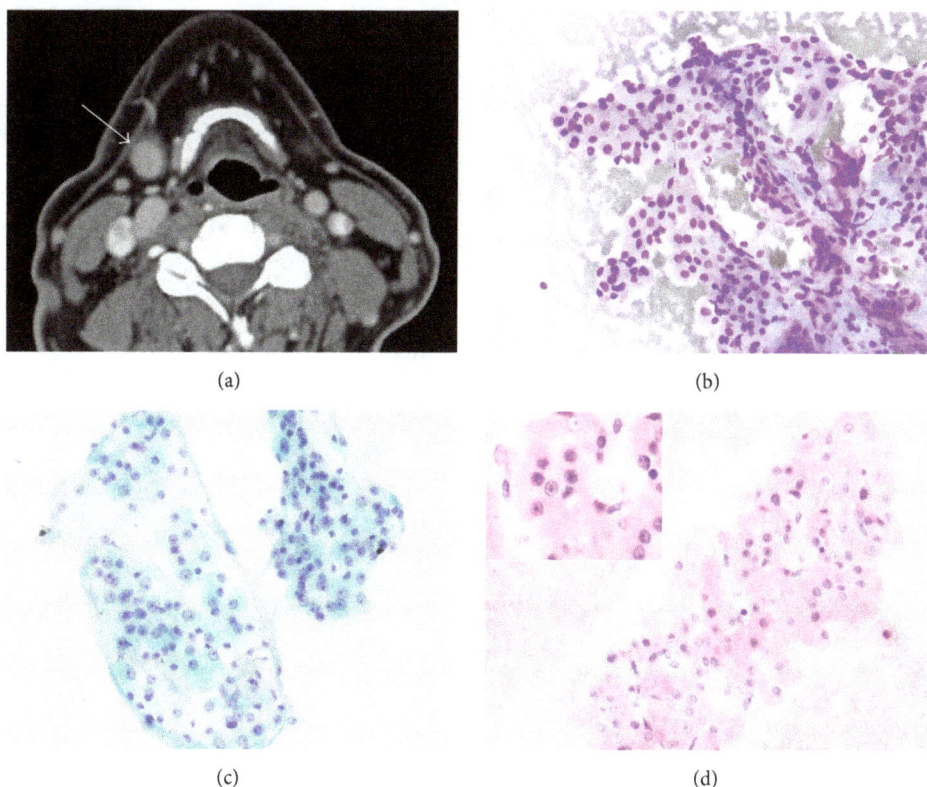

FIGURE 1: Imaging and cytopathology of the submandibular oncocytoma. (a) CT scan showing a well-circumscribed mass (1.6 × 1.3 cm) at the right submandibular space; (b)–(d) FNA of the mass showing clusters of polygonal eosinophilic epithelial cells with low N/C ratio, round nuclei, and prominent nucleoli ((b) Diff-Quik, ×400; (c) pap smear, ×400; and (d) cell block, ×400 (inset, ×600)).

his past medical history was noncontributory. He denied cigarette smoking and tobacco use and reported 15 alcoholic drinks per week. Past surgical surgery included an osteotomy of the clavicle. On physical exam, a 1.5 cm solid nodule was palpated in the right submandibular region above the tip of the hyoid. The presence of the mass was confirmed on CT imaging, which showed a well-defined, homogeneously enhancing 1.6 × 1.3 cm mass in the inferior pole of the submandibular salivary gland (Figure 1(a)).

A fine-needle aspiration (FNA) of the lesion was performed. In cytopathology (Figures 1(b)–1(d)), there were clusters of monotonous, polygonal, eosinophilic (oncocytic) epithelial cells with a low nuclear to cytoplasmic (N/C) ratio. The tumor cells had round nuclei and prominent nucleoli. There was no significant lymphoid population identified, which is commonly seen in Warthin's tumor. No mitotic figures or tumor necrosis were identified. Cytologic features were suggestive of submandibular oncocytoma.

For definitive treatment and pathologic diagnosis, a right submandibular gland resection was performed. Gross examination revealed a weeping tan/yellow mass. The cut surface was coarsely lobulated with focal hemorrhage. Microscopically, the tumor showed a well-circumscribed mass with a thin capsule (Figure 2(a)). The tumor was composed of monotonous epithelial cells with a low N/C ratio, abundant eosinophilic cytoplasm, and round nuclei with prominent

nucleoli (Figure 2(b)). Away from the mass within adjacent submandibular gland tissue were foci of oncocytic hyperplasia (Figures 2(c) and 2(d)). The patient was discharged on the same day following surgery. On the two-week follow-up visit, the patient reported no issues with the wound. On the one-year follow-up, no recurrence was identified.

3. Discussion

Oncocytomas of the salivary gland are rare benign neoplasms that comprise 3-4% of head and neck tumors [5, 20]. The majority of salivary gland tumors arise in the parotid gland (70%), followed by minor salivary glands (22%) and submandibular glands (8%) [5]. Submandibular oncocytoma is a very rare benign tumor that arises primarily in older Caucasian individuals aged 50–70 years. However, there have been cases reported in younger individuals, including a case involving a 19-year-old female [17]. According to previous cases of submandibular oncocytoma listed in Table 1, there is no gender preference, with a male-to-female ratio of approximately 1 : 1. In addition, the average age of diagnosis is comparable for both sexes, with males diagnosed at 59 years and females at 61 years. Submandibular oncocytoma most frequently presents as a painless enlarging mass, which was found in 48% (16/33) of cases, whereas 27% (9/33) involved a tender mass, and the rest had no data on symptoms.

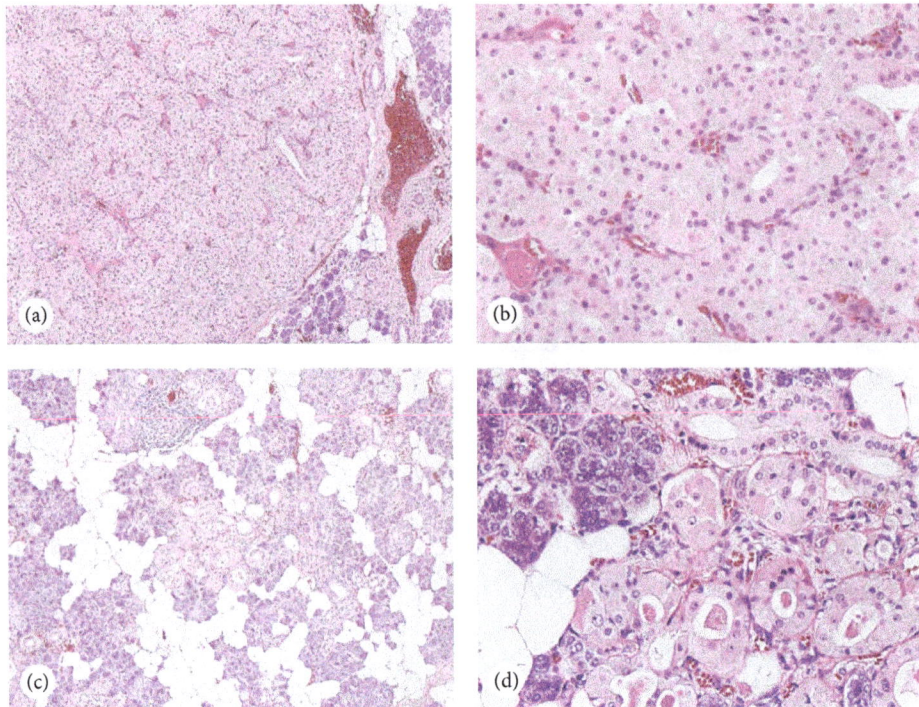

FIGURE 2: Histology of the submandibular oncocytoma. (a-b) The tumor is well circumscribed with a thin capsule ((a) ×100) and is composed of benign appearing oncocytes ((b) ×400); (c)-(d) foci of oncocytes present at the tumor adjacent submandibular tissue ((c) ×100; (d) ×400).

Oncocytosis, marked by increased number of mitochondria, is frequently reported in aged, reactive, inflamed, hyperplastic salivary glands [21]. However, due to its rare incidence in submandibular glands, the etiology of submandibular oncocytomas remains unknown. One theory implicated the role of radiation in the pathogenesis of oncocytomas. In a follow-up study by Brandwein and Huvos, 20% (9/44) of patients with oncocytomas had radiation therapy or prolonged radiation exposure [11]. However, no conclusive evidence exists for the correlation between amount of radiation exposure and development of oncocytomas. Although rare in salivary glands, oncocytomas can be found mainly in the excretory ducts, also known as intercalated ducts, of minor salivary glands and parotid glands. Oncocytomas in the parotid glands may be derived primarily from reserve cells in intercalated ducts [22]. This is supported by immunohistochemistry data, which demonstrated the presence of CK7, CK8, and CK19, which are markers for human duct cells [22]. Submandibular gland oncocytosis may have a similar etiology, although research has mainly been focused on parotid gland oncocytomas.

The differential diagnosis for benign submandibular tumors includes pleomorphic adenoma and Warthin's tumor. Each tumor can be distinguished based on its histopathological characteristics. Oncocytomas are characterized by the presence of monomorphic oncocytes without mitoses and necrosis [11]. Unlike pleomorphic adenomas, which have thick and irregularly margined capsules, oncocytomas have thin capsules, as seen in our case. Warthin's tumor can also be

ruled out on cytology and histology by the lack of lymphatic population [12]. In addition to the primary tumor, surrounding areas of oncocytic metaplasia can be found [3]. This was seen in our patient, who had areas of oncocytic hyperplasia in the adjacent submandibular gland tissue. Submandibular gland oncocytomas have rare malignant potential. In 33 cases to date, only one reported malignant differentiation from a benign lesion [23]. Characteristics of malignant transformation include local invasion into muscular, perineural, and lymphatic structures as well as microscopic features including nuclear atypia, cellular polymorphism, mitoses, and focal necrosis [5].

Due to the similarities in clinical presentation between benign and malignant submandibular oncocytomas, radiologic imaging and fine-needle aspiration cytology (FNAC) are essential in distinguishing between the two entities. Ultrasound is recommended for initial assessment of a mass, but is insufficient because it does not provide information about surrounding structures. Recently, F-18 FDG PET/CT has shown promise in detecting features of salivary gland malignancies. Subramanian and colleagues described the utility of PET/CT in the initial staging and histologic grading of salivary gland malignancies [18]. Despite the superior spatial resolution and functional and anatomic data, there are limitations in using this modality. For instance, due to the lower maximum SUV in salivary glands, the detection accuracy of malignancies with lower F-18 FDG may be variable [18]. In addition, PET/CT is generally not indicated unless initial biopsy is concerning for malignancy. To date, neck CT with

TABLE 1: Summary of clinical characteristics of submandibular oncocytoma.

Case	Age (sex)	Signs/symptoms	Laterality	Size	Mode of diagnosis	Treatment	Follow-up
(1) Eneroth [12]	75 (F)	N/A	N/A	N/A	Aspiration biopsy	N/A	N/A
(2) Dibble and Sanford [13]	79 (M)	Asymptomatic, viral URI	Left	2 × 3 cm, grew to 5.5 × 3 × 2.5 cm	N/A	Excision via external method	N/A
(3) Mukai et al. [14]	61 (M)	N/A	Left	N/A	N/A	N/A	3 years, alive
(4) Goode and Corio [15]	60 (F)	N/A	Unknown	N/A	N/A	N/A	N/A
(5) Brandwein and Huvos [11]	62 (M)	N/A	Left	N/A	N/A	N/A	6 months, alive
(6) Ziegler et al. [16]	56 (F)	N/A	N/A	N/A	N/A	N/A	9 months, alive
(7) Thompson et al.* 22 cases [3]			See descriptions below				
(8) Nakada et al. [2]	68 (M)	Painless, enlarging mass	Left	7 × 4.5 cm	FNA	Radical resection	1.5 years, alive
(9) Sakthikumar et al. [17]	19 (F)	Painless to dull ache	Left	3 × 5 cm	FNA	Excision	8 weeks, comfortable
(10) Subramaniam et al. [18]	85 (M)	Asymptomatic MEN2B, NF1	Left	12 mm	F18 FDG PET/CT	N/A	N/A
(11) Dastaran and Chandu [19]	61 (F)	Long-standing mild tenderness	Bilateral	N/A	Ultrasound, FNA	Bilateral excision	1 year, no recurrence
(12) Chen et al. (present case)	63 (M)	Tender mass	Right	1.6 × 1.3 cm	FNA, CT	Excision	1 year, no recurrence

*Thompson et al. [3] presented 22 cases of submandibular oncocytoma with 50 : 50 female-to-male ratio and an average age of 59 years. Sizes of the tumor ranged from 0.7 cm to 7 cm, averaging 3 cm. More than half of the cases (13/22) involved enlarging asymptomatic painless masses whereas the rest involved tender masses. On follow-up, none of the cases had evidence of recurrent disease.

contrast is the preferred modality for evaluating the extent of invasion and spread of salivary gland tumors [20]. Fine-needle aspiration (FNA) is a common initial diagnostic procedure for investigating salivary gland masses due to its cost-effectiveness, simple technique, and fast results. FNA cytologic features of oncocytomas include uniformly polygonal, cytoplasm-rich cells with characteristic morphological features such as eosinophilic and granulated cells with round centralized nuclei [12]. Generally, no mitotic figures are identified on the cellblock in case other entities cannot be excluded. In addition, a cytology exam of the aspirate can be performed using immunohistochemistry. Benign and malignant tumors have been shown to have different activity of markers such as Ki-67, a nuclear protein expressed in proliferating cells indicative of active mitosis [5].

To date, the first-line treatment for submandibular oncocytomas is surgical excision. Of the cases in Table 1, all known treatments involved surgical resection, including unilateral or bilateral excision and radical resection, with no reported recurrence. Since areas of oncocytic hyperplasia may also be present in the tissue of the adjacent salivary gland, as in this case, resection of the whole gland is recommended. Submandibular oncocytomas have an extremely low potential of malignant transformation, with only one reported case. In addition, no local recurrences have been reported following resection [3, 11, 12, 20, 24]. Thus, radical dissection or adjuvant radiation therapy would not be necessary. Due to the rare incidence of these tumors, alternative methods of treatments such as medical managements have not yet been reported.

In summary, we present a case of submandibular oncocytoma, which is a rare benign salivary gland neoplasm. Distinguishing features of oncocytomas are best seen on preoperative FNA cytology and histology, which include the presence of monotonous oncocytes with low N/C ratio and lack of mitoses and necrosis. The malignant potential of a benign oncocytoma is extremely low at around 3%, with only one previously reported case in literature. CT followed by fine-needle aspiration cytology would be the preferred diagnostic modalities. Treatment is local excision of the tumor with appropriate follow-up as needed.

Competing Interests

The authors declare that there are no competing interests related to this paper.

References

[1] E. Beltaos and W. J. Maurer, "Oncocytoma of the submaxillary salivary gland. Report of a case," Archives of Otolaryngology, vol. 84, no. 2, pp. 193–197, 1966.

[2] M. Nakada, K. Nishizaki, H. Akagi, Y. Masuda, and T. Yoshino, "Oncocytic carcinoma of the submandibular gland: a case report and literature review," Journal of Oral Pathology and Medicine, vol. 27, no. 5, pp. 225–228, 1998.

[3] L. D. Thompson, B. M. Wenig, and G. L. Ellis, "Oncocytomas of the submandibular gland: a series of 22 cases and a review of the literature," Cancer, vol. 78, no. 11, pp. 2281–2287, 1996.

[4] K. Hürthle, "Beiträge zur Kenntniss des Secretionsvorgangs in der Schilddrüse," Archiv für die Gesamte Physiologie des Menschen und der Tiere, vol. 56, no. 1, pp. 1–44, 1894.

[5] T.-H. Lee, Y.-S. Lin, W.-Y. Lee, T.-C. Wu, and S.-L. Chang, "Malignant transformation of a benign oncocytoma of the submandibular gland: a case report," Kaohsiung Journal of Medical Sciences, vol. 26, no. 6, pp. 327–332, 2010.

[6] J. Schaefer, "Beiträge zur Histologie menschlicher Organe: IV. Zunge, V. Mundhöhle-Schlundkopf, VI. Oesophagus, VII. Cardia, Sizungsb," Kaiserlichen Akademie der Wissenschaften, Mathematisch-Naturwissenschaftliche Classe, vol. 106, pp. 353–455, 1897.

[7] H. Hamperl, "Beiträge zur normalen und pathologischen Histologie menschlicher Speicheldrüsen," Zeitschrift für Mikroskopisch-Anatomische Forschung, vol. 27, pp. 1–55, 1931.

[8] J. R. Fernández, M. M. Micas, F. J. M. Tello et al., "Metastatic benign pleomorphic adenoma. Report of a case and review of the literature," Medicina Oral, Patologia Oral y Cirugia Bucal, vol. 13, no. 3, pp. 193–196, 2008.

[9] J. Knight and K. Ratnasingham, "Metastasising pleomorphic adenoma: systematic review," International Journal of Surgery, vol. 19, pp. 137–145, 2015.

[10] F. Allevi and F. Biglioli, "Squamous carcinoma arising in a parotid Warthin's tumour," BMJ Case Reports, 2014.

[11] M. S. Brandwein and A. G. Huvos, "Oncocytic tumors of major salivary glands: a study of 68 cases with follow-up of 44 patients," American Journal of Surgical Pathology, vol. 15, no. 6, pp. 514–528, 1991.

[12] C. M. Eneroth, "Oncocytoma of major salivary glands," The Journal of Laryngology & Otology, vol. 79, no. 12, pp. 1064–1072, 1965.

[13] P. A. Dibble and D. M. Sanford, "Submaxillary oncocytoma. Oxyphil-cell adenoma," Archives of Otolaryngology—Head and Neck Surgery, vol. 74, no. 3, pp. 299–301, 1961.

[14] H. Mukai, K. Sugihara, Y. Dohhara, K. Yamada, and S. Yamashita, "Malignant oncocytoma of the submandibular gland: report of a case," Japanese Journal of Oral & Maxillofacial Surgery, vol. 24, no. 1, pp. 111–116, 1978.

[15] R. K. Goode and R. L. Corio, "Oncocytic adenocarcinoma of salivary glands," Oral Surgery, Oral Medicine, Oral Pathology, vol. 65, no. 1, pp. 61–66, 1988.

[16] M. Ziegler, E.-A. Maibach, and J. Ussmuller, "Malignant oncocytoma of the submandibular gland," Laryngo- Rhino- Otologie, vol. 71, no. 8, pp. 423–425, 1992.

[17] K. R. V. Sakthikumar, S. Mohanty, and K. Dineshkumar, "Solitary oncocytoma of the submandibular salivary gland in an adolescent female: a case report," Indian Journal of Otolaryngology and Head and Neck Surgery, vol. 59, no. 2, pp. 171–173, 2007.

[18] R. M. Subramaniam, D. K. Durnick, and P. J. Peller, "F-18 FDG PET/CT imaging of submandibular gland oncocytoma," Clinical Nuclear Medicine, vol. 33, no. 7, pp. 472–474, 2008.

[19] M. Dastaran and A. Chandu, "Bilateral submandibular gland oncocytoma in a patient with multiple endocrine neoplasia 2B syndrome and neurofibromatosis type 1: an unusual case," International Journal of Oral and Maxillofacial Surgery, vol. 40, no. 7, pp. 764–767, 2011.

[20] P. Ziglinas, A. Arnold, M. Arnold, and P. Zbären, "Primary tumors of the submandibular glands: a retrospective study based on 41 cases," Oral Oncology, vol. 46, no. 4, pp. 287–291, 2010.

[21] P. M. McLoughlin, A. W. Barrett, and P. M. Speight, "Oncocytoma of the submandibular gland," *International Journal of Oral & Maxillofacial Surgery*, vol. 23, no. 5, pp. 294–295, 1994.

[22] T. Muramatsu, S. Hashimoto, M.-W. Lee et al., "Oncocytic carcinoma arising in submandibular gland with immunohistochemical observations and review of the literature," *Oral Oncology*, vol. 39, no. 2, pp. 199–203, 2003.

[23] W.-Y. Lee and S.-L. Chang, "Fine needle aspiration cytology of oncocytic carcinoma of the submandibular gland with pre-existing oncocytoma: a case report," *Cytopathology*, vol. 21, no. 5, pp. 339–341, 2010.

[24] T. J. Palmer, M. J. Gleeson, J. W. Eveson, and R. A. Cawson, "Oncocytic adenomas and oncocytic hyperplasia of salivary glands: a clinicopathological study of 26 cases," *Histopathology*, vol. 16, no. 5, pp. 487–493, 1990.

41

Laryngeal Fracture after Blunt Cervical Trauma in Motorcycle Accident and Its Management

Nuno Ribeiro-Costa, Pedro Carneiro Sousa, Diogo Abreu Pereira, Paula Azevedo, and Delfim Duarte

Hospital Pedro Hispano, Rua Dr. Eduardo Torres, Senhora da Hora, 4464-513 Matosinhos, Portugal

Correspondence should be addressed to Nuno Ribeiro-Costa; nunodanielcosta@gmail.com

Academic Editor: Andrea Gallo

Laryngeal fracture is a rare traumatic injury, potentially fatal, with an estimated incidence of 1 in 30,000 patients admitted to severe trauma centers. Because of the rarity of this injury, physician may be not aware of its existence, leading to a late diagnosis of this entity. We report a case of a 59-year-old woman admitted to the emergency room after a motorcycle accident with cervical trauma. The patient presented with dysphonia, hemoptysis, cervical subcutaneous emphysema, and increasing respiratory distress that led to the intubation of the patient. CT-scan demonstrated displaced fracture of the cricoid and thyroid cartilage. The patient was submitted to tracheostomy and the fracture was surgically repaired. Tracheostomy was removed in third postoperative month. The patient presented a good recovery, reporting only hoarseness but without swallowing or breathing problems at 6-month follow-up.

1. Introduction

Laryngeal fracture is a rare traumatic injury, potentially fatal, with an estimated incidence of 1 in 30,000 patients admitted to severe trauma centers [1–4]. Factors such as mobility and elasticity of the larynx and its protection by the mandible and the sternum make it able to withstand severe trauma [2]. The rarity of this type of injury often leads to a delay in diagnosis which may contribute to airway patency problems, vocal production and swallowing [5]. Therefore it is important for clinicians who treat it to have a comprehensive understanding of its diagnosis and treatment in order to improve the patient outcome.

2. Case Presentation

A 59-year-old woman is admitted in the emergency room after a motorcycle accident with cervical trauma. The patient was conscious and oriented, presenting dysphonia, hemoptysis, and increasing respiratory distress that led to the intubation of the patient by an anesthetist in the emergency room. Her physical examination revealed a subcutaneous emphysema, edema, and tenderness in the cervical area, and other facial and extremity abrasions and ecchymosis. The cervical and thorax CT-scan demonstrated an anterior traumatic lesion of the larynx with severe emphysema of the cervical and supraclavicular area and fracture of the cricoid and thyroid cartilage (Figure 1).

After the patient stabilization, the patient was evaluated by otolaryngology and immediately admitted to the operating room. During surgery, a transversal fracture of thyroid and cricoid cartilage was found. The thyroid fracture was repaired and the cricoid cartilage was fixed to the thyroid cartilage with 3-0 prolene and tracheostomy was performed (Figure 2). The patency of the laryngeal lumen was maintained with an endotracheal tube, which was removed one week later.

The patient was initially admitted in intermediary care unit and fed through a nasogastric tube. The postoperative evaluation with flexible endoscopy revealed a bilateral paresis of the vocal cords and significant reduction of laryngeal sensibility and saliva aspiration. During her stay in the intermediary care unit the patient case was complicated with a pulmonary infection with multisensitive *Pseudomonas aeruginosa* which was successfully treated with piperacillin-tazobactam for 21 days. During this period the patient started sessions of speech therapy to help improved vocalization and

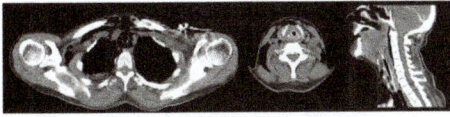

FIGURE 1: Neck and thorax CT-scan at admittance. It reveals anterior traumatic lesion of the larynx with severe emphysema of the cervical and supraclavicular area and displaced fracture of the thyroid cartilage. No laryngotracheal separation was observed.

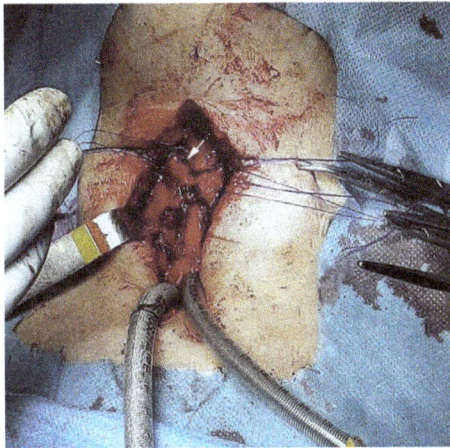

FIGURE 2: Intraoperative view of the laryngeal fracture (marked with a white arrow), with suture of the laryngeal framework.

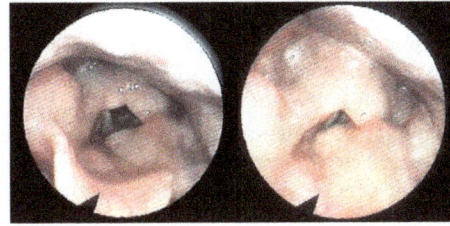

FIGURE 3: Flexible endoscopy demonstrating the postoperative view of the larynx.

deglutition. Before discharge the patient was submitted to surgical gastrostomy because of persistent food aspiration.

At 3-month follow-up the flexible endoscopy revealed a normal mobilization of both vocal cords (Figure 3). However, during the swallowing evaluation, the patient still could not tolerate liquid food with occasional episodes of aspiration. At this time the tracheostomy was removed, and progressive oral feeding with creamy and solid food was started. Subsequently, at 6-month follow-up, the patient presented no evidence of secretions or food aspiration and the gastrostomy was removed. Although improved, her hoarseness still persists.

3. Discussion

Laryngeal fracture is an infrequent injury, most frequently resulting from anterior, blunt trauma to the neck from motor vehicles accidents, sports-related trauma, assault, or strangulation [4, 6]. Other causes include penetrating trauma due to gunshot or stab wounds to the neck [7]. Laryngeal trauma has a high mortality rate (17,9% to 40%), with many patients dying before reaching the emergency room because of severe airway injury or multiple organ injury [1, 4, 8].

In our case the patient presented with some of the classical, but not pathognomonic, symptoms such as hoarseness, anterior neck pain, progressive respiratory distress, hemoptysis, and cervical subcutaneous emphysema [5, 7]. However, some patients with laryngeal fracture may not present such symptoms, and a high level of suspicion is required of all anterior neck trauma [4, 6]. About 37% of the patients in reported series had delayed diagnosis [8]. CT-scan of the neck

is considered the gold standard for diagnosing such injuries [3, 7, 9].

The primary objective in treating laryngeal trauma is maintaining the airway patency. Early airway management and aggressive physiologic compensation performed in the initial phase are an important determinant in the laryngeal trauma mortality [3, 10]. However, the most appropriate method for airway management is controversial. Both endotracheal intubation and tracheostomy have been recommended [2, 4, 6, 9]. Our patient was successfully intubated in the emergency room, but when severe trauma has been inflicted to the larynx, intubating can be extremely difficult because of distorted anatomy and poor visualization. The posterior conversion to tracheostomy after endotracheal intubation is also a good method, being recommended within 24 h because it decreases the length of hospitalization [3, 7, 8].

After safeguarding the airway, laryngeal treatment should be considered to improve the long-term voice and swallowing outcomes in these patients. Nondisplaced fractures can be managed nonoperatively, while surgical reduction of laryngeal framework should be performed in patients with displaced fractures [1, 7]. The timing of such repair is subject of debate but recent evidence suggests that early treatment within 48 hours resulted in a higher recovery rate than that of the delayed treatment group [6].

Competing Interests

The authors declare that there is no conflict of interests regarding the publication of this paper.

References

[1] G. S. Gussack, G. J. Jurkovich, and A. Luterman, "Laryngotracheal trauma: a protocol approach to a rare injury," *Laryngoscope*, vol. 96, no. 6, pp. 660–665, 1986.

[2] S. D. Schaefer, "The acute management of external laryngeal trauma. A 27-year experience," *Archives of Otolaryngology—Head and Neck Surgery*, vol. 118, no. 6, pp. 598–604, 1992.

[3] J. P. Kim, S. J. Cho, H. Y. Son, J. J. Park, and S. H. Woo, "Analysis of clinical feature and management of laryngeal fracture: recent 22 case review," *Yonsei Medical Journal*, vol. 53, no. 5, pp. 992–998, 2012.

[4] S. Jalisi and M. Zoccoli, "Management of laryngeal fractures—a 10-year experience," *Journal of Voice*, vol. 25, no. 4, pp. 473–479, 2011.

[5] A. Narci, D. B. Embleton, A. Ayçiçek, F. Yücedağ, and S. Çetinkurşun, "Laryngeal fracture due to blunt trauma presenting with pneumothorax and pneumomediastinum," *ORL*, vol. 73, no. 5, pp. 246–248, 2011.

[6] A. P. Butler, A. K. O'Rourke, B. P. Wood, and E. S. Porubsky, "Acute external laryngeal trauma: experience with 112 patients," *Annals of Otology, Rhinology and Laryngology*, vol. 114, no. 5, pp. 361–368, 2005.

[7] N. Schaefer, A. Griffin, B. Gerhardy, and P. Gochee, "Early recognition and management of laryngeal fracture: a case report," *Ochsner Journal*, vol. 14, no. 2, pp. 264–265, 2014.

[8] A. H. Mendelsohn, D. R. Sidell, G. S. Berke, and M. S. John, "Optimal timing of surgical intervention following adult laryngeal trauma," *Laryngoscope*, vol. 121, no. 10, pp. 2122–2127, 2011.

[9] J. P. Bent, J. R. Silver, and E. S. Porubsky, "Acute laryngeal trauma: a review of 77 patients," *Otolaryngology-Head and Neck Surgery*, vol. 109, no. 3, pp. 441–449, 1993.

[10] C.-H. Liao, J.-F. Huang, S.-W. Chen et al., "Impact of deferred surgical intervention on the outcome of external laryngeal trauma," *Annals of Thoracic Surgery*, vol. 98, no. 2, pp. 477–483, 2014.

42

Response to: Comment on "Original Solution for Middle Ear Implant and Anesthetic/Surgical Management in a Child with Severe Craniofacial Dysmorphism"

Giovanni Bianchin,[1] Lorenzo Tribi,[1] Aronne Reverzani,[2] Patrizia Formigoni,[1] and Valeria Polizzi[1]

[1]MD Otolaryngology and Audiology Department, Santa Maria Nuova Hospital, Viale Risorgimento, No. 80, 42100 Reggio Emilia, Italy
[2]MD Emergency Medicine Department, Santa Maria Nuova Hospital, Viale Risorgimento, No. 80, 42100 Reggio Emilia, Italy

Correspondence should be addressed to Lorenzo Tribi; lorenzo.tribi@asmn.re.it

Academic Editor: Richard T. Miyamoto

We thank Kruyt et al. [1], for their interest in our publication titled "Original Solution for Middle Ear Implant and Anesthetic/Surgical Management in a Child with Severe Craniofacial Dysmorphism" [2]. In response to their comments, we would like to offer clarification as to the choice of treatment for our five-year-old patient with Van Maldergem syndrome, affected by severe bilateral malformation of the external auditory canal and middle ear.

It is important to reiterate the fact that we are independent authors working for a public hospital. We do not have any conflict of interests nor are we financially supported by any company.

The goal of our case report was to present an example of a multidisciplinary approach for the treatment of congenital aural atresia with severe craniofacial dysmorphism. As stated in the article, the multidisciplinary team was formed by speech therapists, audiologists, medical doctors, neuropsychiatrists, anaesthesiologists, surgeons, radiologists, and, of course, the parents. In our article, we aimed to emphasize the importance of a multidisciplinary approach, as there are currently no guidelines available for syndromic children. Only after a careful evaluation of the pros and cons of all available treatment options, including those the patient had already trialled, was a consensus reached. The parents

themselves rejected percutaneous bone conduction devices for their child, not because of the (suboptimal) pre-op hearing impression or discomfort of the test steel spring headband but due to the permanent wound and the aesthetics of the externally worn device. The bone conductor trial showed more than satisfactory results.

As the child's malformation has a grade of 6 on the Jahrsdoerfer score, surgical reconstruction of the EAC was not considered a possibility. Publications report that patients with a higher score than 6 have a significantly better hearing outcome after surgery [3].

Bone-anchored hearing aids have been considered as first option [4]. A literature review looking into postoperative complications with the percutaneous bone conduction implants confirms a high incidence of complications related to the percutaneous system.

What follows are outcomes from a systematic study review by Kiringonda and Lusting [5], illustrating the complication rates from bone conduction hearing aid.

The article analysed 20 articles and 2,134 patients who underwent a total of 2,310 osseoimplants. Failure of osseointegration ranged from 0% to 18% in adult and mixed populations and 0% to 14.3% in the paediatric population. The rate of revision surgery ranged from 0.0% to 44.4% in pediatric patients, whereas the total rate of implant loss ranged from 0.0% to 25% in pediatric patients.

Ernst et al. [6] reported postoperative complications with percutaneous bone conductions devices as well: in a total of 543 patients who received 609 implants, the occurrence of adverse skin reactions of grade 1 or 2 according to Holger's grading was as high as 29.4%. Revision surgery was required in 29.9%.

In addition to the above outcomes, scientific evidence proves increased complication rates following paediatric percutaneous bone conduction device surgery [7–11]. Loss of the fixture due to failure of osseointegration is significantly higher in younger children [9, 12]. Compromised bone quality or immature and abnormal bone structure presents an additional burden to osseointegration of the screw. Cass and Mudd (2010) [13] consider this a relative contraindication for a percutaneous bone conductor implant. The presented case is made more complex by the fact that our patient is not only a child but is also suffering from a syndrome. Recent literature shows that complication rates are particularly common in syndromic children [14–19]. The skull bone thickness was less than 3 mm (measured on the axial CT slices at 1 cm posterior to the sigmoid sinus, at the superior margin of the bony canal). As trauma to the head is always a possibility and the bone is very thin, the additional risk of percutaneous bone conduction implants causing intracranial intrusion of fixture or other severe risks also needed to be considered [20–23].

Due to the increased incidence of complications with percutaneous bone conduction devices mentioned above and due to the parent's decision, our multidisciplinary team opted to look into intact skin solutions such as the Vibrant Soundbridge.

An important aspect considered has been binaural hearing. The cranial malformation of the 5-year-old affects hearing on both sides. The transducer of the VSB stimulates the only implanted ear. Therefore a contralateral implantation could reestablish a bilateral hearing sensation.

Another key aspect is the wide amplification range of middle ear transducers. It is shown that the Vibrant Soundbridge provides high gain especially in the high frequencies leading to better speech comprehension in noise [24, 25].

We would also like to comment on the reversibility of the performed treatment and the risk of the anesthesia.

The Vibrant Soundbridge is a reversible procedure as no structures of the middle ear have been harmed. The intervention is not compromising any future treatment opportunity including the aesthetical reconstruction of the auricle. We mentioned in the article that the surgery was performed respecting the skin needed for auricle reconstruction. Special care was taken while performing the skin incision in order to enable the aesthetic surgeons to reconstruct the auricle [26].

The additional risk of anaesthesia for maxillofacial malformations is related to the intubation itself, while no additional risk is represented by the prolonged duration of the surgery. In our hospital, all implantable devices require intubation. Therefore the chosen treatment did not increase the risk for the patient.

Regarding MRI incompatibility, in the last years, results from extensive testing for MRI safety were published and a 1.5 T MRI examination can be performed on VSB users at a calculated risk [27]. The patient's parents were extensively informed of the possibility of transducer dislocation after exposure to a magnetic field over 1.5 T, and the choice to proceed with an MRI was made with all of the risks considered. If the patient will undergo an MRI examination image artefacts will be seen in proximity of the implant. This is a known issue that even cochlear implant users need to face. We would like to emphasize that the patient does not have a neurological development disorder or a pathology which would require regular MRIs.

Competing Interests

To reiterate, we had no conflict of interests and no funding from private companies.

References

[1] I. J. Kruyt, A. L. Mc Dermott, and M. K. S. Hol, "Comment on 'original solution for middle ear implant and anesthetic/surgical management in a child with severe craniofacial dysmorphism,'" *Case Reports in Otolaryngology*, vol. 2016, Article ID 2859051, 6 pages, 2016.

[2] G. Bianchin, L. Tribi, A. Reverzani, P. Formigoni, and V. Polizzi, "Original solution for middle ear implant and anesthetic/surgical management in a child with severe craniofacial dysmorphism," *Case Reports in Otolaryngology*, vol. 2015, Article ID 205972, 4 pages, 2015.

[3] D. C. Shonka Jr., W. J. Livingston III, and B. W. Kesser, "The Jahrsdoerfer grading scale in surgery to repair congenital aural atresia," *Archives of Otolaryngology—Head and Neck Surgery*, vol. 134, no. 8, pp. 873–877, 2008.

[4] K. Amonoo-Kuofi, A. Kelly, M. Neeff, and C. R. S. Brown, "Experience of bone-anchored hearing aid implantation in children younger than 5 years of age," *International Journal of Pediatric Otorhinolaryngology*, vol. 79, no. 4, pp. 474–480, 2015.

[5] R. Kiringoda and L. R. Lustig, "A meta-analysis of the complications associated with osseointegrated hearing aids," *Otology and Neurotology*, vol. 34, no. 5, pp. 790–794, 2013.

[6] A. Ernst, I. Todt, and J. Wagner, "Safety and effectiveness of the Vibrant Soundbridge in treating conductive and mixed hearing loss: a systematic review," *Laryngoscope*, vol. 6, pp. 1451–1457, 126.

[7] L. Tietze and B. Papsin, "Utilization of bone-anchored hearing aids in children," *International Journal of Pediatric Otorhinolaryngology*, vol. 58, no. 1, pp. 75–80, 2001.

[8] S. Lloyd, J. Almeyda, K. S. Sirimanna, D. M. Albert, and C. M. Bailey, "Updated surgical experience with bone-anchored hearing aids in children," *Journal of Laryngology and Otology*, vol. 121, no. 9, pp. 826–831, 2007.

[9] A.-L. McDermott, J. Williams, M. Kuo, A. Reid, and D. Proops, "The birmingham pediatric bone-anchored hearing aid program: a 15-year experience," *Otology and Neurotology*, vol. 30, no. 2, pp. 178–183, 2009.

[10] T. Davids, K. A. Gordon, D. Clutton, and B. C. Papsin, "Bone-anchored hearing aids in infants and children younger than 5 years," *Archives of Otolaryngology—Head and Neck Surgery*, vol. 133, no. 1, pp. 51–55, 2007.

[11] A. Tjellstrom, J. Lindstrom, O. Hallen, T. Albrektsson, and P. I. Brånemark, "Osseointegrated titanium implants in the

temporal bone. A clinical study on bone-anchored hearing aids," *American Journal of Otology*, vol. 2, no. 4, pp. 304–310, 1981.

[12] M. J. F. De Wolf, M. K. S. Hol, P. L. M. Huygen, E. A. M. Mylanus, and C. W. R. J. Cremers, "Nijmegen results with application of a bone-anchored hearing aid in children: simplified surgical technique," *Annals of Otology, Rhinology and Laryngology*, vol. 117, no. 11, pp. 805–814, 2008.

[13] S. P. Cass and P. A. Mudd, "Bone-anchored hearing devices: indications, outcomes, and the linear surgical technique," *Operative Techniques in Otolaryngology—Head and Neck Surgery*, vol. 21, no. 3, pp. 197–206, 2010.

[14] G. Santarelli, R. E. Redfern, and A. G. Benson, "Bone-anchored hearing aid implantation in a patient with Goldenhar syndrome," *Ear, Nose & Throat Journal*, vol. 94, no. 12, pp. E1–E3, 2015.

[15] N. C. Bodnia, S. Foghsgaard, M. N. Møller, and P. Cayé-Thomasen, "Long-term results of 185 consecutive osseointegrated hearing device implantations: a comparison among children, adults, and elderly," *Otology and Neurotology*, vol. 35, no. 10, pp. e301–e306, 2014.

[16] C. A. den Besten, E. Harterink, A.-L. McDermott, and M. K. S. Hol, "Clinical results of Cochlear™ BIA300 in children: experience in two tertiary referral centers," *International Journal of Pediatric Otorhinolaryngology*, vol. 79, no. 12, pp. 2050–2055, 2015.

[17] W. Gawęcki, O. M. Stieler, A. Balcerowiak et al., "Surgical, functional and audiological evaluation of new Baha Attract system implantations," *European Archives of Oto-Rhino-Laryngology*, vol. 273, no. 10, pp. 3123–3130, 2016.

[18] P. Z. Sheehan and P. S. Hans, "UK and Ireland experience of bone anchored hearing aids (BAHA®) in individuals with Down syndrome," *International Journal of Pediatric Otorhinolaryngology*, vol. 70, no. 6, pp. 981–986, 2006.

[19] A.-L. McDermott, J. Williams, M. J. Kuo, A. P. Reid, and D. W. Proops, "The role of bone anchored hearing aids in children with Down syndrome," *International Journal of Pediatric Otorhinolaryngology*, vol. 72, no. 6, pp. 751–757, 2008.

[20] A.-L. McDermott, J. Barraclough, and A. P. Reid, "Unusual complication following trauma to a bone-anchored hearing aid: case report and literature review," *The Journal of Laryngology & Otology*, vol. 123, no. 3, pp. 348–350, 2009.

[21] T. Deitmer, M. Kraßort, and S. Hartmann, "Two rare complications in patients with bone-anchored hearing aids," *Laryngo-Rhino-Otologie*, vol. 82, no. 3, pp. 162–165, 2003.

[22] M. Scholz, H. Eufinger, A. Anders et al., "Intracerebral abscess after abutment change of a bone anchored hearing aid (BAHA)," *Otology and Neurotology*, vol. 24, no. 6, pp. 896–899, 2003.

[23] F. B. Mesfin, N. W. Perkins, C. Brook, D. Foyt, and J. W. German, "Epidural hematoma after tympanomastoidectomy and bone-anchored hearing aid (BAHA) placement: case report," *Neurosurgery*, vol. 67, no. 5, pp. E1451–E1453, 2010.

[24] M. Leinung, E. Zaretsky, B. P. Lange, V. Hoffmann, T. Stöver, and C. Hey, "Vibrant Soundbridge® in preschool children with unilateral aural atresia: acceptance and benefit," *European Archives of Oto-Rhino-Laryngology*, 2016.

[25] K. Böheim, A. Nahler, and M. Schlögel, "Rehabilitation of high frequency hearing loss: use of an active middle ear implant," *HNO*, vol. 55, no. 9, pp. 690–695, 2007.

[26] H. Frenzel, F. Hanke, M. Beltrame, and B. Wollenberg, "Application of the vibrant soundbridge in bilateral congenital atresia in toddlers," *Acta Oto-Laryngologica*, vol. 130, no. 8, pp. 966–970, 2010.

[27] J. H. Wagner, A. Ernst, and I. Todt, "Magnet resonance imaging safety of the vibrant soundbridge system: a review," *Otology and Neurotology*, vol. 32, no. 7, pp. 1040–1046, 2011.

43

Osteoradionecrosis of the Temporal Bone Leading to Cerebellar Abscess

Thomas B. Layton

Faculty of Life Sciences, University of Manchester, Manchester M13 9PL, UK

Correspondence should be addressed to Thomas B. Layton; thomasbenjaminlayton@gmail.com

Academic Editor: Frank R. Miller

Squamous cell carcinoma of the temporal bone is a rare and destructive malignancy and represents both diagnostic and therapeutic challenge. The complex regional anatomy of the temporal bone requires equally intricate surgical techniques to adequately resect the tumour mass during surgical excision. Adjuvant radiotherapy is offered to patients with advanced disease and has been showed to confer a survival benefit in carefully selected patients. One feared complication of radiotherapy is osteoradionecrosis and is a major obstacle faced in the treatment of head and neck cancers. The case presented here is a rare example of a patient who was successfully treated for SCC of the temporal with both surgical resection and adjuvant radiotherapy who subsequently developed two major complications: first, osteoradionecrosis of the temporal bone that leads to penetrating osteomyelitis; second, the formation of a large cerebellar abscess that required surgical drainage. This case is a rare example of the complications that are possible following radiotherapy to the head and the close follow-up that is required in patients.

1. Introduction

Squamous cell carcinoma (SCC) of the temporal bone was first described by Schwartze and Wilde in 1775, but it was not until 1917 when the first large scale review was published by Newhart [1, 2]. SCC of the temporal bone is a rare tumour with a reported incidence of between 1 and 6 cases per million population per year [3]. It accounts for less than 0.2% of all tumours of the head and neck but is the most common neoplasm in the external auditory canal [3]. SSC of the temporal bone is a tumour known for its relatively late and nebulous clinical presentation, as well as an aggressive tendency for local invasion [3]. Although strict risk factors for the disease have not been well established, chronic suppurative otitis media, cholesteatoma, and a history of radiation exposure have all been implicated [3]. Other putative risk factors are smoking and alcohol abuse. In a large study of patients diagnosed between 1945 and 2005 Gidley et al. (2009) stated that the mean patient age was 62 years (median, 63 years; range 21–89 years) and that the 5-year overall survival rate was 48% for early-stage disease and 28% for patients with late-stage disease [3]. In addition, Moffat et al. (2005) reported 80–100% five-year survival rates in patients who had successful primary surgical resection, with or without adjuvant radiotherapy [4].

In terms of management, a plethora of surgical techniques are available to combat the variable locations and sizes of the tumour mass: mastoidectomy, lateral and extended lateral temporal bone resection, and pinnectomy. The standard description is one of either standard or extended mastoidectomy with the later including a parotidectomy [5]. It has been suggested that a parotidectomy is mandatory for control of occult parotid node metastases and for optimizing adequate resection margins [5].

Adjuvant radiotherapy is offered to patients with locally advanced disease and has been shown to be beneficial [5]. The mean postoperative adjuvant radiotherapy given is 58.0 Gy (range, 29.6–75.0 Gy) to the primary tumour site and 49.5 Gy (range, 10.5–75.0 Gy) to the neck. Although radiotherapy offers a survival advantage in some well-selected patients it is not without the potential for significant morbidity [5]. One of feared sequelae of radiotherapy is radiation-induced bone injury, the most serious of which is osteoradionecrosis. This disease leads to the destruction of bone and by forming necrotic areas produces an ideal environment for bacterial colonisation and infection. It can also produce debilitating symptoms for patients including profuse and pulsatile otor-rhoea and significant pain as well as leading to rare but potentially life threatening intracranial complication such as meningitis and abscess formation [6].

2. Case Report

A 50-year-old female presented with a four-month history right-sided headaches with occasional bloody otorrhoea. The patient had been treated with a mastoidectomy twenty years previous to chronic suppurative otitis media and a cholesteatoma but had no symptoms following her surgery. Past medical history included a schizophreniform disor-der and Barrett's oesophagus under surveillance. Otoscopy revealed a mass within the middle ear and a biopsy confirmed moderately differentiated squamous cell carcinoma. A stag-ing CT scan established that there was no distant metastatic disease and that the tumour was confined to the temporal bone. The TNM staging of the tumour was T3N2M0. A radical right mastoidectomy was performed that involved the removal of posterior and superior canal wall, meatoplasty, and exteriorisation of middle ear. At the time of surgery it appeared that the carcinoma was arising from the middle ear cleft and extending up to an eroded patch of tegmen. This was easily cleared but the eustachian tube orifice appeared widened and biopsy confirmed the presence of squamous carcinoma. In the hope of clearing residual disease the patient was offered adjuvant radiotherapy. The patient exhibited a good response to radiotherapy and showed a complete remission.

After treatment the patient was reviewed regularly at follow-up. Eleven months later the area of irradiated mastoid bone developed osteoradionecrosis (ORN) and periodically became infected. The initial diagnosis was made following a head and neck CT scan with intravenous contrast. The indica-tion for imaging was a two- to three-week history of increas-ing pain adjacent to the surgical site and it was initially feared that this might have represented recurrent malignant disease. The radiological features included slight erosion and sclerosis of the adjacent temporal bone, no mass lesions, and mastoid opacification. It must be noted that the radiological features of ORN are often challenging to discriminate between malig-nancies, particularly in patients with a past history of cancer. The ORN was initially treated conservatively with regular local irrigation, analgesia, and antibiotics for episodes of infection. Repeated local cultures and blood cultures did not grow any organisms. After several months a CT head revealed a sequestrum in the temporal bone overlying the facial nerve and the patient suffered intermittent pain in the area of her ear that was treated with various analgesics including Tylex and amitriptyline. In addition a Tri-Adcortyl was inserted and Optomize was instilled into the external ear during episodes of infection. In addition, her mastoid cavity was periodically cleared through irrigation. The patient also suffered from recurrent episodes of labyrinthitis proposed to be caused by an exposed section of a semicircular canal adjacent to the sequestra of bone. These episodes were managed with vestibular sedatives and lasted only a few days. However, she did not suffer any significant hearing loss in either ear and

between attacks of labyrinthitis her vestibular function was preserved without any associated symptoms. Stemetil was prescribed and these attacks became less and less frequent over the next 12 months.

Two years after the patient's initial surgery the area of necrotic temporal bone developed into penetrating osteomy-elitis that lead to the formation of a $2\,cm^3$ cerebellar abscess abutting the area of infected bone. The initial presentation was one of worsening headaches and an urgent MRI head revealed the presence of the abscess. In addition, the MRI revealed the sequestrum within the temporal bone opacifica-tion of the temporal bone adjacent to the abscess. No mass lesions were noted on imaging. The patient had no other features of raised intracranial pressure. The temporal bone osteomyelitis and cerebellar abscess were treated with broad-spectrum IV antibiotics and surgical drainage and irrigation through a burr hole. Local wound cultures and peripheral blood cultures were negative but local wound cultures grew fully sensitive *Pseudomonas aeruginosa*. The procedure was uneventful and the patient made a full recovery without any lasting neurological deficit.

At the time of writing the patient has repeated foul smelling otorrhoea. Repeated microsuction and toileting of the mastoid is performed during follow-up appointments every 3 to 6 months. Moreover, antibiotics are given when infections develop including Augmentin.

3. Discussion

Squamous cell carcinoma of the temporal bone is a rare and invasive tumour. Surgical resection is crucial as a treatment modality, and early surgical intervention is associated with an increased survival [3]. The patient presented here was treated with a radical mastoidectomy and adjuvant radiotherapy. At 17 years postoperatively there is no evidence of tumour recurrence so it appears that treatment was sufficient in controlling the disease. The plethora of surgical techniques available mandate a clear rationale when selecting a treatment strategy that aims to balance postoperative morbidity with adequate resection of the tumour.

An interesting feature of this care report is the patient's past history of chronic suppurative otitis media (CSOM) and previous mastoidectomy 13 years ago. Wierzbick et al. (2008) described a similar case in which a 67-year-old patient developed SCC in the postoperative cave 50 years after being operated on for a cholesteatoma [7]. CSOM has been pro-posed as a potential aetiological factor in middle ear cancer and the case here is an example that supports this hypothesis. The association between the two remains unclear and is yet to be studied in detail [8]. An important point is the need to con-sider any new symptoms such as severe earache and bleeding with suspicion in a patient with a history of CSOM. Early diagnosis of malignancy in such a case rests on a high index of suspicion and a thorough investigation that should always include multiple biopsies of the abnormal areas. Vikram et al. (2006) described three patients that had SCC of the middle ear with concurrent cholesteatoma and otitis media. This illustrates the importance of obtaining a sufficient histological specimen, as malignant cells can be found adjacent to area of both inflammation and infection [8].

SCC of the temporal bone is a tumour capable of significant local invasion and the use of adjuvant radiotherapy can lead to further weakening of the bone. The complexity of the anatomy of this region means that several delicate structures can be damaged including the middle and inner ear. This can produce debilitating symptoms for patients including hearing loss, vertigo, and tinnitus. The patient presented is a clear example of how disease complications arising from the temporal bone affected by radiotherapy can be significant morbidity. The patient suffered from recurrent episodes of severe labyrinthitis with one episode requiring hospital admission. Moreover, she developed recurrent headaches that were debilitating and significantly impacted upon her quality of life. She also has had multiple episodes of otitis and at present has a chronically discharging ear that requires repeated treatment. A challenge in managing patients with temporal bone SCC is balancing adequate surgical resection with the need for adjuvant radiotherapy. A more extensive surgical resection may reduce the need for radiotherapy but may also comprise the integrity of the remaining temporal bone structures. It is likely that surgical excision is likely to be tailored to an individual patient and will reflect not only the experience of the surgeon, but also the grade and stage of the tumour.

The most severe consequence of this was the development of osteomyelitis of the temporal bone that leads to the formation of a cerebellar abscess. Otogenic brain abscesses carry a high mortality rate and are one of many intracranial complications of osteoradionecrosis including meningitis, sigmoid sinus thrombosis, subdural empyema, perisinus abscess, and transverse and cavernous sinus thrombosis [6]. As part of the patient's follow-up it is paramount to screen for evidence not only of recurrence of the tumour, but also of any burgeoning infection and if detected antibiotics must be considered promptly.

4. Conclusion

Squamous cell carcinoma of the middle ear represents both diagnostic and surgical challenge and the case presented here provides a positive outcome with regard to the long-term survival following treatment. However, it also illustrates the significant impact that can follow this malignancy and its treatment. Osteoradionecrosis can have a great impact on a patient's well-being acutely with the potential for life threatening intracranial complications but also chronic symptoms that can severely hinder a patient's quality of life.

Competing Interests

The author declares that there is no conflict of interests regarding the publication of this paper.

References

[1] J. C. Peele and C. H. Hauser, "Primary carcinoma of the external auditory canal and middle ear," *Archives of Otolaryngology*, vol. 34, no. 2, pp. 254–266, 1941.

[2] H. Newhart, "Primary carcinoma of the middue-ear; report of a case," *Laryngoscope*, vol. 27, no. 7, pp. 543–555, 1917.

[3] P. W. Gidley, D. B. Roberts, and E. M. Sturgis, "Squamous cell carcinoma of the temporal bone," *Laryngoscope*, vol. 120, no. 6, pp. 1144–1151, 2009.

[4] D. A. Moffat, S. A. Wagstaff, and D. G. Hardy, "The outcome of radical surgery and postoperative radiotherapy for squamous carcinoma of the temporal bone," *Laryngoscope*, vol. 115, no. 2, pp. 341–347, 2005.

[5] S. C. Leong, A. Youssef, and T. H. Lesser, "Squamous cell carcinoma of the temporal bone: outcomes of radical surgery and postoperative radiotherapy," *Laryngoscope*, vol. 123, no. 10, pp. 2442–2448, 2013.

[6] L. Migirov, S. Duvdevani, and J. Kronenberg, "Otogenic intracranial complications: a review of 28 cases," *Acta Oto-Laryngologica*, vol. 125, no. 8, pp. 819–822, 2005.

[7] M. Wierzbick, W. Gawecki, M. Leszczyńska, and T. Kopeć, "Middle ear cancer hidden by chronic otitis media—a case report," *Otolaryngologia Polska*, vol. 62, no. 6, pp. 797–799, 2008.

[8] B. Vikram, S. Saimanohar, and G. Narayanaswamy, "Is squamous cell carcinoma of the middle ear a complication of chronic suppurative otitis media?" *The Internet Journal of Otorhinolaryngology*, vol. 6, no. 1, 2006.

44

Nonodontogenic Cervical Necrotizing Fasciitis Caused by Sialadenitis

Alper Yenigun,[1] **Bayram Veyseller,**[2] **Omer Vural,**[1] **and Orhan Ozturan**[1]

[1]*Department of Otorhinolaryngology, Faculty of Medicine, Bezmialem Vakif University, Fatih, Istanbul, Turkey*
[2]*Department of Otorhinolaryngology, Faculty of Medicine, Acibadem University, Istanbul, Turkey*

Correspondence should be addressed to Alper Yenigun; alperyenigun@gmail.com

Academic Editor: M. Tayyar Kalcioglu

Necrotizing fasciitis is a rapidly progressive infectious disease of the soft tissue with high mortality and morbidity rates. Necrotizing fasciitis is occasionally located in the head and neck region and develops after odontogenic infections. Factors affecting treatment success rates are early diagnosis, appropriate antibiotic treatment, and surgical debridement. We present a necrotizing fasciitis case located in the neck region that developed after sialoadenitis. It is important to emphasize that necrotizing fasciitis to be seen in the neck region is very rare. Nonodontogenic necrotizing fasciitis is even more rare.

1. Introduction

The term necrotizing fasciitis was described initially by Wilson in the 1950s [1]. Necrotizing fasciitis is a rapid spreading disease of the soft tissue, which includes the superficial fascia and subcutaneous layer of tissue [2–4]. Necrotizing fasciitis is associated with some situations in which the immune system is compromised, including diabetes mellitus (DM), elderly, acute, or chronic renal disease, postpartum period, alcoholism, intravenous (IV) drug use, malnutrition, malignancy, peripheral vascular disease, and radiation exposure [5]. Necrotizing fasciitis diagnosis is based on certain clinical features that include fulminant progression, presence of grey-black necrotic area, and easy separation of the superficial layers of the underlying tissue [2, 6]. Necrotizing fasciitis can emerge from a local infection region after a minor trauma, which leads to the entrance of site of the infection. The exact etiology of one-third of the necrotizing fasciitis patients is not clear [2, 3, 6]. If necrotizing fasciitis is not diagnosed and treated early, it is potentially a fatal disease [4, 7, 8]. This situation is based on the absence of early clinical findings, rapid progression of the disease, and the delay of surgical intervention [9]. Therefore, experience in the diagnosis and treatment of necrotizing fasciitis is quite limited. Involvement of the head and neck region is quite rare

for necrotizing fasciitis patients [2]. In this region there are two types of necrotizing fasciitis and they include cervical and craniofacial involvement [10]. Mortality rates of cervical necrotizing fasciitis range from 7% to 20% depending on the width of the cervical lesion [11]. This case report is presented because, unlike most of the others, this case of necrotizing fasciitis is nonodontogenic, sialoadenitis induced cervical necrotizing fasciitis.

2. Case Report

A 66-year-old male patient with complaints of fever, neck swelling, redness, and shortness of breath was admitted to the emergency department and on examination an edematous area was seen in the hyperemic region starting from the right submandibular area, spreading to the mastoid apex, right neck, and sternum. There was no known diabetes or immune deficiency in this case. Physical examination revealed a medium hard and crepitating swelling that was approximately 10 cm in dimension and was larger in the right side of the neck. On laryngoscope examination the vocal cords were edematous and had normal movement. Laboratory examination revealed a white blood cell (WBC) count of 24000/mm^3 (neutrophils were prominent); sedimentation rate of 76 mm/h; C-reactive protein (CRP) of

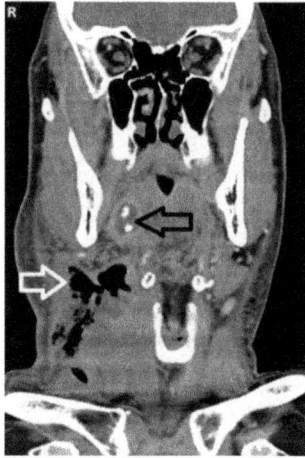

FIGURE 1: Coronal neck CT image showing cervical subcutaneous gas (white arrow) and right inflamed submandibular gland region with ductal stones (black arrow).

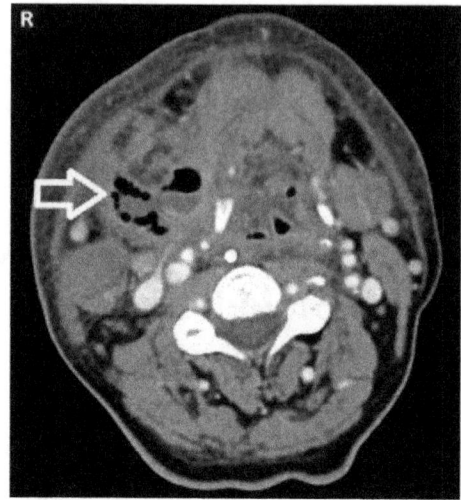

FIGURE 2: Axial neck CT image showing cervical subcutaneous gas (white arrow).

31.9 mg/dL. Noticeably soft tissue edema was found in the neck ultrasound. Neck and thorax computed tomography (CT) showed right submandibular sialoadenitis and abscess induced by an intraductal stone. Widespread emphysema and edema were seen in the neck and mediastinum (Figures 1–3). Considering these findings, necrotizing fasciitis was thought to be the diagnosis and the patient underwent wide cervical and thoracic debridement with exploration of the neck after the initiation of parenteral ampicillin 4 * 1 gr for Gram-positive and Gram-negative bacteria, metronidazole 4 * 0.5 gr for anaerobic organisms, and supportive therapy. The right submandibular gland was excised. After debridement the defect was left for secondary healing. In addition, 20 sessions of hyperbaric oxygen therapy were applied at 2.5 atmospheres (ATA) for 150 minutes. Mixed oropharyngeal flora prominent with anaerobic organisms was seen in the microbiologic examination of the pathology specimen. The patient did not develop any complications and the skin defects were covered completely with secondary healing during follow-up.

3. Discussion

Meleney described subcutaneous tissue necrosis caused by streptococcus in 1924 and used the term of "streptococcal gangrene" [12]. It is known that necrotizing fasciitis shows different behavior in each area. Necrotizing fasciitis is divided into two subgroups in the head and neck region. The first group involves the eyelids and scalp, with infection generally developing after trauma. The second group is seen rarely and shows involvement of the face and neck. Although the most common etiologic cause is dental infections, other reasons include trauma, peritonsillar abscess, osteoradionecrosis, infections of the tonsils or the pharynx, injury, foreign bodies, cervical adenitis, surgical wounds, tumors, and salivary glands [11, 13]. In addition to these, sialoadenitis with ductal stones may lead to necrotizing fasciitis by forming abscess [11]. In our case, sialoadenitis with ductal stones was

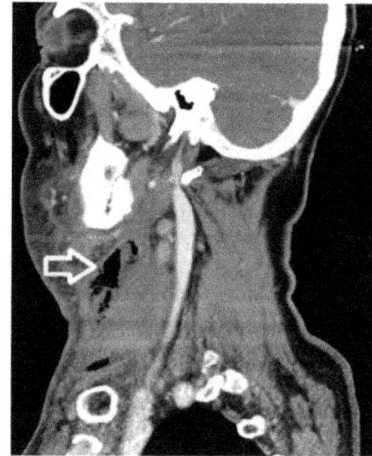

FIGURE 3: Sagittal neck CT image showing cervical subcutaneous gas (white arrow).

also responsible for the necrotizing fasciitis causing abscess formation.

In this group of patients the disease extends to the chest wall and mediastinum at a rate of 65%, while 27% are fatal [7, 14–17]. Necrotizing fasciitis can affect people of all age groups regardless of gender or race [14]. Appropriate radiological examination and thorough assessment of the airway should be done without delay in order to determine the severity of the disease. Subcutaneous gas and abscess formation can be seen by CT [18]. Surgical treatment includes drainage and excision of all necrotic tissue with a wide fasciotomy incision and exploration of facial region [18]. Medical treatment required is broad spectrum antibiotics with fluid and electrolyte replacement [18]. Taking the anaerobic microorganisms into consideration, the hyperbaric oxygen treatment can be applied as support. In our case, after extensive surgical debridement, 20 sessions of hyperbaric oxygen therapy were given at 2.5 ATA for 150 minutes.

In conclusion, it is important to emphasize that necrotizing fasciitis to be seen in the neck region is very rare. Nonodontogenic necrotizing fasciitis is even more rare. It should be kept in mind that necrotizing fasciitis can be progressive and lead to deadly complications; the medical and surgical treatment should be applied without wasting time.

Competing Interests

The authors declare that they have no competing interests.

References

[1] B. Wilson, "Necrotizing fasciitis," *The American Surgeon*, vol. 18, no. 4, pp. 416–431, 1952.

[2] V. Fung, Y. Rajapakse, and P. Longhi, "Periorbital necrotising fasciitis following cutaneous herpes zoster," *Journal of Plastic, Reconstructive & Aesthetic Surgery*, vol. 65, no. 1, pp. 106–109, 2012.

[3] G. Benavides, P. Blanco, and R. Pinedo, "Necrotizing fasciitis of the face: a report of one successfully treated case," *Otolaryngology—Head and Neck Surgery*, vol. 128, no. 6, pp. 894–896, 2003.

[4] R. A. Dale, D. S. Hoffman, R. O. Crichton, and S. B. Johnson, "Necrotizing fasciitis of the head and neck: review of the literature and report of a case," *Special Care in Dentistry*, vol. 19, no. 6, pp. 267–274, 2016.

[5] D. B. Safran and W. G. Sullivan, "Necrotizing fasciitis of the chest wall," *The Annals of Thoracic Surgery*, vol. 72, no. 4, pp. 1362–1364, 2001.

[6] G. Marioni, R. Bottin, A. Tregnaghi, M. Boninsegna, and A. Staffieri, "Craniocervical necrotizing fasciitis secondary to parotid gland abscess," *Acta Oto-Laryngologica*, vol. 123, no. 6, pp. 737–740, 2003.

[7] M. Umeda, T. Minamikawa, H. Komatsubara, Y. Shibuya, S. Yokoo, and T. Komori, "Necrotizing fasciitis caused by dental infection: a retrospective analysis of 9 cases and a review of the literature," *Oral Surgery, Oral Medicine, Oral Pathology, Oral Radiology, and Endodontics*, vol. 95, no. 3, pp. 283–290, 2003.

[8] Y. M. Liu, C. Y. Chi, M. W. Ho et al., "Microbiology and factors affecting mortality in necrotizing fasciitis," *Journal of Microbiology, Immunology, and Infection*, vol. 38, no. 6, pp. 430–435, 2005.

[9] C.-H. Wong and Y.-S. Wang, "The diagnosis of necrotizing fasciitis," *Current Opinion in Infectious Diseases*, vol. 18, no. 2, pp. 101–106, 2005.

[10] W.-J. Zhang, X.-Y. Cai, C. Yang et al., "Cervical necrotizing fasciitis due to methicillin-resistant *Staphylococcus aureus*: a case report," *International Journal of Oral and Maxillofacial Surgery*, vol. 39, no. 8, pp. 830–834, 2010.

[11] A. Suárez, M. Vicente, J. A. Tomás, L. M. Floría, J. Delhom, and M. C. Baquero, "Cervical necrotizing fasciitis of nonodontogenic origin: case report and review of literature," *The American Journal of Emergency Medicine*, vol. 32, no. 11, pp. 1441.e5–1441.e6, 2014.

[12] P. G. Djupesland, "Necrotizing fascitis of the head and neck—report of three cases and review of the literature," *Acta Oto-Laryngologica. Supplementum*, vol. 543, pp. 186–189, 2000.

[13] I. L. Feinerman, H. K. K. Tan, D. W. Roberson, R. Malley, and M. A. Kenna, "Necrotizing fasciitis of the pharynx following adenotonsillectomy," *International Journal of Pediatric Otorhinolaryngology*, vol. 48, no. 1, pp. 1–7, 1999.

[14] V. Sasindran and A. Joseph, "Necrotizing fasciitis: an unusual presentation," *Indian Journal of Otolaryngology and Head & Neck Surgery*, vol. 63, no. 4, pp. 390–392, 2011.

[15] M. Bulut, V. Balci, S. Akköse, and E. Armağan, "Fatal descending necrotising mediastinitis," *Emergency Medicine Journal*, vol. 21, no. 1, pp. 122–123, 2004.

[16] L. Krenk, H. U. Nielsen, and M. E. Christensen, "Necrotizing fasciitis in the head and neck region: an analysis of standard treatment effectiveness," *European Archives of Oto-Rhino-Laryngology*, vol. 264, no. 8, pp. 917–922, 2007.

[17] W. Tung-Yiu, H. Jehn-Shyun, C. Ching-Hung, and C. Hung-An, "Cervical necrotizing fasciitis of odontogenic origin: a report of 11 cases," *Journal of Oral and Maxillofacial Surgery*, vol. 58, no. 12, pp. 1347–1352, 2000.

[18] R. L. Scher, "Hyperbaric oxygen therapy for necrotizing cervical infections," *Advances in Oto-Rhino-Laryngology*, vol. 54, pp. 50–58, 1998.

45

Recurrent Massive Epistaxis from an Anomalous Posterior Ethmoid Artery

Marco Giuseppe Greco, Francesco Mattioli, Maria Paola Alberici, and Livio Presutti

Unità Operativa Complessa di Otorinolaringoiatria, Azienda Ospedaliero-Universitaria Policlinico di Modena, Italy Via del Pozzo 71, 41124 Modena, Italy

Correspondence should be addressed to Marco Giuseppe Greco; marcogreco81@libero.it

Academic Editor: Marco Berlucchi

A 50-year-old man, with no previous history of epistaxis, was hospitalized at our facility for left recurrent posterior epistaxis. The patient underwent surgical treatment three times and only the operator's experience and radiological support (cranial angiography) allowed us to control the epistaxis and stop the bleeding. The difficult bleeding management and control was attributed to an abnormal course of the left posterior ethmoidal artery. When bleeding seems to come from the roof of the nasal cavity, it is important to identify the ethmoid arteries always bearing in mind the possible existence of anomalous courses.

1. Introduction

Epistaxis is the most common emergency encountered by the otolaryngologist-head and neck surgeon and affects all age groups, although with different incidence rates. It is most common before age 10 and between ages 45 and 65 years [1, 2].

Nasal packing usually provides good control of epistaxis but sometimes, especially in arterial bleeding, surgical treatment represents the only available treatment and can be particularly troublesome, even for experienced surgeons [3].

We report an unusual case of epistaxis arising from the left posterior ethmoid artery, which presented an abnormal course.

Control of epistaxis was particularly difficult and was only achieved after three surgical interventions.

2. Case Report

We report the case of a 50-year-old man affected by hypertension and chronic ischemic heart disease with no previous history of epistaxis and who we hospitalized at our facility for left recurrent posterior epistaxis.

During the 6 days before hospitalization, the patient had attended the emergency room of our otolaryngology department on a number of occasions for recurrent left

epistaxis: two times for left nasal packing with two Merocel® Standard dressings; once for nasal packing with one Merocel Standard dressing in the right fossa and one Rapid Rhino® + Tabotamp® in the left fossa. On the following day, after further bleeding, he was hospitalized after nasal packing with one Merocel Standard dressing in the right fossa and a Bivona® Silicone Epistaxis Catheter in the left fossa.

During the previous epistaxis, we noted a major source of bleeding that seemed to come from the roof of the nasal fossa. Another significant element was the onset of bleeding: it was sudden and violent but discontinuous. The patient did not present any coagulation disorders and blood pressure had always remained in the normal range.

On the following day, the patient first underwent cerebral and maxillofacial computed tomography (CT) with normal results. Angio-CT of the carotid and cerebral circulation did not reveal intracranial vascular malformations or the presence of vascular aneurysms.

Meanwhile, as a result of the violent nose bleeding, the patient's hemoglobin level continued to fall until it reached 8.9 g/dL; for this reason, he underwent surgery. We removed the nasal swabs previously placed. From nasal endoscopy, we noticed the presence of widespread mucosal bleeding from the roof of the left nasal cavity but could not identify the source of bleeding. We aspirated clots and cauterized the

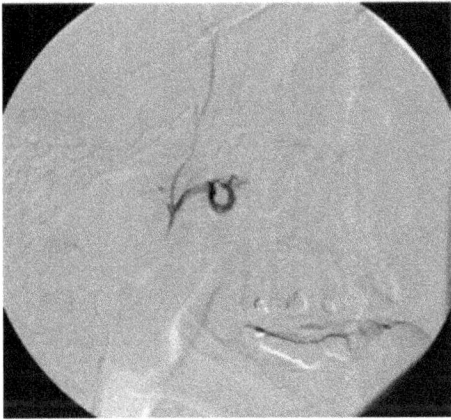

FIGURE 1: Left internal maxillary artery embolization.

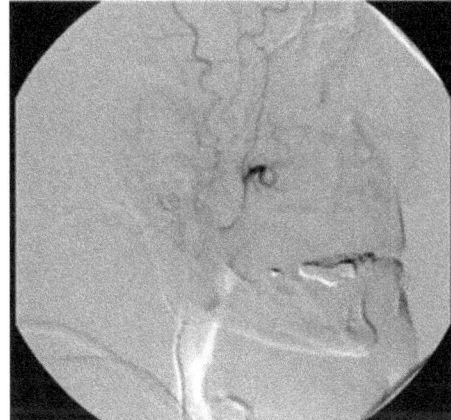

FIGURE 2: Persistent nosebleeds after embolization.

inferior turbinate. We then removed the head of the middle turbinate to better visualize the back of the nasal cavity. We performed middle meatal antrostomy, identification of the posterior wall of the maxillary sinus, and identification of the sphenopalatine artery and its cauterization. Anterior ethmoidectomy with nasal packing was then carried out. There was no bleeding upon awakening.

The next day, further surgical treatment was required for left recurrent epistaxis. Under endoscopic control, the surgeon removed the nasal swabs and several washes were performed to remove clots. Left posterior ethmoidectomy was completed. The arterial bleeding seemed to originate from the ethmoid roof. The anterior ethmoid artery was isolated from its bony shell so as to perform accurate cauterization of the artery. At the end of the procedure, there was no further epistaxis and blood pressure was normal (120/80 mmHg).

On the following day, a new violent left epistaxis occurred which resolved spontaneously after a few minutes. Given the context, we planned urgent angiography to exclude the presence of vascular malformations, abnormal arterial courses, or serious injury to the internal carotid artery in the sphenoid sinus.

The exam was performed 2 days later by femoral selective catheterization of the internal and external carotid arteries bilaterally. The onset of epistaxis was noted during the exam, and so the radiologist performed embolization of both internal maxillary arteries (Figures 1 and 2) and the left facial artery with injection of polyvinyl alcohol particles (500 μm) but did not achieve control of the bleeding. Selective catheterization of the internal carotid artery bilaterally showed significant ethmoid vascularization by branches from the ophthalmic artery (anterior and posterior ethmoid arteries) with small irregularities of the branches (Figure 3).

On the same day, the patient underwent surgery a further time. Also on this occasion, bleeding seemed to originate from the ethmoid roof. During this last revision surgery we found the remains of the anterior ethmoid artery cauterized above the roof of the ethmoid; we closed the anterior ethmoid artery with clips (Figure 4), then, using an endoscope, we explored the sphenoid sinus. Here we found that the posterior ethmoid artery presented an abnormal path, located between

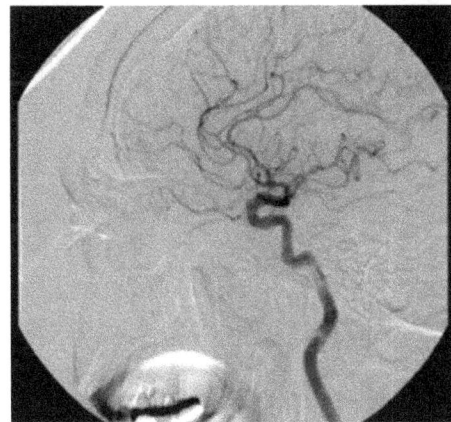

FIGURE 3: Ethmoid vascularization by branches from the left ophthalmic artery.

the canal of the optic nerve and the carotid canal (Figures 5 and 6); at this level, there was a small dehiscence responsible for the bleeding. The artery was covered by a bony shell along its intrasinual course which made thermal cauterization with bipolar forceps impractical so the artery was cauterized using a diamond drill and this achieved control of the bleeding (Figures 7 and 8).

3. Discussion

Posterior bleeding (10%) usually originates from the sphenopalatine artery (terminal branch of the internal maxillary artery) or from its branches or, more rarely, from the anterior or posterior ethmoid arteries, branches of the ophthalmic artery [4, 5].

The posterior ethmoidal artery (PEA) originates from the ophthalmic artery, but in the posterior third of the orbit. Many anatomical variations frequently occur at the origin of the PEA (86%) [6, 7]. The PEA can also originate from the third part of the ophthalmic artery (5%), or from the second part of the ophthalmic artery (5%). At its origin, it runs between the rectus superior and the superior oblique muscle and then emerges from the myofascial cone of the orbit to finally pass perpendicular to the medial wall and enter

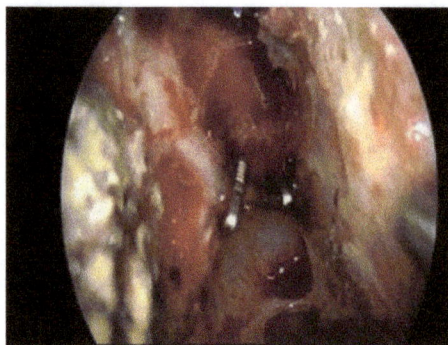

FIGURE 4: Endoscopic image: anterior ethmoid artery: closure with metal clips.

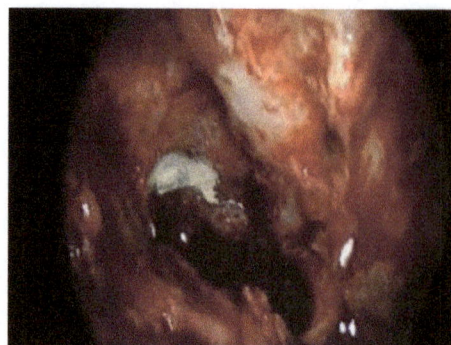

FIGURE 5: Endoscopic image: posterior ethmoidal artery in its bony shell.

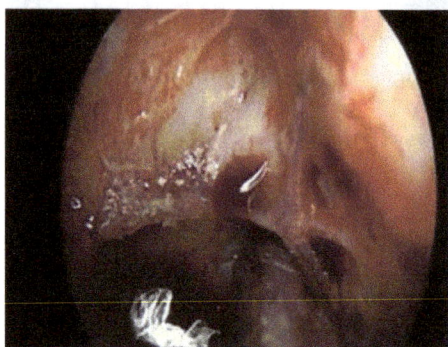

FIGURE 6: Endoscopic image: posterior ethmoidal artery between the optic nerve and the carotid canal.

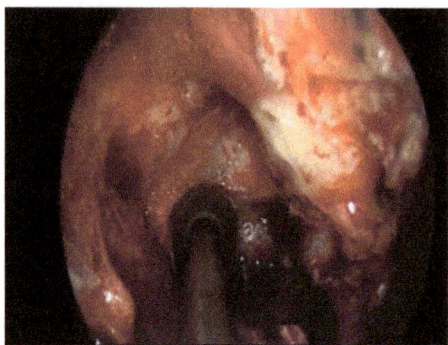

FIGURE 7: Endoscopic image: posterior ethmoidal artery: hemostasis with diamond drill.

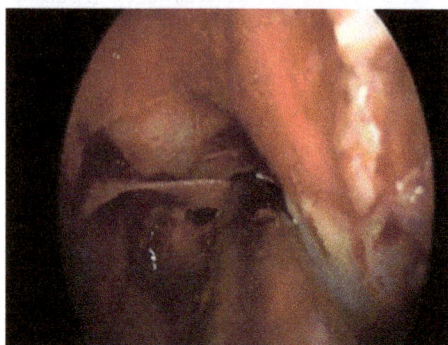

FIGURE 8: Endoscopic image: posterior ethmoidal artery: hemostasis with diamond drill.

the posterior ethmoidal canal (PEC); the PEA runs toward the medial orbital wall, crossing obliquely from the upper part of the superior oblique muscle and trochlear nerve [8]. On its intraorbital course, it follows a superior convex loop and ends up above the oblique muscle. The PEA has a small caliber, usually less than 1 mm, which makes its identification difficult in CT studies; the intraorbital part has a 0.66 ± 0.21 mm diameter and the intracranial part has a 0.45 ± 0.12 mm (range, 0.32 to 0.57 mm) diameter. In the study by Tomkinson et al. [1, 2], they could identify the PEA in only 14/40 nasal fossae.

Then PEA crosses the roof of the ethmoid labyrinth inside the homonymous canal 2-3 mm from the anterior wall of the sphenoid sinus. PEA into its canal presents a more horizontal orientation than that of the AEA with an entry angle into the skull base of between 0° and 18° [9]. During nasal surgery, it is very important to remember that the PEA runs very close to the optic nerve: the distance between the two structures is variable and can range from 4 to 16 mm; for this reason, extreme care is required during approaches that require working in this territory. A damage to the artery may cause hemorrhages resulting in a surgical eye emergency in cases where an orbital hematoma forms rapidly as a result of retraction of the lacerated artery into the orbit.

PEA is usually identified in its bony canal at the insertion of the partitioning roof of the middle turbinate but in our patient it presented an abnormal path: we found it into the lateral wall of the sphenoid sinus located between the canal of the optic nerve and the carotid canal; at this level, there was a small dehiscence responsible for the bleeding.

Surgical experience is very important especially in the management of complex cases of posterior epistaxis.

Radiological examinations represent an important aid but only if surgeons require specific and useful investigations: in our patient, angio-CT did not contribute to resolution of the case; on the contrary, it slowed the diagnostic process and subsequent surgical resolution.

On the contrary, the anatomical findings of the radiologist during angiography allowed the surgeon to focus his attention on the branches of the ophthalmic artery (anterior and posterior ethmoid arteries) and to identify the origin of the bleeding.

We must also emphasize that, in addition to its indisputable diagnostic value, angiography is the only radiological investigation that may be used for therapeutic purposes through selective catheterization and embolization of the bleeding vessel.

Finally, it is worth remembering the role of clinical observation. In most cases, arterial bleeding originates from the sphenopalatine artery or its branches, and its cauterization solves the problem. When bleeding seems to come from the roof of the nasal cavity, it is important to identify the ethmoid arteries always bearing in mind the possible existence of anomalous courses.

Ethical Approval

For this type of study, formal consent is not required. This article does not contain any studies with animals performed by any of the authors.

Consent

Informed consent was obtained from all individual participants included in the study.

Competing Interests

The authors declare that they have no conflict of interests.

References

[1] A. Tomkinson, D. G. Roblin, P. Flanagan et al., "Patterns of hospital attendance with epistaxis," *Rhinology*, vol. 35, pp. 129–135, 1997.

[2] L. Nikoyan and S. Matthews, "Epistaxis and hemostatic devices," *Oral and Maxillofacial Surgery Clinics of North America*, vol. 24, no. 2, pp. 219–228, 2012.

[3] R. Douglas and P.-J. Wormald, "Update on epistaxis," *Current Opinion in Otolaryngology and Head and Neck Surgery*, vol. 15, no. 3, pp. 180–183, 2007.

[4] M. Supriya, M. Shakeel, D. Veitch, and K. W. Ah-See, "Epistaxis: prospective evaluation of bleeding site and its impact on patient outcome," *Journal of Laryngology and Otology*, vol. 124, no. 7, pp. 744–749, 2010.

[5] S. W. McClurg and R. L. Carrau, "Endoscopic management of posterior epistaxis: a review," *Acta Otorhinolaryngologica Italica*, vol. 34, no. 1, pp. 1–8, 2014.

[6] J. Lang and K. Schäfer, "Arteriae ethmoidales: ursprung, verlauf versorgungsgebiete und anastomosen," *Cells Tissues Organs*, vol. 104, no. 2, pp. 183–197, 1979.

[7] I. Monjas-Cánovas, E. García-Garrigós, J. J. Arenas-Jiménez, J. Abarca-Olivas, F. Sánchez-Del Campo, and J. R. Gras-Albert, "Radiological anatomy of the ethmoidal arteries: CT cadaver study," *Acta Otorrinolaringologica Espanola*, vol. 62, no. 5, pp. 367–374, 2011.

[8] S. Erdogmus and F. Govsa, "The anatomic landmarks of ethmoidal arteries for the surgical approaches," *Journal of Craniofacial Surgery*, vol. 17, no. 2, pp. 280–285, 2006.

[9] J. K. Han, S. S. Becker, S. R. Bomeli, and C. W. Gross, "Endoscopic localization of the anterior and posterior ethmoid arteries," *Annals of Otology, Rhinology and Laryngology*, vol. 117, no. 12, pp. 931–935, 2008.

Filariasis of Stensen's Duct: An Index Case

Eishaan K. Bhargava,[1] **Nikhil Arora,**[1] **Varun Rai,**[1] **Ravi Meher,**[1]
Prerna Arora,[2] **and Ruchika Juneja**[1]

[1]*Department of Ent and Head and Neck Surgery, Maulana Azad Medical College, New Delhi, India*
[2]*Department of Pathology, Maulana Azad Medical College, New Delhi, India*

Correspondence should be addressed to Nikhil Arora; for_nikhilarora@yahoo.com

Academic Editor: Nicolas Perez-Fernandez

Filariasis, a neglected tropical disease, is a global health problem and is endemic to 73 countries including India. It is caused by nematodes of Filariodidea family, namely, *W. bancrofti* and *B. malayi* in India, which have a predilection for the lower limbs and testis. We report a never before reported case of filariasis of the main parotid duct in a 25-year-old male that resolved on medical management, exemplifying the importance of maintaining a high index of suspicion and careful examination of cytological smears in endemic countries, allowing for an early diagnosis and treatment, decreasing the morbidity of this debilitating disease.

1. Introduction

Filariasis, a neglected tropical disease, is a global health problem affecting 73 countries, including India, with a population of over 1.2 billion at risk for infection [1]. It is caused by infection with nematodes of the family Filariodidea, namely, *Wuchereria bancrofti* (90% cases), *Brugia malayi* (majority of remainder cases), and *B. timori* (rare), of which the former two are found in India. Although these parasites have a marked predilection for lower limb lymphatics, the epididymis, and the spermatic cord [2], they have also been reported to occur at unusual sites such as the thyroid gland [3], body fluids [4], skin [5], breast [6], and the oral or perioral region [7]. Salivary gland involvement is very rare and has been reported only once previously [8]. Here, we report a previously unreported case of filariasis of the parotid duct in a young adult male.

2. Case Report

A 25-year-old man, resident of Uttar Pradesh, presented to the otorhinolaryngology outpatient department with a painless swelling of the left cheek, gradually increasing in size since he first noticed it 1 year earlier. He gave a history of temporary increase in size of the swelling while eating, with subsequent return to previous size on completion of a meal. On examination, a 2 cm × 1.5 cm globular swelling was present just below the left malar prominence, which, on palpation, was nontender, euthermic, firm, and mobile in all directions with no fixity to skin or underlying tissues and a grossly normal overlying skin. The swelling increased in prominence when the patient was made to clench his teeth. He was afebrile, with no lymphadenopathy or organomegaly. His complete blood counts revealed absolute eosinophilia ($1100/mm^3$), with an essentially normal peripheral smear.

On ultrasonography, a cystic dilatation of the middle part of the left Stensen's duct was seen with minimal lobulated soft tissue contents and a mildly thickened duct wall. A contrast enhanced computed tomography scan was done that showed a small, well defined, hypodense cystic lesion superficial to the anterolateral aspect of the left masseter muscle indenting its surface, communicating with a tubular hypodense structure communicating with the parotid gland, suggestive of a dilated Stensen's duct with a sialocele formation (Figures 1(a) and 1(b)).

After clinical and radiological examination, the differential diagnosis that came to our mind was that it is either a sialolith blocking the duct that has lead to the inflammatory swelling or cysticercosis but further investigations showed a diagnosis which was very different and rare.

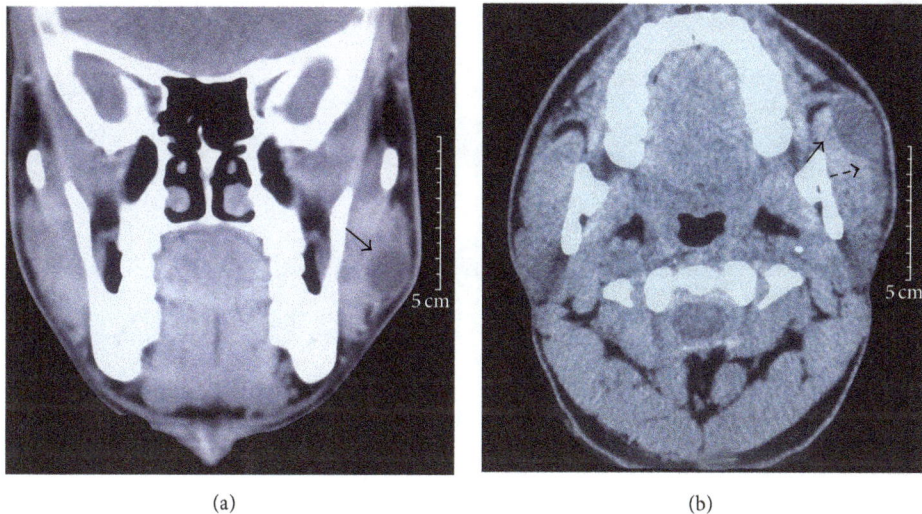

(a)   (b)

FIGURE 1: Coronal (a) and axial (b) cuts of computed tomography scan showing a small 2.2 cm × 1.5 cm, well defined, hypodense cystic lesion superficial to the anterolateral aspect of the left masseter muscle indenting its surface (solid arrow), communicating with a tubular hypodense structure (dashed arrow) communicating with the parotid gland, suggestive of a dilated Stensen's duct with a sialocele formation.

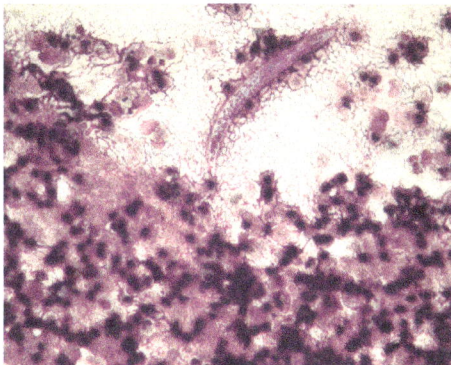

FIGURE 2: Fine needle aspiration cytology showing macrophages and nucleated squamous cells in a dense acute suppurative background with degenerated microfilariae.

Fine needle aspiration cytology (FNAC) revealed macrophages and nucleated squamous cells in a dense acute suppurative background with degenerated microfilariae, with no acid-fast bacilli (Figure 2).

On the basis of the radiological and cytological findings, a final diagnosis of filariasis of the parotid duct was made, and the patient was started on a two-week course of diethyl carbamazine, along with a five-day adjunctive course of albendazole.

On completion of the medical management, the patients symptoms were completely resolved, and he remains asymptomatic after 10 months of regular follow-up.

3. Discussion

Filariasis is a disfiguring and debilitating disease endemic to 73 nations worldwide, including India, with an estimated 600 million people at risk in 250 endemic districts of India, with the highest burden of disease in the states of Uttar Pradesh, Bihar, Jharkhand, Andhra Pradesh, Kerala, and Gujarat [9]. The causative organisms in India are mainly *W. bancrofti* and *B. malayi*, with subcutaneous filariasis caused by *Loa loa*, *Onchocerca volvulus*, and *Mansonella* [7].

Clinically apparent infection occurs only in a small proportion of infected individuals and may be classified either as *lymphatic filariasis*, caused by the presence of the parasite in the lymphatic system, or *occult filariasis*, due to an immune hyperresponsiveness of the host towards the parasite. In lymphatic filariasis, microfilariae may be found circulating in the bloodstream and may present in the acute phase as filarial fever, lymphangitis, lymphadenitis, and lymphedema. This would progress to the chronic phase over years, leading to permanent structural changes. Occult or cryptic filariasis refers to cases like ours where classical clinical signs of filariasis are absent with no circulating microfilariae. It is believed to be due to a hypersensitivity reaction to filarial antigens derived from microfilariae [8].

In the past, diagnosis of filariasis rested solely upon the demonstration of microfilariae in blood, making the definitive diagnosis tedious since blood samples would have to be taken at night between 2200 and 0400 hours [7].

FNAC has emerged as a useful diagnostic tool, used for the confirmatory diagnosis of suspected cases of filariasis, especially in cryptic cases where circulating microfilariae are absent, affecting the testis, epididymis, thyroid, breast, and subcutaneous nodules [7, 10]. The typical cytological picture comprises the detection of an adult worm or microfilarial form in a background of eosinophils, mononuclear cells, and neutrophils. It is usual to find associated epithelioid cell granulomas and giant cells, resulting in a diagnostic conundrum where mycobacterial infection needs to be ruled out using 20 and 5% Ziehl-Neelsen staining [7].

Filariasis may present in an unusual fashion in many different sites, ranging from subcutaneous nodules and thyroid gland filariasis to extremely rare cases like ours where salivary glands or their ducts are involved. This wide spectrum of unusual presentation necessitates a high index of suspicion and careful examination of cytological smears in endemic countries like ours. This rings true especially in this era of elimination of lymphatic filariasis (ELF), where the world is making extraordinary efforts to eliminate, and eventually eradicate, this disfiguring and debilitating disease that has been the cause for great mental, social, and economic loss to patients, contributing to stigma and poverty in the affected nations, including India. A timely diagnosis and management, as was done in the reported case, can not only alleviate one patient's suffering but also prevent the transmission of infection to many others, a small but important step towards the final goal of ELF.

Competing Interests

The authors declare that they have no competing interests.

References

[1] World Health Organisation, Fact sheet no. 102: Lymphatic filariasis, 2015, http://www.who.int/mediacentre/factsheets/fs102/en/.

[2] E. C. Faust, P. F. Russell, and R. C. Jung, *Craig and Faust's Clinical Parasitology*, Lea and Febiger, Philadelphia, Pa, USA, 7th edition, 1970.

[3] R. Meher, A. Garg, and S. Singh, "Microfilaria in thyroid gland fine needle aspiration cytology—an unusual finding," *Nigerian Journal of Otorhinolaryngology*, vol. 3, no. 1, pp. 36–38, 2006.

[4] R. Varghese, C. V. Raghuveer, M. R. Pai, and R. Bansal, "Microfilariae in cytologic smears: a report of six cases," *Acta Cytologica*, vol. 40, no. 2, pp. 299–301, 1996.

[5] A. G. Valand, B. S. Pandya, Y. V. Patil, and L. G. Patel, "Subcutaneous filariasis: an unusual case report," *Indian Journal of Dermatology*, vol. 52, no. 1, pp. 48–49, 2007.

[6] N. G. Singh and L. Chatterjee, "Filariasis of the breast, diagnosed by fine needle aspiration cytology," *Annals of Saudi Medicine*, vol. 29, no. 5, pp. 414–415, 2009.

[7] P. S. Naik, S. S. Tamboli, S. R. Agashe, P. P. Patil, and Y. Kale, "Cheek swelling: an unusual presentation of filariasis," *Journal of Vector Borne Diseases*, vol. 52, no. 3, pp. 270–272, 2015.

[8] K. K. Sahu, P. Pai, C. V. Raghuveer, and R. R. Pai, "Microfilaria in a fine needle aspirate from the salivary gland," *Acta Cytologica*, vol. 41, no. 3, p. 954, 1997.

[9] K. Park, *Park's Textbook of Preventive and Social Medicine*, Banrsidas Bhanot, Jabalpur, India, 23rd edition, 2015.

[10] S. K. Mitra, R. K. Mishra, and P. Verma, "Cytological diagnosis of microfilariae in filariasis endemic areas of eastern Uttar Pradesh," *Journal of Cytology*, vol. 26, no. 1, pp. 11–14, 2009.

Permissions

All chapters in this book were first published in CRIO, by Hindawi Publishing Corporation; hereby published with permission under the Creative Commons Attribution License or equivalent. Every chapter published in this book has been scrutinized by our experts. Their significance has been extensively debated. The topics covered herein carry significant findings which will fuel the growth of the discipline. They may even be implemented as practical applications or may be referred to as a beginning point for another development.

The contributors of this book come from diverse backgrounds, making this book a truly international effort. This book will bring forth new frontiers with its revolutionizing research information and detailed analysis of the nascent developments around the world.

We would like to thank all the contributing authors for lending their expertise to make the book truly unique. They have played a crucial role in the development of this book. Without their invaluable contributions this book wouldn't have been possible. They have made vital efforts to compile up to date information on the varied aspects of this subject to make this book a valuable addition to the collection of many professionals and students.

This book was conceptualized with the vision of imparting up-to-date information and advanced data in this field. To ensure the same, a matchless editorial board was set up. Every individual on the board went through rigorous rounds of assessment to prove their worth. After which they invested a large part of their time researching and compiling the most relevant data for our readers.

The editorial board has been involved in producing this book since its inception. They have spent rigorous hours researching and exploring the diverse topics which have resulted in the successful publishing of this book. They have passed on their knowledge of decades through this book. To expedite this challenging task, the publisher supported the team at every step. A small team of assistant editors was also appointed to further simplify the editing procedure and attain best results for the readers.

Apart from the editorial board, the designing team has also invested a significant amount of their time in understanding the subject and creating the most relevant covers. They scrutinized every image to scout for the most suitable representation of the subject and create an appropriate cover for the book.

The publishing team has been an ardent support to the editorial, designing and production team. Their endless efforts to recruit the best for this project, has resulted in the accomplishment of this book. They are a veteran in the field of academics and their pool of knowledge is as vast as their experience in printing. Their expertise and guidance has proved useful at every step. Their uncompromising quality standards have made this book an exceptional effort. Their encouragement from time to time has been an inspiration for everyone.

The publisher and the editorial board hope that this book will prove to be a valuable piece of knowledge for researchers, students, practitioners and scholars across the globe.

List of Contributors

Koji Otsuka
Department of Otorhinolaryngology, Tokyo Medical University, 6-7-1 Nishishinjuku, Shinjuku-ku, Tokyo 160-0023, Japan

Akihide Ichimura
Department of Otorhinolaryngology, Tokyo Medical University, 6-7-1 Nishishinjuku, Shinjuku-ku, Tokyo 160-0023, Japan
Ichimura ENT Clinic, 2-11-10 Nishiwaseda, Shinjuku-ku, Tokyo 169-0051, Japan

Richard Heyes, Ramkishan Balakumar, Krishan Ramdoo and Taran Tatla
Department of Otolaryngology-Head and Neck Surgery, Northwick Park Hospital,
London NorthWest Healthcare NHS Trust, London, UK

Ryan J. Bickley
Johns Hopkins University School of Medicine, Baltimore, MD, USA

Erik Cohen
Department of Otolaryngology, Morristown Medical Center, Morristown, NJ, USA

Danya Wenzler
Department of Infectious Diseases, Morristown Medical Center, Morristown, NJ, USA

Nancy Hunter
Department of Pathology, Morristown Medical Center, Morristown, NJ, USA

Donna Astiz
Department of Internal Medicine, Morristown Medical Center, Morristown, NJ, USA

Chikoti Wheat
Department of Dermatology, Johns Hopkins University, Baltimore, MD, USA
Department of Internal Medicine, Morristown Medical Center, Morristown, NJ, USA

Diego Escobar Montatixe, José Miguel Villacampa Aubá, Álvaro Sánchez Barrueco and Carlos Cenjor Español
Department of Otolaryngology, Head and Neck Surgery, Hospital Universitario Fundación Jiménez Díaz, Madrid, Spain

Beatriz Sobrino Guijarro
Department of Neuroradiology, Hospital Universitario Fundación Jiménez Díaz, Madrid, Spain

Kholoud A. Alhysoni, Sumaiyah M. Bukhari and Mutawakel F. Hajjaj
Otolaryngology Department, Ohud Hospital, Medina, Saudi Arabia

Kevin Hur and Changxing Liu
Caruso Department of Otolaryngology, Keck School of Medicine, University of Southern California, Los Angeles, CA 90033, USA

Jeffrey A. Koempel
Division of Otolaryngology, Head and Neck Surgery, Children's Hospital Los Angeles, Los Angeles, CA 90027, USA

Dana Lucila Lucarelli
Vestibular Argentina Institute, Buenos Aires, Argentina

Ana Carolina Binetti and Andrea Ximena Varela
Vestibular Argentina Institute, Buenos Aires, Argentina
Department of Otolaryngology, British Hospital of Buenos Aires, Buenos Aires, Argentina

Daniel Héctor Verdecchia
Vestibular Argentina Institute, Buenos Aires, Argentina
Center for Medical Research on Human Movement (CIMMHU), Maimónides University, Buenos Aires, Argentina

Joe Iwanaga, Koichi Watanabe, Saga Tsuyoshi, Yoko Tabira and Koh-ichi Yamaki
Department of Anatomy, Kurume University School of Medicine, Kurume, Fukuoka 830-0011, Japan

Ivan Keogh, Rohana O'Connell and John Lang
Otorhinolaryngology Department, University College Hospital Galway and Academic Department of Otorhinolaryngology, National University of Ireland Galway, Newcastle Road, Galway, Ireland

Sean Hynes
Department of Pathology, University College Hospital Galway, Newcastle Road, Galway, Ireland

Takahito Kondo, Toru Sasaki, Kazuyoshi Kawabata, Hiroki Mitani, Hiroyuki Yonekawa, Hirofumi Fukushima and Wataru Shimbashi
Department of Head and Neck Oncology, Cancer Institute Hospital of Japanese Foundation for Cancer Research, 3-8-31 Ariake, Koutou-ku, Tokyo 135-8550, Japan

Yukiko Sato
Department of Pathology, Cancer Institute Hospital of Japanese Foundation for Cancer Research, 3-8-31 Ariake, Koutou-ku, Tokyo 135-8550, Japan

Hiroko Tanaka
Department of Diagnostic Imaging, Cancer Institute Hospital of Japanese Foundation for Cancer Research, 3-8-31 Ariake, Koutou-ku, Tokyo 135-8550, Japan

Kenro Kawada, Tatsuyuki Kawano, Kazuya Yamaguchi, Yuudai Kawamura, Toshihiro Matsui, Masafumi Okuda, Taichi Ogo, Yuuichiro Kume, Yutaka Nakajima, Andres Mora, Takuya Okada, Akihiro Hoshino, Yutaka Tokairin and Yasuaki Nakajima
Department of Gastrointestinal Surgery, Tokyo Medical and Dental University, Tokyo, Japan

Taro Sugimoto, Ryuhei Okada, Yusuke Kiyokawa and Takahiro Asakage
Department of Head and Neck Surgery, Tokyo Medical and Dental University, Tokyo, Japan

Fuminori Nomura
Department of Otorhinolaryngology, Tokyo Medical and Dental University, Tokyo, Japan

Ryo Shimoda
Department of InternalMedicine and Gastrointestinal Endoscopy, Saga Medical School, Saga, Japan

Takashi Ito
Department of Human Pathology, Tokyo Medical and Dental University, Tokyo, Japan

Dario A. Yacovino
Department of Neurology, Cesar Milstein Hospital, Buenos Aires, Argentina
Memory and Balance Clinic, Buenos Aires, Argentina

John B. Finlay
Department of Neurology, Cesar Milstein Hospital, Buenos Aires, Argentina
Princeton University, Princeton, NJ, USA

Praveenkumar Ramdurg and Naveen Srinivas
Department of Oral Medicine and Radiology, PMNM Dental College and Hospital, Bagalkot, Karnataka, India

Vijaylaxmi Mendigeri
Department of Orthodontics, PMNM Dental College and Hospital, Bagalkot, Karnataka, India

Surekha R. Puranik
Department of Oral Medicine and Radiology, PMNM Dental College and Hospital, Bagalkot, Bagalkot District, India

Ozan Erol, Alper Koycu and Erdinc Aydin
Department of Otorhinolaryngology, Baskent University Faculty of Medicine, 06500 Ankara, Turkey

I. M. Villarreal, D. Méndez, J. M. Duque Silva and P. Ortega del Álamo
Otorhinolaryngology Department, "Móstoles" University Hospital, Madrid, Spain

Eleftheria Iliadou, Nektarios Papapetropoulos, Eleftherios Karamatzanis and Konstantinos Saravakos
Department of Otorhinolaryngology, Head and Neck Surgery, Penteli Children Hospital, Athens, Greece

Panagiotis Saravakos
Department of Otorhinolaryngology, Head and Neck Surgery, Siloah St. Trudpert Hospital, Pforzheim, Germany

Gilberto Acquaviva, Stefano Badia, Francesco Casorati and Gianluca Bellocchi
Department of Otolaryngology and Head & Neck Surgery, "San Camillo-Forlanini" Hospital, Rome, Italy

Alberto Eibenstein
Department of Applied Clinical Sciences and Biotechnology (DISCAB), L'Aquila University, L'Aquila, Italy

Theodoros Varakliotis
Department of Otolaryngology and Head & Neck Surgery, "San Camillo-Forlanini" Hospital, Rome, Italy
Department of Applied Clinical Sciences and Biotechnology (DISCAB), L'Aquila University, L'Aquila, Italy

Geetha Narayanan
Department of Medical Oncology, Regional Cancer Centre, Trivandrum 695011, India

Anto Baby
St. Gregorios Medical Mission Hospital, Parumala, Pathanamthitta 689626, India

Thara Somanathan
Department of Pathology, Regional Cancer Centre, Trivandrum 695011, India

Sreedevi Konoth
Department of Radiology, Lourdes Hospital, Kochi 682012, India

Amit Kumar Dey, Rajaram Sharma, Kartik Mittal, Puneeth Kumar,
Vivek Murumkar, Sumit Mitkar, and Priya Hira
Department of Radiology, King Edward Memorial Hospital and Seth G.S. Medical College, Room No. 107, KEM Main Boy's Hostel, Parel, Mumbai 400012, India

Serena Byrd, Adnan S. Hussaini and Jastin Antisdel
Department of Otolaryngology-Head and Neck Surgery, Saint Louis University School of Medicine, Saint Louis, MO, USA

Taha A. Mur
Lewis Katz School of Medicine, Temple University, Philadelphia, PA, USA

Ronald Miick
Department of Pathology and Laboratory Medicine, Einstein Medical Center, Philadelphia, PA, USA

Natasha Pollak
Department of Otolaryngology-Head & Neck Surgery, Lewis Katz School of Medicine, Temple University, Philadelphia, PA, USA

Sanjay Vaid, Jyoti Jadhav and Aparna Chandorkar
Head and Neck Imaging Division, Star Imaging and Research Center, Pune 411001, India

Neelam Vaid
Department of Otorhinolaryngology, KEM Hospital, Pune 411011, India

Fatih Bingöl, Buket Özel Bingöl and Korhan Kılıç
Erzurum Research and Training Hospital, Department of Otorhinolaryngology, Erzurum, Turkey

Hilal Balta
Erzurum Research and Training Hospital, Department of Pathology, Erzurum, Turkey

Recai Muhammet Mazlumğlu
Palandöken State Hospital, Department of Otorhinolaryngology, Erzurum, Turkey

Hiroto Moriwaki, Nana Hayama, Shouko Morozumi, Mika Nakano, Akari Nakayama, Yoshiomi Takahata, Yuusuke Sakaguchi, Natsuki Inoue, Toshiki Kubota, Akiko Takenoya, Yoshiko Ishii, Haruka Okubo, Souta Yamaguchi and Mamoru Yoshikawa
Department of Otorhinolaryngology, Toho University Ohashi Medical Center, Tokyo, Japan

Tsuyoshi Ono
Division of Cardiovascular Medicine, Toho University Ohashi Medical Center, Tokyo, Japan

Toshiaki Oharaseki
Department of Pathology, Toho University Ohashi Medical Center, Tokyo, Japan

Justin A. Edward, Ryan A. Williams and Jayakar V. Nayak
Division of Rhinology, Department of Otolaryngology-Head and Neck Surgery, Stanford University School of Medicine, Stanford, CA 94305, USA

Alkis J. Psaltis
Department of Surgery-Otorhinolaryngology, Head and Neck Surgery, University of Adelaide, Adelaide, SA, Australia

Gregory W. Charville
Department of Pathology, Stanford University School of Medicine, Stanford, CA 94305, USA

Robert L. Dodd
Department of Neurosurgery, Stanford University School of Medicine, Stanford, CA 94305, USA

Uzeyir Yildizoglu
Department of Otorhinolaryngology Head and Neck Surgery, Beytepe Military Hospital, Ankara, Turkey

Fatih Arslan
Department of Otolaryngology, Head and Neck Surgery, Ankara Mevki Military Hospital, Ankara, Turkey

Bahtiyar Polat
Department of Otorhinolaryngology Head and Neck Surgery, Gelibolu Military Hospital, Çanakkale, Turkey

Abdullah Durmaz
Department of Otolaryngology, Head and Neck Surgery, Gulhane Military Medical Academy, Ankara, Turkey

Colleen F. Perez and Curtis W. Gaball
Naval Medical Center San Diego, SanDiego, CA, USA

Kohei Nishimoto, Ryosei Minoda and Eiji Yumoto
Department of Otolaryngology Head and Neck Surgery, Graduate School of Medicine, Kumamoto University, Kumamoto, Japan

Ryoji Yoshida
Department of Oral and Maxillofacial Surgery, Graduate School of Medicine, Kumamoto University, Kumamoto, Japan

Toshinori Hirai
Department of Diagnostic Radiology, Graduate School of Medicine, Kumamoto University, Kumamoto, Japan

Ara Darakjian
Department of Psychiatry and Behavioral Sciences, Keck School of Medicine, 1975 Zonal Ave, Los Angeles, CA 90033, USA

Ani B. Darakjian
Department of Radiology, Southern California Permanente Medical Group, 4867W. Sunset Blvd, Los Angeles, CA 90027, USA

Edward T. Chang
Division of Otolaryngology-Head and Neck Surgery, Tripler Army Medical Center, 1 JarrettWhite Rd, Honolulu, HI 96859, USA

Macario Camacho
Division of Otolaryngology-Head and Neck Surgery, Tripler Army Medical Center, 1 JarrettWhite Rd, Honolulu, HI 96859, USA
Department of Psychiatry and Behavioral Sciences, Sleep Medicine Division, Stanford Hospital and Clinics, 450 Broadway St, Pavillion B., Redwood City, CA 94063, USA

Jeffrey C. Yeung, Shaun J. Kilty and Kristian Macdonald
1Department of Otolaryngology-Head & Neck Surgery, University of Ottawa, Ottawa, ON, Canada

C. Elizabeth Pringle
Division of Neurology, Department of Medicine, University of Ottawa, Ottawa, ON, Canada

Harmanjatinder S. Sekhon
Department of Pathology & Laboratory Medicine, University of Ottawa, Ottawa, ON, Canada

Jacob F. Lentz
Department of Emergency Medicine, David Geffen School of Medicine at UCLA, Los Angeles, CA 90095, USA

Edward C. Kuan
Department of Head and Neck Surgery, David Geffen School of Medicine at UCLA, Los Angeles, CA 90095, USA

Hiwot H. Araya and Mohammad Kamgar
Department of Medicine, David Geffen School of Medicine at UCLA, Los Angeles, CA 90095, USA

Albert Y. Han
Department of Medicine, David Geffen School of Medicine at UCLA, Los Angeles, CA 90095, USA

Medical Scientist Training Program, David Geffen School of Medicine at UCLA, Los Angeles, CA 90095, USA

Ashraf Nabeel Mahmood and Sarah Ashkanani
Rhinology Section, Otorhinolaryngology, Head & Neck Surgery (ORL-HNS) Department, Rumailah Hospital, Hamad Medical Corporation, Doha, Qatar

Rashid Sheikh
Otorhinolaryngology, Head & Neck Surgery (ORL-HNS) Department, Rumailah Hospital, Hamad Medical Corporation, Doha, Qatar

Hamad Al Saey
Rhinology Section, Otorhinolaryngology, Head & Neck Surgery (ORL-HNS) Department, Rumailah Hospital, Hamad Medical Corporation, Doha, Qatar
Weill Cornell Medical College, Ar-Rayyan, Qatar

Shanmugam Ganesan
Otorhinolaryngology, Head & Neck Surgery (ORL-HNS) Department, Rumailah Hospital, Hamad Medical Corporation, Doha, Qatar
Weill Cornell Medical College, Ar-Rayyan, Qatar

Ozge Turhan
Department of Infectious Diseases, Akdeniz University School of Medicine, Antalya, Turkey

Asli Bostanci and Murat Turhan
Department of Otolaryngology, Head and Neck Surgery, Akdeniz University School of Medicine, Antalya, Turkey

Irem Hicran Ozbudak
Department of Pathology, Akdeniz University School of Medicine, Antalya, Turkey

Massimo Ralli
Department of Oral and Maxillofacial Sciences, Sapienza University of Rome, Rome, Italy

Giancarlo Altissimi and Rosaria Turchetta
Department of Sense Organs, Audiology Section, Policlinico Umberto I, Sapienza University of Rome, Rome, Italy

Mario Rigante
Department of Otorhinolaryngology, Catholic University of Sacred Heart, Rome, Italy

X. Y. Yeoh, P. S. Lim and K. C. Pua
Department of Otorhinolaryngology, Penang General Hospital, Jalan Residensi, 10990 Penang, Malaysia

Mustafa Aslıer, Mustafa Cenk Ecevit and Semih Sütay
Department of Otorhinolaryngology, Dokuz Eylul University School of Medicine, Izmir, Turkey

Sülen Sarıoğlu
Department of Pathology, Dokuz Eylul University School of Medicine, Izmir, Turkey

Kemal Koray Bal, Onur Ismi, Helen Bucioglu, Yusuf Vayısoğlu and Kemal Gorur
Department of Otorhinolaryngology, Faculty of Medicine, University of Mersin, Mersin, Turkey

Gustavo Barreto da Cunha, Tatiane Costa Camurugy, Thiago Cavalcante Ribeiro, Nara Nunes Barbosa Costa, Amanda Canário Andrade Azevedo, Eriko Soares de Azevedo Vinhaes and Nilvano Alves de Andrade
Santa Casa de Misericórdia da Bahia, Hospital Santa Izabel, Salvador, BA, Brazil

Michael Coulter
Health Science Center, Stony Brook University School of Medicine, Stony Brook, NY 11794, USA

Jingxuan Liu
Department of Pathology, Stony Brook University Hospital, 101 Nicolls Road, Stony Brook, NY 11794, USA

Mark Marzouk
Department of Otolaryngology, Upstate University Hospital, 750 E. Adams, Syracuse, NY 13210, USA

Betty Chen, Joshua I. Hentzelman and Ronald J. Walker
Department of Otolaryngology-Head and Neck Surgery, Saint Louis University School of Medicine, St. Louis, MO 63104, USA

Jin-Ping Lai
Department of Pathology, Saint Louis University School of Medicine, St. Louis, MO 63104, USA

Nuno Ribeiro-Costa, Pedro Carneiro Sousa, Diogo Abreu Pereira, Paula Azevedo and Delfim Duarte
Hospital Pedro Hispano, Rua Dr. Eduardo Torres, Senhora da Hora, 4464-513 Matosinhos, Portugal

Giovanni Bianchin, Lorenzo Tribi, Patrizia Formigoni and Valeria Polizzi
MD Otolaryngology and Audiology Department, Santa Maria Nuova Hospital, Viale Risorgimento, No. 80, 42100 Reggio Emilia, Italy

Aronne Reverzani
MD Emergency Medicine Department, Santa Maria Nuova Hospital, Viale Risorgimento, No. 80, 42100 Reggio Emilia, Italy

Thomas B. Layton
Faculty of Life Sciences, University of Manchester, Manchester M13 9PL, UK

Alper Yenigun, Omer Vural and Orhan Ozturan
Department of Otorhinolaryngology, Faculty of Medicine, Bezmialem Vakif University, Fatih, Istanbul, Turkey

Bayram Veyseller
Department of Otorhinolaryngology, Faculty of Medicine, Acibadem University, Istanbul, Turkey

Marco Giuseppe Greco, Francesco Mattioli, Maria Paola Alberici and Livio Presutti
Unità Operativa Complessa di Otorinolaringoiatria, Azienda Ospedaliero-Universitaria Policlinico di Modena, Italy Via del Pozzo 71, 41124 Modena, Italy

Eishaan K. Bhargava, Nikhil Arora, Varun Rai, Ravi Meher and Ruchika Juneja
Department of Ent and Head and Neck Surgery, Maulana AzadMedical College, NewDelhi, India

Prerna Arora
Department of Pathology,Maulana AzadMedical College, NewDelhi, India

Index